HANDBOOK OF FRACTURES

Third Edition

EDITORS

John A. Elstrom, M.D.
Clinical Assistant Professor
University of Illinois
Chicago, Illinois
Department of Surgery
Northern Illinois Medical Center
McHenry, Illinois

Walter W. Virkus, M.D.
Assistant Professor
Department of Orthopaedic Surgery
Rush University Medical Center
Senior Attending Physician
Cook County Hospital
Chicago, Illinois

Arsen M. Pankovich, M.D.
Clinical Professor of Orthopaedic Surgery
New York University Medical Center and
Hospital for Joint Diseases
New York, New York

Illustrated by
Arsen M. Pankovich, M.D.

McGRAW-HILL
Medical Publishing Division
New York   Chicago   San Francisco   Lisbon   London
Madrid   Mexico City   Milan   New Delhi   San Juan
Seoul   Singapore   Sydney   Toronto

HANDBOOK OF FRACTURES, THIRD EDITION

1 2 3 4 5 6 7 8 9 0   DOC/DOC   0 9 8 7 6 5

ISBN   0-07-144377-0

This book was set in Times Roman by MidAtlantic Books and Journals.
The editors were Hilarie Surrena, Robert Pancotti, and Lester A. Sheinis.
The production supervisors were Sherri Souffrance and Richard C. Ruzycka.
The cover designer was Janice Bielawa.
The indexer was Alexandra Nickerson.
RR Donnelley was printer and binder.

This book is printed on acid-free paper.

Library of Congress Cataloging-in-Publication Data

Handbook of fractures / editors, John A. Elstrom, Walter W. Virkus, Arsen M. Pankovich.—3rd ed.
      p.;   cm.
   Includes bibliographical references and index.
   ISBN   0-07-144377-0 (alk. paper)
      1. Fractures—Handbooks, manuals, etc. 2. Orthopedics—Handbooks, manuals, etc. I. Elstrom, John A. II.Virkus, Walter W. III. Pankovich, Arsen M.
      [DNLM: 1. Fractures—therapy—Handbooks. 2. Dislocations—therapy—Handbooks. 3. Orthopedics—methods—Handbooks.
WE 39 H236 2005]
RD101.H24 2005
617.19 5—dc22
                                                              2005043878

Contents

Contributors

EDWARD R. ABRAHAM, M.D.
Professor and Chairman
Department of Orthopedics
University of Illinois at Chicago
Chicago, Illinois
(Chapter 10)

PAUL APPLETON, M.D.
Registrar in Orthopaedic
    Trauma
Edinburgh Orthopaedic Trauma
    Unit
Royal Infirmary of Edinburgh at
    Little France
Edinburgh, Scotland
(Chapter 24)

KEITH H. BRIDWELL, M.D.
Professor
Department of Orthopaedic
    Surgery
Washington University School
    of Medicine
St. Louis, Missouri
(Chapter 15)

CHARLES M. COURT-BROWN, M.D., F.R.C.S.
Professor of Orthopaedic
    Trauma Surgery
Edinburgh Orthopaedic Trauma
    Unit
Royal Infirmary of Edinburgh
    at Little France
Edinburgh, Scotland
(Chapters 7 and 24)

CHRIS JOHN DANGLES, M.D.
Clinical Assistant Professor
University of Illinois at Urbana-
    Champaign
Carle Foundation Hospital
Urbana, Illinois
(Chapter 25)

KENNETH A. DAVENPORT, M.D.
Chief of Staff
Marquette General Hospital
Marquette, Michigan
(Chapter 19)

THOMAS A. EINHORN, M.D.
Professor and Chairman
Department of Orthopedic
    Surgery
Boston University School of
    Medicine
Chief, Orthopaedic Surgery
Boston Medical Center
Boston, Massachusetts
(Chapter 6)

JOHN A. ELSTROM, M.D.
Clinical Assistant Professor
University of Illinois
Chicago, Illinois
Department of Surgery
Northern Illinois Medical Center
McHenry, Illinois
(Chapters 1, 3, 8, 11, 14, 17,
    and 25)

xi

JOHN J. FERNANDEZ, M.D., F.A.A.O.S.
Assistant Professor
Department of Orthopaedic Surgery
Rush University Medical Center
Chicago, Illinois
(Chapter 13)

RON C. GABA, M.D.
Department of Radiology
University of Illinois Medical Center at Chicago
Chicago, Illinois
(Chapter 5)

MARK R. HUTCHINSON, M.D.
Associate Professor of Orthopaedic Surgery and Sports Medicine
Director of Sports Medicine Services
Department of Orthopaedics
University of Illinois at Chicago
Chicago, Illinois
(Chapter 28)

JESSE BERNARD JUPITER, M.D.
Chief of the Orthopaedic Hand Service
Massachusetts General Hospital
Hansjörg Wyss AO Professor of Orthopaedic Surgery
Harvard Medical School
Boston, Massachusetts
(Chapter 12)

SANJEEV KAKAR, M.D.
Research Associate, Orthopaedic Surgery
Boston Medical Center
Boston, Massachusetts
(Chapter 6)

ENES M. KANLIC, M.D., Ph.D.
Associate Professor
Orthopaedic Surgery Department
Texas Tech University Health Science Center
El Paso, Texas
(Chapters 18, 23, and 27)

RAYMOND KLUG, M.D.
Department of Orthopedics
University of Illinois at Chicago
Chicago, Illinois
(Chapter 28)

LAWRENCE G. LENKE, M.D.
Department of Orthopedic Surgery
Washington University School of Medicine
St. Louis, Missouri
(Chapter 15)

JOHN L. LIN, M.D.
Department of Orthopedic Surgery
Rush University Medical Center
Chicago, Illinois
(Chapter 26)

SANTIAGO A. LOZANO-CALDRON, M.D.
Research Fellow, Orthopaedic Hand Service
Massachusetts General Hospital
Research Fellow, Orthopaedic Surgery
Harvard Medical School
Boston, Massachusetts
(Chapter 12)

CARL H. NIELSEN, M.D.
Associate Professor
Department of Anesthesiology
Washington University School of Medicine
St. Louis, Missouri
(Chapter 4)

GBOLAHAN O. OKUBADEJO, M.D.
Department of Orthopedic
    Surgery
Washington University School
    of Medicine
St. Louis, Missouri
(Chapter 15)

ARSEN M. PANKOVICH, M.D.
Clinical Professor of
    Orthopaedic Surgery
New York University Medical
    Center and Hospital for
    Joint Diseases
New York, New York
(Chapters 17, 19, and 25)

MIGUEL A. PIRELA-CRUZ, M.D.
Professor and Director
Orthopedic Surgery Department
Texas Tech University Health
    Science Center
El Paso, Texas
(Chapters 18, 23, and 27)

PRAHLAD S. PYATI, M.D.
Clinical Professor of Surgery
Rosalind Franklin University/
    Chicago Medical School
Chief, Division of Orthopedics
Mount Sinai Medical Center at
    Chicago
Chicago, Illinois
(Chapter 9)

C. M. ROBINSON
Senior Lecturer and Consultant
Orthopaedic Trauma Surgeon
Edinburgh Orthopaedic Trauma
    Unit
Royal Infirmary of Edinburgh at
    Little France
Edinburgh, Scotland
(Chapter 7)

D. KEVIN SCHEID, M.D.
Director of Orthopedic Trauma
Methodist Hospital
Indianapolis, Indiana
(Chapter 16)

ROBERT C. SCHENCK, JR., M.D.
Professor of Orthopedic
    Surgery
University of New Mexico
    Health Science Center
Albuquerque, New Mexico
(Chapters 20, 21, and 22)

JAMES P. STANNARD, M.D.
Associate Professor of Surgery
Division of Orthopaedic
    Surgery
University of Alabama at
    Birmingham
Birmingham, Alabama
(Chapters 20, 21, and 22)

MARGARET A. STULL, M.D.
Associate Professor of Clinical
    Radiology
Department of Diagnostic
    Radiology
University of Illinois Medical
    Center at Chicago
Chicago, Illinois
(Chapter 5)

BRETT A. TAYLOR, M.D.
Assistant Professor
Department of Orthopedic
    Surgery
Washington University School
    of Medicine
Adult Spine Specialist
Barnes-Jewish Hospital
St. Louis, Missouri
(Chapter 15)

ELEFTHERIOS TSIRIDIS, M.D., M.Sc., F.R.C.S.
Research Fellow, Orthopaedic Surgery
Boston Medical Center
Boston, Massachusetts
(Chapter 6)

WALTER W. VIRKUS, M.D.
Assistant Professor
Department of Orthopaedic Surgery
Rush University Medical Center
Senior Attending Physician
Cook County Hospital
Chicago, Illinois
(Chapters 1, 2, and 26)

EMILE P. WAKIM, M.D.
Department of Orthopedic Surgery
Rush University Medical Center
Chicago, Illinois
(Chapter 2)

Preface

Just over ten years ago, McGraw-Hill approached Dr. Arsen Pankovich and asked him to prepare a pocket-sized *Handbook of Fractures*, which would be a portable reference on fracture management written for the practicing orthopedic surgeon. In 1995, the first edition of the *Handbook* was published. The contributing authors, with few exceptions, had obtained their trauma management experience at the Cook County Hospital in Chicago or through their affiliation with the Washington University School of Medicine in St. Louis, Missouri. A second edition of the *Handbook* was published in 2000. Dr. Clayton R. Perry served as the senior editor for the first two editions.

Although the purpose of the third edition remains the same as that of the first two editions—to bring together the basic information that the reader must have to classify, diagnose, and manage specific fractures—the text and illustrations have been extensively revised and the trim size of the book has been increased to accommodate additional chapters. Since the first edition was published, chapters on radiologic evaluation and on injuries related to athletic competition have been added. The single chapter "Injuries about the Knee" has been divided into four chapters dealing with fractures of the distal femur, fractures of the patella, fractures of the proximal tibia, and dislocations of the knee. A new chapter on injuries of the tibial pilon has been separated from the chapter on lower-energy fractures of the ankle.

The organization of the book remains straightforward. The book begins with general chapters, four of which have been extensively rewritten, dealing with evaluation and initial management of patients with multiple injuries, methods of fixation, nonoperative techniques, anesthetic techniques, radiologic evaluation, and fracture healing and bone grafting. The subsequent chapters are organized according to the injured anatomy, starting with the shoulder and proceeding distally to the foot. Each chapter contains introductory anatomic information, fracture classification, diagnostic and radiologic considerations, and recommendations for management based on current practice and the author's experience. The Orthopaedic Trauma Association (OTA) fracture classification method has been nearly universally adopted. The highlighting with bold type for key words in the text continues to help the reader to identify quickly material for which he or she is searching.

Since the publication of the second edition, the number of contributing authors has increased by twenty. This increase provides not only additional material but also fresh perspectives on current fracture management. The editors gratefully acknowledge the efforts and expertise of all of the contributing authors. We are also deeply appreciative of the support given to us by our publisher, McGraw-Hill, and their senior editor, Hilarie Surrena. The reader will find that many new illustrations have been added to this edition. The format of the illustrations has been standardized, and the selected readings have been extensively updated. As with the previous editions, our goal is to provide a pertinent, practical, portable reference for all persons involved in fracture management.

Acknowledgments

I would like to acknowledge my indebtedness to the following persons: Lu Boorman, for her perseverance in preparing the manuscript for submission to the publisher; and Dr. Mohamad T. Kassab,* Dr. Arsen M. Pankovich, and Dr. Robert F. Hall, Jr., for their progressive and positive influence on me and many others by the example that they set in their care for patients with fracture problems.

John A. Elstrom, M.D.

*Deceased.

HANDBOOK
OF
FRACTURES

1 | Evaluation and Management of the Multiply Injured Patient

Walter W. Virkus   John A. Elstrom

Although most orthopedic fracture care involves patients with isolated injuries, orthopedists must be familiar with the evaluation and management of patients with multisystem or multiextremity trauma. This requires an assessment and understanding of the patient's overall condition, an examination for additional injuries, and an understanding of the factors directing the prioritization and management of these injuries.

The care of patients with multiple extremity injuries requires the establishment of priorities and the answer to the following questions: (1) Which injuries require surgery? (2) If surgery is required, when, by what methods, and in what order should it be done? and (3) How much surgery can the patient tolerate?

Immediate emergency surgery with an unfamiliar team in the middle of the night can risk more, accomplish less, and take more time than would be the case in a better-controlled situation. The treatment of orthopedic injuries must take its proper place in the treatment algorithm behind potentially life-threatening injuries.

Patients with multiple-system injuries (extremity plus head, neck, thorax, abdomen, pelvis, and/or spine) require the same considerations as those with injuries isolated to a single extremity, restrained by the knowledge that treatment of these other injuries will most likely have priority, that the metabolic state of the patient will be more severely compromised, and that ideal fracture treatment may be of a lesser priority than the treatment of immediate life-threatening injuries. Alternative initial treatment methods and the delay of definitive treatment until homeostasis has been restored is often prudent for all involved.

The crucial issues in assessing systemic injuries include (1) head or cervical spine injury (increased intracranial pressure, major neurologic deficit), (2) shock (hypovolemia, ongoing blood loss, hypothermia, coagulopathy, acidosis), (3) thoracic injury (aortic tear, pneumothorax, pulmonary contusion, decreased cardiac output, hypoxia), and (4) abdominal injury (hypovolemia, ruptured or perforated viscus).

The care of the multiply injured patient requires an emergency room staff, intensive care unit, and trauma surgeon familiar with the resuscitation and pathophysiology of these severe injuries. Modern trauma systems provide triage and expeditious transportation to these hospitals; this has dramatically improved the condition of the patient on reaching the emergency department.

CARE OF THE MULTIPLY INJURED PATIENT

Victims of severe trauma are evaluated with a protocol developed to prioritize treatment and avoid oversights in the assessment. This evaluation is divided into primary, secondary, and tertiary surveys of the patient. The primary survey begins as soon as the patient arrives in the emergency department and follows the acronym **ABCDE**.

The presence of a functioning **airway** must be assured. If any concern exists on admission, the patient may be intubated to prevent loss of the airway at a critical time. Indications for intubation include decreased mental status, severe pulmonary injury, facial fractures, and laryngeal injury.

After establishment of the airway, it must be confirmed that the patient is **breathing** independently. If there is any question concerning the patient's ability to maintain this, intubation with ventilator-assisted respiration should be instituted.

Circulation is the last of the ABCs and is quickly assessed by palpation of peripheral pulses. Blood pressure is also assessed during this portion of the evaluation and gives an indication of whether the patient is in shock. Hypotension in a trauma patient indicates that the patient's circulatory system has lost the ability to maintain a normal intravascular pressure. This can occur in the presence of a severe neurologic injury, where the loss of sympathetic control of vasoconstriction in the peripheral vascular system leads to a relative intravascular hypovolemia (**neurogenic shock**). Hypotension can also result from a cardiac injury or myocardial infarction (**cardiogenic shock**). Most common in the trauma patient, however, is **hypovolemic shock** secondary to hemorrhage. While hemorrhage can be external and visible, severe hemorrhage leading to shock is usually internal and not readily apparent on inspection of the patient.

In patients without severe medical comorbidities, a significant amount of hemorrhage must occur before the compensatory mechanisms of the circulatory system are overwhelmed and hypotension results. This is why **shock is such a poor prognostic finding in the trauma patient**. The search for the source of hemorrhage goes on concurrently with fluid resuscitation during the primary survey and continues into the secondary survey. Balanced saline solutions such as Ringer's lactate are given in liter boluses during the primary survey and then adjusted based on the patient's response as measured by heart rate, blood pressure, and urine output. If hemorrhage is present and the patient's hematocrit/hemoglobin decreases significantly or ongoing hemorrhage is anticipated, crossmatched or even type-specific packed RBC transfusions are needed.

After the ABCs, **disability** and **exposure** are evaluated. **Disability** refers to the initial evaluation of the neurologic system, including level of consciousness and gross extremity neurologic exam. **Exposure** refers to the complete visual inspection of the patient, requiring the complete removal of all clothing in order to inspect for signs of injury of the extremities, torso, and perineum. This is an important **requirement**, and is the responsibility of the physician who undertakes the patient's care.

After completion of the primary survey, the secondary survey is initiated. This includes obtaining the "trauma series" radiographs: lateral cervical spine, AP chest, and AP pelvis. If the cervical spine radiograph does not adequately visualize the C7/T1 junction, a swimmer's view or CT scan is necessary to clear the cervical spine radiographically. Additional studies for determining the extent of abdominal injuries are performed as necessary, including ultrasound, diagnostic peritoneal lavage (DPL), or abdominal CT scan. Assessment for urgent injuries such as pneumothorax/hemothorax (diminished breath sounds), tension pneumothorax (hypotension, tracheal deviation, and decreased breath sounds), cardiac tamponade (hypotension and diminished heart sounds), and rectal and urethral injuries (blood visible on rectal exam or at urethral meatus) must be performed. The initial musculoskeletal exam of the spine and extremities is performed at this time and radiographs are obtained of areas that demonstrate substantial tenderness, swelling, deformity, or crepitus.

A tertiary survey is performed in the days following admission of the multiply injured patient. This ideally occurs after the patient's mental status has returned to normal. In the tertiary survey, the orthopedist should repalpate every bone. This is an occasion to detect fractures in small bones such as those of the hand, foot, and clavicle and ligamentous injuries to the knee and ankle.

Evaluation and Care of the Patient with Regard to Orthopedic Injuries

The history-taking portion of the assessment depends on the condition of the patient but should include the mechanism of injury. A history of a fall should prompt questions about the cause of the fall, the distance of the fall, and the position in which the patient landed. Additional questions should elicit complaints of back or foot pain due to the frequent association of spinal and calcaneal fractures in patients who have experienced severe axial loads.

For patients involved in a motor vehicle accident (MVA), the patient's location in the car, direction and speed of impact, and use of seat belts and the deployment of airbags are important. Patients involved in head-on collisions can sustain high-energy deceleration forces as well as significant direct forces to the knee, leading to knee or hip dislocation, fracture of the femur, and pelvic and acetabular fractures. The foot and wrist are also often traumatized. Side-impact accidents can lead to similar injuries and shoulder girdle involvement. Determination of the severity of the accident is essential: were there fatalities, was extraction from a vehicle required, was resuscitation needed, was the patient ejected? Certain occult life-threatening injuries are associated with a high-energy type of MVA.

Past medical and surgical history can reveal details that will affect the treatment plan or surgical approach. Diabetes, coronary artery or peripheral vascular disease, or the use of systemic steroids may increase the risks of certain open procedures. The existing use of anticoagulants must be addressed. Pertinent details of the social history include the use of tobacco, occupation, handedness, and living situation.

The physical examination should look for findings that may signal systemic compromise while also evaluating the entire injured extremity. Confusion, coma, agitation, pallor, tachypnea, tachycardia, and hypotension need explanation and treatment and are signs for caution for those considering a major orthopedic procedure.

Critical areas for assessment include the skin and soft tissue, muscle compartments, alignment and stability of the joints of the extremity, and the vascular and neurologic status.

The skin over and around a fracture must be thoroughly assessed. Lacerations should be carefully examined to determine if they communicate with the fracture, indicating an open fracture. It should be determined if foreign material and devitalized tissue will need to be debrided from wounds.

The vascular examination is important to assure adequate perfusion of the injured extremity. Is bone or joint displacement affecting perfusion of the limb? These should be rectified immediately by closed reduction and splinting. Are there signs of a compartment syndrome or vascular disruption? Are compartment pressure measurements indicated (unconscious patient, tense compartment), or do we just go ahead with a fasciotomy? Ankle-brachial indices (ABI) are useful in determining the likelihood of a vascular injury. An ABI of less than 0.8 should be evaluated with an angiogram.

Fractures are often associated with ligamentous injuries of adjacent joints. Signs such as effusion and ecchymosis should be sought. While a ligamentous exam may be difficult in the presence of a nearby fracture, it is important to confirm joint stability before or after fracture stabilization.

Neurologic testing is a critical part of the initial exam, and this is the best time to accurately document the neurologic status. Procedures for fracture treatment can be complicated by neurologic injury; therefore documentation of a preoperative neurologic deficit is critical to avoid the question of iatrogenic injury.

The neurologic exam of the lower extremity should include specific evaluation of the femoral nerve (knee extension), superficial peroneal nerve (foot eversion), deep peroneal nerve (ankle and big toe dorsiflexion), and tibial nerve (ankle plantarflexion). Upper extremity evaluation should include evaluation of the axillary nerve (shoulder abduction), radial nerve (elbow and wrist extension), ulnar nerve (thumb adduction, little finger abduction and flexion), median nerve (thumb opposition and flexion), posterior interosseous nerve (thumb, index finger extension), and anterior interosseous nerve (index DIP flexion).

By the end of the physical examination, the following question should have been answered: Is this a multiply injured patient with substantial alterations in basic physiology that are life-threatening? If so, how are the objectives of treatment limited? (1) Vascular impairment needs to be corrected. (2) Wounds need exploration, cleaning, debridement, dressing, tetanus prophylaxis, and antibiotic coverage. (3) Long bone fractures need stabilization, often by a temporary external fixator, traction, or splinting. (4) Joint dislocations are reduced and intraarticular fractures splinted or stabilized by joint-spanning external fixation. (5) Neurologic impairment (involuntary movements, coma, and paralysis) will be a consideration in the timing and choice of treatment alternatives.

The orthopedist involved in the care of the multiple trauma victim must be careful to prioritize the management of spine and extremity injuries based on the patient's other injuries and overall condition. Studies in the 1980s suggested that early fixation of major long bone fractures, femoral shaft fractures in particular, resulted in the improved survival of victims of multiple trauma. It was felt that early definitive fixation led to a decrease in systemic inflammatory mediators, decreased analgesic needs, and allowed earlier mobilization. This resulted in a decreased incidence of adult respiratory distress syndrome (ARDS) and multisystem organ failure.

Over the last 10 years, questions have arisen as to whether early definitive fixation of extremity fractures can actually exacerbate tenuous systemic physiology. It has been suggested that patients with multisystem injury are in a tenuous equilibrium after their initial resuscitation and that prolonged fracture surgeries or instrumentation of the intramedullary canal of a long bone can deliver a **"second hit,"** resulting in a dangerous downturn in the patient's overall status. Some theories suggest that ARDS and other systemic insults can be limited by delaying definitive fixation until the patient is stable. This has led to the term *damage-control orthopedics*, which describes a rationale whereby temporary fracture stabilization is obtained, usually by external fixation, and definitive fixation performed when the patient's overall condition improves. Patients with external femoral fixation can be converted to an intramedullary nail up to 4 weeks after external fixation placement without an increased risk of infection. It is important to understand that the concern about early definitive internal fixation applies only to patients with systemic injuries in addition to their orthopedic injuries. **Patients without systemic injury are best treated by early fixation of long bone fractures**.

Damage-control orthopedics also refers to a method of staged periarticular fracture fixation in which open reduction and internal fixation (ORIF) is either delayed, allowing restitution of homeostasis and resolution of soft tissue swelling, or abandoned in favor of definitive external fixation combined with **limited** internal fixation. The use of a staged or less invasive protocol for periarticular injuries such as those around the knee or ankle has resulted in a lower incidence of wound-related complications.

HEAD INJURY

The timing of fracture fixation is also controversial when a concurrent **head injury** is present. Neurosurgeons are often reluctant to allow **early internal fracture fixation**, in particular intramedullary nailing, in patients with closed head injuries. Their concern is that positioning (supine without the head elevated), pain, and anesthetics could lead to transient increases in blood pressure, which would lead to elevated intracranial pressure and exacerbate the long-term damage caused by closed head injury. Alternatively, blood loss during surgery could result in hypotension, with a reduction in cerebral perfusion. Studies looking into this issue have not only been unable to demonstrate a deleterious effect of intramedullary nailing but have actually suggested that obtaining a stable fracture may lead to lower intracranial pressures, presumably due to decreased pain. There is no doubt that early internal femoral (or pelvic) fracture fixation facilitates the mobilization of the patient with a head injury. Collegial communication between the neurosurgeon and orthopedic surgeon is essential for the optimal care of the patient.

COMPARTMENT SYNDROME

The diagnosis of compartment syndrome is of critical importance. Compartment syndrome can occur in any muscle compartment but is most common in the leg, thigh, and forearm. Less common locations include the foot, buttock, and abdomen. The diagnosis in an alert patient is straightforward. Pain is due to ischemia and is out of proportion to the injury; often it is not relieved by narcotic pain medication. The involved compartments are tense and tender to palpation. Passive stretch of the involved muscles is extremely painful. Paresthesias are common, but a decrease in the pulse or alteration of sensation or motor function is a late finding. Diagnosis in the unconscious or mentally altered patient is more difficult. A high index of suspicion must be maintained.

In the presence of firm compartments and any of the aforementioned symptoms, intracompartmental pressures must be measured or surgical decompression carried out. Direct measurement of intracompartmental pressures confirms the diagnosis. The exact pressure criterion defining compartment syndrome is controversial. A pressure of 40 mmHg has been used as the defining criterion. More recently, the relationship of the intracompartmental pressure to the patient's blood pressure has been shown to be a more objective measure. By this method, compartment syndrome is felt to be present if the intracompartmental pressure is within 30 mmHg of the diastolic blood pressure. If elevated compartmental pressures are obtained, an urgent open fasciotomy of the involved muscle compartments is indicated. Failure to perform fasciotomy in a timely manner can result in permanent ischemia of the muscles and nerves in the involved compartment, with myonecrosis and severe limb dysfunction.

OPEN FRACTURES

An open fracture requires prompt assessment and treatment even when it occurs as an isolated extremity injury. Open fractures require a timely and thorough exploration, debridement of foreign material and necrotic tissue, and irrigation to minimize the chance of acute infection, gas gangrene, and osteomyelitis. The method of fracture management may need to be modified depending on the degree of contamination and fracture pattern. The historic 6-h time frame for the debridement of open fractures has been extended by the prompt administration of appropriate antibiotics. The successful treatment of open fractures is more likely related to the adequacy of the debridement rather than an arbitrary time frame in which the debridement occurs.

Open fractures are classified by the **Gustillo-Anderson classification**. In this system, **grade I fractures** are low-energy fractures with a wound less than 1 cm in length. This is often a wound caused by the bone tearing through the soft tissue from inside the extremity. **Grade II fractures** are slightly higher energy fractures, generally heralded by a wound less than 10 cm that can be closed primarily. **Grade III fractures** result from high-energy trauma. **Grade IIIA fractures** include segmental fractures, fractures with gross contamination, fractures with extensive periosteal stripping, and fractures with a soft tissue injury longer than 10 cm but not requiring flap coverage. **Grade IIIB fractures** require flap coverage for closure, and **grade IIIC fractures** have an associated arterial injury that requires repair.

Open fractures require early irrigation and debridement prior to definitive fracture fixation. **Most open fractures above grade I should have a second irrigation and debridement 24 to 72 h after initial debridement to allow removal of tissue that has become necrotic in the days following the injury.** Debridement must include all nonarticular bone fragments that are without soft tissue attachment, even if this results in a bone defect. Temporary use of antibiotic polymethylmethacrylate beads placed under closed skin or under a synthetic dressing as a "bead pouch" can deliver high levels of antibiotics locally. Patients with open fractures should also receive immediate parenteral antibiotic coverage using a first-generation cephalosporin in grade I and II fractures and adding an aminoglycoside for grade III fractures. Penicillin is added for wounds with extensive soil contamination or for barnyard injuries. It is also important to make sure that the patient has an updated tetanus prophylaxis or receives tetanus toxoid. Antibiotic coverage and due respect for open injuries is associated with reduced rates of infection.

Fracture management for open fractures depends on the location, fracture pattern, and grade of injury. In general, low-grade fractures can be treated similarly to closed fractures after adequate irrigation and debridement have been performed. In grade III injuries, temporary external fixation is prudent until wound healing is assured, at which time conversion to internal fixation is often beneficial.

MANGLED EXTREMITY

Treatment of the patient with a mangled extremity is another difficult scenario for the orthopedist. The mangled extremity is defined by the presence of a high-energy open fracture of a long bone (usually the tibia) with a grade

III wound that cannot be closed with local tissues and at least one additional confounding characteristic: vascular injury, major nerve injury with loss of tactile or protective sensation, and/or a second complex osseous injury in the limb.

Advances in microvascular surgery, soft tissue coverage, bone grafting techniques, and implant metallurgy have made salvage of almost any extremity injury technically possible. However, the financial, physical, and emotional investment on the part of the patient can be overwhelming. The following questions need to be addressed: what are the prospects for a *functioning, pain-free* limb, how much time will it take, and what will be the cost to the patient financially and emotionally in time lost from employment and separation from family?

Limb salvage often necessitates multiple surgical procedures for soft tissue problems, infection, and fracture nonunion; the patient suffers economic damage, pain, and stress-related issues that often result in narcotic addiction, depression, and divorce. Early amputation and prosthetic rehabilitation has been shown to achieve a faster, more predictable recovery with reduced long-term impairment. The prosthesis will often function better than the salvaged limb. The physical and psychosocial effects of the injury and amputation are, however, substantial in spite of advances in prosthetics.

The difficulty for the surgeon is to determine when to attempt salvage and when to amputate. A variety of scoring systems have been devised (such as The Mangled Extremity Severity Score) based on the presence of risk factors such as time of ischemia and shock, neurologic injury, patient age, and wound characteristics (type of energy of injury and contamination). These systems have been shown not to be completely reliable.

Indications for early tibial fracture amputation include (1) grade IIIC fractures with a poor prognosis with complete tibial nerve injury and/or a severe foot injury and (2) an open fracture crush injury with an ischemia time of more than 6 h.

In the upper extremity, complete disruption of the brachial plexus combined with a grade III fracture is often the indication for amputation.

The decision whether to proceed with amputation or limb salvage must be made on an individual basis and undertaken with consideration for the patient's overall physical and psychosocial milieu and the injury. Older patients with medical or social comorbidities such as diabetes, peripheral vascular disease, or smoking are poor candidates for attempts at reconstruction of large osseous and soft tissue defects. A discussion with the patient and family of the options, likely course of treatment, and risks and benefits is crucial prior to final decision making. Unfortunately, the patient who is unable to deal with amputation and move ahead will be equally poorly equipped to deal with the trials of limb salvage.

SELECTED READINGS

Bosse MJ, Kellam JF. Orthopaedic management decisions in the multiple-trauma patient. In Browner BD, Jupiter JB, Levine AM, Trafton PG (eds): *Skeletal Trauma*, 3d ed. Philadelphia: Saunders, 2003: chap 6.

Georgiadis GM, Behrens FF, Joyce MJ, et al. Open tibial fractures with severe soft-tissue loss. *J Bone Joint Surg* 75A:1431–1441, 1993.

MacKenzie EJ, Bosse MJ, Castillo BC, et al. Functional outcomes following trauma-related lower-extremity amputation. *J Bone Joint Surg* 86A:1636–1645, 2004.

Nowotarski PJ, Turen CH, Brumback RJ, Scarboro JM. Conversion of external fixation to intramedullary nailing for fractures of the shaft of the femur in multiply injured patients. *J Bone Joint Surg* 82A:781–788, 2000.

Pape HC, Hildebrand F, Pertschy S, et al. Changes in the management of femoral shaft fractures in polytrauma patients: from early total care to damage control orthopedic surgery. *J Orthop Trauma* 18(8 suppl):S13–S22, 2004.

Reynolds MA, Richardson JD, Spain DA, et al. Is the timing of fracture fixation important for the patient with multiple trauma? *Ann Surg* 222:470–478, 1995.

Scalea TM, Boswell SA, Scott JD, et al. External fixation as a bridge to intramedullary nailing for patients with multiple injuries and with femur fractures: damage control orthopaedics. *J Trauma* 48:613–621, 2000.

Starr AJ, Hunt JL, Chason DP, et al. Treatment of femur fracture with associated head injury. *J Orthop Trauma* 12(1):38–45, 1998.

2 | Methods of Fixation

Walter W. Virkus   Emile P. Wakim

Fracture healing requires stability at the fracture site. Stability can be obtained with both operative and nonoperative methods. The advantage of most operative methods is that they eliminate the need for postoperative bracing, which allows earlier motion and limits stiffness and disuse osteopenia. Stability can be either absolute, in which case there is no motion at the fracture site, or relative, where there is a slight amount of motion at the fracture site. The fracture fixation employed depends on the stability desired and the nature of the injury. Generally, absolute stability requires rigid fixation with plates and screws, which generate compression across the fracture site. Compression of the fracture ends increases stability. Relative stability can be achieved with multiple methods, including casting, external fixation, and various types of internal fixation. Fractures stabilized with rigid fixation heal by primary bone healing, whereas fractures stabilized with relative stability methods heal by secondary bone healing (formation of callus).

There are two general methods of operative fracture fixation: internal fixation and external fixation. Internal fixation involves the placement of screws, plates, wires, or intramedullary rods through open means, across fracture fragments to impart stability. External fixation implies the use of percutaneously placed pins and wires attached to external bars or rings to stabilize the fracture.

INTERNAL FIXATION

The main benefit of internal fixation is that it provides stable fixation, allowing postoperative mobilization. Healing can occur via primary or secondary bone healing, depending on the stability obtained at surgery. It is important to understand that plate fixation can be used to obtain both absolute and relative stability, depending on how it is applied. Internal fixation methods include plates and screws, Kirschner wires, intramedullary nails, and tension-band constructs.

Implant Metallurgy

Orthopedic implants used for fracture fixation are generally made of one of two types of metal. Historically, stainless steel has been the most commonly used metal for fracture implants. It has the advantage of being relatively inexpensive, easy to machine, and strong. It is fairly stiff compared to the modulus of elasticity of cortical bone. Titanium fracture implants are becoming more common. Compared to stainless steel, they are softer, less stiff, and more expensive. One advantage is that they have higher fatigue strength. However, if they become nicked or scratched during implantation, the nick serves as a stress riser, dramatically decreasing the strength of the implant. Titanium can also be more difficult to work with because it is softer, and screw heads tend to strip or shear off more easily. Studies have not shown any significant clinical advantage of titanium versus stainless steel implants for most fracture scenarios.

Screw Anatomy

Screws vary based on certain specifics of their construction. The core diameter of a screw is the diameter of the shaft of the screw without the threads (Fig. 2-1). This corresponds to the drill bit size used to create a pilot hole for the screw. The outer diameter of a screw is the diameter across the threads. This corresponds to the drill bit size used to create a glide hole. Screw sizes are named according to their outer diameter. The pitch of a screw is the distance between the threads. This is the distance a screw will advance with one full revolution. Cortical screws have a shallow thread (smaller difference between the core and outer diameter) and finer pitch to increase the contact area within hard cortical bone. Cancellous screws are designed with deep threads (larger difference between the core and outer diameter) and a coarse pitch (large distance between threads) to maximize their purchase in softer cancellous bone. Screws are further differentiated by whether they are fully or partially threaded. Holding strength is increased and insertional torque decreased when grooves for the screw threads are created prior to screw insertion, a process called *tapping*. Self-tapping screws have cutting flutes at their ends, which cut grooves in the bone at the same time the screw is inserted.

Screw Applications

Screws can be used to provide compression across a fracture or to secure a plate to the involved bone. Interfragmentary compression can be accomplished

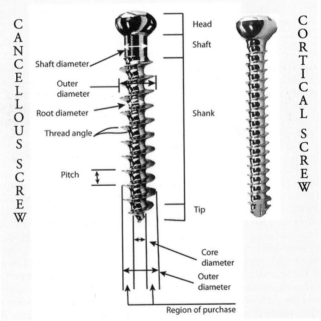

FIG. 2-1   Schematic showing the differences between a cortical and a cancellous screw.

2 METHODS OF FIXATION

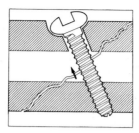

FIG. 2-2   Lag screw technique.

with a partially threaded screw or, more classically, with a fully threaded screw placed through a glide hole (a hole of the same diameter as the screw) (Fig. 2-2). The best compression is obtained when the screw is placed perpendicular to the fracture. Lag screws should not be placed less than three screw diameters from the nearest cortical margin so as to minimize the risk of fragmentation of the nearby cortex and screw hole. Self-tapping screws and non–self-tapping screws offer nearly the same holding power. The advantage of a standard screw in a tapped hole is that it can be inserted into bone with greater ease and precision, especially when lagging obliquely through a thick cortex. Self-tapping screws cut new grooves into the bone each time they are inserted; this can result in loosening of the screw if it is loosened or reinserted. Thus, self-tapping screws should be used with caution as lag screws. Self-tapping screws are best suited for the fixation of plates to bone because of their relatively fast placement.

Plate Fixation

Many different plate designs are available today. Dynamic compression plates (DCPs) offer a ramped hole that allows the plate to generate compression across a fracture without the use of a lag screw (Fig. 2-3).

Limited-contact dynamic compression plates (LC-DCPs) have grooves on their undersurface; these limit the interference with periosteal blood supply and allow easier contouring between the plate holes. All plates, including DC plates, can also be used to apply compression by using additional devices such as clamps or tensioners. LC-DC plates come in small-fragment (3.5 mm) and large-fragment (4.5 mm) sizes. Broad LC-DC 4.5-mm plates have staggered holes designed to minimize the placement of multiple screws in a single plane, thus possibly causing splintering or cracks in large, thick cortical bones. These plates are used for the femur, tibia, and humerus. Narrow LC-DC 4.5-mm plates are used for smaller tibiae and humerii. The LC-DC 3.5-mm plate is used for fractures of the forearm, fibula, clavicle, and pelvis. Semitubular plates are thinner, rounded plates. They come in large-fragment (one-half tubular) and small-fragment (one-third tubular) varieties. The one-third tubular plate is less stiff and thinner than an LC-DC plate and is typically used in regions with minimal soft tissue coverage, such as the lateral malleolus of the ankle. Reconstruction plates are less stiff than compression plates but allow for greater contouring. These plates are especially useful in pelvic, distal humeral, and clavicular fractures because they can be bent on a flat axis to better conform to the osseous anatomy. Anatomy and fracture-specific plates are

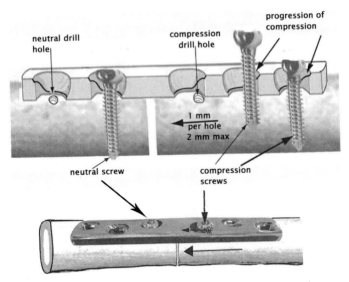

FIG. 2-3   The ramped hole of a DC plate can apply compression across a transverse fracture.

newer designs. Theoretically, these plates can be applied more easily than plates that need contouring, with enhanced fixation and little alteration in their biomechanics.

Plating Methods

Plates can be used in many ways to obtain the ideal fixation for a given fracture. **Compression plating**, with the screws applied eccentrically in an oblong hole, can be used to compress the ends of a simple transverse fracture together. The plate is applied to the first fragment in neutral position and then to the second fragment in compression mode. In plating transverse, diaphyseal fractures, prebending of the plate approximately 1 mm will prevent a fracture gap from forming on the far cortex (compressive forces are greater at the near cortex than the far cortex with placement of a straight plate on a straight bone). **Neutralization plating** occurs when a plate is used to provide protection to lag-screw fixation. Although lag screws provide excellent compression across an oblique fracture, they are weak in resisting torsional forces. A neutralization plate neutralizes these torsional forces (Fig. 2-4). The lag screw can be placed either through the neutralization plate (preferred) or outside the plate. **Buttress plates** are used to hold up or buttress an elevated fracture fragment (Fig. 2-5). **Antiglide plating** is used to reduce or prevent the shortening of oblique fractures (Fig. 2-6).

   Bridge plating is a technique whereby a long plate is fixed to either side of a long segmental fracture (Fig. 2-7). The fracture site is minimally violated, with plate fixation occurring at opposite ends of the plate remote from the zone of injury. This provides relative stability and preserves the relative length and alignment of the extremity without disturbing the biology of a comminuted fracture.

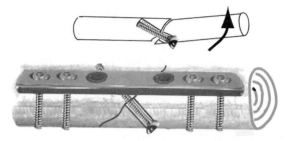

FIG. 2-4   A neutralization plate protects a lag screw against torsional failure.

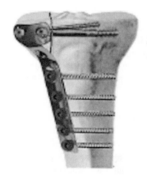

FIG. 2-5   A buttress plate holds up fractures that have been depressed or tend to collapse.

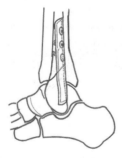

FIG. 2-6   An antiglide plate prevents shortening of an oblique fracture line.

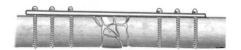

FIG. 2-7   A bridge plate is a long plate applied to a comminuted fracture; it is affixed to the bone only on either side of the area of comminution.

Percutaneous plating with less dissection of soft tissue and percutaneous screw fixation is an advanced plating technique that minimizes soft tissue disruption and optimizes the biology of fracture healing.

It is important to understand that all these techniques can be utilized with a variety of different plates. The names used above describe the plating technique, not the type of plate.

Locking plates are a new addition to the inventory of internal fixation. The stability of the plate-screw-bone unit with these plates is maintained by the screws threading into the plate, as opposed to the frictional force created by screws compressing the plate to the bone, as in standard plates. Additionally, the screws locking into the plate create a fixed-angle device that provides additional stability to the side of the fracture opposite the plate (Fig. 2-8A). This is because the screws do not toggle at their junction with the plate. The fixed-angle construct is also much stronger in resisting pullout than conventional plating, because locked plates require the simultaneous pullout of all the screws from the bone before the plate fails; with conventional plating, on the other hand, the screws loosen individually. Moreover, because the locking fixation relies less on purchase in the bone, these plates can maintain good fixation with only unicortical screws. In general, the stability of a unicortical locked screw approximates the stability of a bicortical standard screw.

Thus, locked plating has a definite advantage over conventional plating in treating fractures in osteoporotic bone, fractures with no inherent axial stability, and periarticular fractures. Most of these plates have oblong holes that allow a locking screw on one side of the hole or a standard screw on the other side. This allows the use of both locking and standard plating techniques in obtaining optimal reduction and fixation. In summary, the locking plates are advantageous when they are used to treat osteoporotic patients, periprosthetic fractures, periarticular fractures, and in connection with minimally invasive fixation techniques.

The less invasive stabilization system (LISS) is a specific type of locking plate for percutaneous insertion (Fig 2-8B). It is made of titanium, uses only unicortical screws, and has an outrigger guide for placing the screws through the plate. Its uses are similar to those of the standard locking plate.

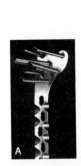
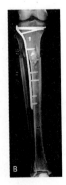

FIG. 2-8 *A.* A locking plate with divergent and convergent screws that lock into the plate, making it a modular fixed-angle plate. *B.* An AP radiograph demonstrating the use of an LISS plate on a fracture of the proximal tibia.

Cerclage Wires

Cerclage wires are used for adjunctive fixation in fracture care. The wires can be tensioned to hold a plate or bone strut against the fractured bone. However, cerclage wires offer minimal rotational control of the fracture and can severely disrupt the vascular supply to the bone in the region of the fracture. They can also loosen quickly if necrosis occurs under the wires. Therefore they should not be used as primary fixation. Their use should be limited to situations where screws cannot be used to fix a plate to the involved bone, as in periprosthetic fractures.

Tension Band

Tension-band constructs function by converting tension forces at the near cortex (under the tension band) into compressive forces at the far cortex (Fig. 2-9). Tension bands provide only active compression when applied to a mobile joint, allowing active motion during fracture healing; otherwise the tension band will apply static compressive forces (i.e., fixation of the medial malleolus). Olecranon and patellar fractures are ideal for converting distracting (tension) forces into compressive forces. Avulsion fractures are often fixed well with tension-band constructs (i.e., medial malleolus, greater tuberosity of the humerus, and greater trochanter of the femur).

Dynamic Compression Screw

Sliding compression screws are an excellent choice for fixation of intertrochanteric femoral fractures. These implants function by allowing controlled shortening of the fracture due to the sliding mechanism of the lag screw through the side plate. This sliding motion allows the fracture ends to settle until bone-to-bone contact prevents further shortening and provides stability to the construct (Fig. 2-10). The controlled shortening of the fracture decreases the possibility that the lag screw will cut out of the femoral head, which is often osteoporotic. These devices require an intact lateral cortex and posteromedial cortical buttress to function optimally and avoid failure.

Intramedullary Nails

Intramedullary nailing of long bone diaphyseal fractures is a widely accepted and successful form of treatment. The advantages of intramedullary nailing

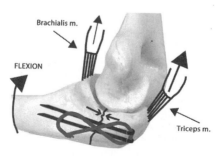

FIG. 2-9   A tension band converts tensile forces across a fracture into compression forces.

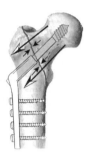

FIG. 2-10   A dynamic compression screw allows controlled shortening at the fracture site.

include minimal soft tissue disruption, ease of insertion, preservation of fracture hematoma, and the potential for load sharing between the injured bone and the nail. Variables in intramedullary nailing include nail stiffness (rigid vs. flexible), insertion method (reamed vs. unreamed), insertion direction (antegrade vs. retrograde), and locking mode (static vs. dynamic).

Flexible intramedullary nails have historically been used in patients with axially stable fractures and more recently in pediatric fractures. These nails are inserted through portals in the metaphysis and therefore do not disrupt growth plates. Usually multiple nails are placed so as to provide sufficient stability. They are fairly easy to remove because they are not statically locked. They provide good bending stability in more stable fracture patterns but are less stable against torsional forces or in comminuted fractures. Examples include Rush rods, Enders nails, and newer flexible titanium nails.

Rigid nails provide greater stiffness and mechanical strength than flexible nails. The design of the rigid nail mirrors the anatomy of the bone it is stabilizing (i.e., providing anterior bow to the femur) to re-create normal biomechanics. Nails can be inserted after reaming the intramedullary canal, to increase its diameter, or without reaming. The advantage of reaming is that it allows a nail of greater diameter to be inserted. The strength of a nail is exponentially related to its diameter. The insertion of larger nails and their corresponding larger locking screws has been shown to minimize implant breakage. Reaming may also generate an autografting effect. There are theoretical disadvantages to reaming. Vascular studies have shown that reaming destroys the endosteal blood supply, which feeds the inner cortex of the bone. This was thought to be detrimental to fracture healing and potentially to increase the incidence of infection due to the presence of necrotic bone. Additionally, reaming leads to embolization of the marrow contents, which may adversely affect pulmonary function in patients with preexisting lung injury. Current literature, however, supports the use of reaming in the insertion of intramedullary nails into all fractures except those with high-grade open injuries.

Some long bones, notably the femur and humerus, are amenable to either proximal-to-distal (antegrade) or distal-to-proximal (retrograde) nail insertion. In both these bones, there are advantages and disadvantages to each method. These are best demonstrated in the femur. Antegrade nailing traditionally uses a starting point in the piriformis fossa. Newer nails are being introduced that utilize a starting point in the greater trochanter. This starting point is not in line with the intramedullary canal of the femur and can lead to iatrogenic fracture of the femur or malalignment. Retrograde nailing uses a starting point in the distal femoral articular cartilage, just anterior to the intercondylar notch. The advantage of retrograde nails is that they are easier for the surgeon to place, especially in obese patients or in distal femoral fractures. They can also be inserted with the patient in the supine position, without a fracture table, which can be important in patients with multiple injuries. Commonly accepted indications for **retrograde femoral nailing** include **obese patients**, patients with **very distal femoral fractures**, and those with **multiple injuries**.

Statically locking an intramedullary nail prevents rotation and shortening at the fracture site but does not allow additional impaction at the fracture (Fig. 2-11). As a result, the nail and locking screws are required to bear a higher load until fracture healing. Dynamic locking of a nail allows for axial compression at the fracture site with weight bearing. The nail is either left unlocked proximal or distal to the fracture or a locking screw is placed in the oblong hole on the side opposite the fracture, allowing translation of the nail down the slot in axial compression. Dynamically locking the nail through an oblong hole has the advantage of controlling rotation and is preferred over the use of no locking screw. Dynamization is optimally utilized in fracture patterns that have some inherent axial stability, but nails should have at least one locking screw on each side of the fracture when acute fractures are being nailed. Reconstruction nails, also called cephalomedullary nails, are of a specific kind in which the proximal locking screw is placed up the femoral neck into the head for proximal femoral fractures.

External Fixation

External fixation is the percutaneous placement, above and below a fracture, of wires or half pins that are connected to bars and tubes to provide stability. The advantages of external fixation include minimal soft tissue trauma, avoidance of hardware in a contaminated wound, rapidity of application, and modularity to adapt to many injury patterns. An external fixator can be used for temporary or long-term fixation; it is a good option in situations where the risk of infection is high or the soft tissue is compromised. The disadvantages include the cumbersome nature of the fixator, complications related to the pin

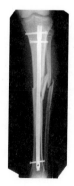

FIG. 2-11   A statically locked nail stabilizes a comminuted fracture of the tibial shaft.

sites (infection, loosening), and varying degrees of stability, which can result in malunion or nonunion. External fixators can vary from very simple frames consisting of two pins connected by two bars to very complex frames with wires and rings that have the ability to correct deformities or lengthen bones.

External fixation components vary slightly, but the basic sets include transfixation pins (5- or 6-mm pins, often with threads in the central portion, designed to be inserted much like a traction pin, protruding from both sides of the bone), half pins or Shanz pins (protruding from only one side of the bone), bars, and clamps to attach pins to bars or bars to bars. Pins vary in diameter from 2.0 to 6.0 mm. For tibial, femoral, and pelvic fixation, the pins should be at least 5 mm in diameter. For the humerus, forearm/wrist, and fingers, the pins should be at least 4, 3, and 2 mm, respectively. If a pin is too small in diameter, the tension across it can cause micromotion and eventual loosening. If the pin's diameter is too large, the bone can fracture at this stress riser. Thin wires can also be used for external fixation. These are particularly useful in very small segments, where there is limited room for multiple pins. When placed under high tension, thin wires have a strength and stiffness similar to that of half pins. The wires used in external fixation range from 1.5 to 2.0 mm in diameter, and they are typically attached to rings.

The ability of an external fixator to provide sufficient stability for fracture healing depends on multiple factors. In approximate order of importance, these factors include:

- Pin diameter (larger is stiffer)
- Pin location close to the fracture site on either side of the fracture
- Pin spread (distance between adjacent pins maximized)
- Pin number (an increased number of pins means less stress at each individual pin-bone interface; the minimum number of pins on each side of the fracture is two)
- Placing bars as close to the bone without impinging on soft tissues
- Placing at least one rod in the same axis as the applied load
- Double stacking of bars is stiffer than single-bar constructs
- Multiple planes of fixation are stiffer than single plane

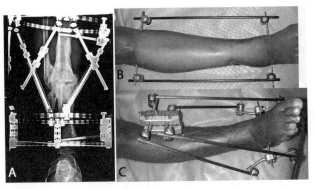

FIG. 2-12   *A.* AP radiograph of a ring external fixator on a tibial nonunion, *B.* uniplanar external fixator, and *C.* delta frame external fixator.

The term *uniplanar external fixator* indicates that all pins are placed in the same plane. Biplanar fixators have pins in two or more planes (Fig. 2-12). The construction of an external fixator depends on the goals of treatment. Fixators placed for short-term restoration of limb length and alignment can be very simple. Fixators placed for definitive fixation of a fracture require additional pins or wires and bar attachments to increase the stability of the frame and limit motion at the fracture site.

SELECTED READINGS

Gautier E, Sommer C. Guidelines for the clinical application of the LCP injury. *Int J Care Injured* 34(suppl 12):63–76, 2003.

Mazzacca AD, Caputo AE, Browner BD, et al. Principles of internal fixation. In Browner BD, Jupiter JB, Levine AM, Trafton PG (eds): *Skeletal Trauma: Basic Science, Management, and Reconstruction,* Vol I, 3d ed. Philadelphia: Saunders, 2003.

Reudi TP, Murphy WM. *AO Principles of Fracture Management.* Stuttgart: Thieme, 2000.

Texhammar R, Colton C. *AO/ASIF Instruments and Implant: A Technical Manual.* Berlin: Springer-Verlag, 1994.

3 | Nonoperative Techniques

John A. Elstrom

The nonoperative techniques covered in this chapter are splints and casts, traction, and arthrocentesis. Fractures that are undisplaced and fractures that can be reduced and stabilized by external means are suitable for casting, splinting, traction, or a combination of casting and traction.

SPLINTS AND CASTS

Splints and casts support and immobilize the injured extremity and thereby reduce pain, prevent further injury of tissues in proximity to a fracture, and maintain alignment. Splinting and casting are also used postoperatively to reduce swelling, maintain surrounding joints in a position of function (e.g., after open reduction of an ankle fracture to prevent equinus deformity), and provide additional stabilization when fracture fixation is tenuous. Splinting and casting are accomplished with plaster or synthetic materials such as fiberglass. Splints differ from casts in that they are not circumferential and thus allow swelling of the extremity with less increase in pressure. Casts are circumferential and swelling within the cast increases pressure, potentially resulting in increased compartment pressures or pressure sores. Casts tend to immobilize an extremity more completely than splints.

Fundamental Rules of Splinting and Casting

The rules for splinting and casting are essentially identical:

1. At least one joint distal to the injury is immobilized. Immobilization of both joints, proximal and distal to the injury, is often beneficial if the fracture is below the elbow or the knee.
2. Prior to immobilization, deformity is corrected and fractures are reduced and, if possible, the extremity is placed in a position of function (e.g., the hand is immobilized in the clam-digger position, with the metacarpophalangeal joints in flexion and the interphalangeal joints in extension).
3. The extremity is padded to prevent skin breakdown and neurovascular compression. Incisions or wounds are covered with a sterile dressing. A layer of stockinette is applied, followed by cast padding appropriate to the type of material being used. Bony prominences (e.g., the posterior aspect of the heel and malleoli) and areas where nerves pass over bone (e.g., the medial elbow and the fibular neck) are protected with extra padding, foam, or felt.
4. The splint or cast material is moistened with cold or room-temperature water to provide a prolonged setting time and decrease the heat of reaction, which could burn the skin as the material sets. This is especially important if the patient is anesthetized and cannot complain of pain. Fingertip indentation is avoided because it can result in pressure necrosis of the skin. Splints and casts covering damaged skin or surgical wounds should not be allowed to get wet.

Techniques of Cast Application

Plaster and fiberglass have different physical properties. It has been demonstrated that the intrinsic recoil of fiberglass results in potentially greater pressures on the skin. Plaster casts are undoubtedly safer in situations where swelling is apt to be significant and the patient's skin is vulnerable (as in those with diabetes, stasis dermatitis, or peripheral vascular disease). It has been suggested that fiberglass casts be applied with a stretch-relax technique to address this potential pitfall. The polyurethane resin can be tacky, making it difficult to unwind the roll, and when the mesh is applied with the standard technique, the material may be applied around the limb under substantial tension; this could lead to increased pressure. The stretch-relax technique involves pulling the fiberglass roll away from the limb to unwind the mesh. After the segment is unwound, the tension is relaxed and the mesh is laid on and around the limb. Only slight restretching is needed for contouring. To reduce pressure further, an anterior longitudinal cut can be made and the cast spread.

Fatigue prevents the patient from holding the upper extremity in the desired position during cast application. If an assistant is not available, a short or long arm cast can be applied by using fingertip traction to the index and long fingers, with countertraction over the flexed elbow. The material is rolled on and carefully molded to prevent the cast from slipping or the fracture from displacing.

Short arm casts are applied far enough proximally and with appropriate three-point molding to create an oval cross section, preventing the cast from sliding down the forearm like a glove. To prevent forearm rotation, the cast is extended above the elbow. To prevent elbow flexion and extension, the cast is extended to the proximal arm.

Lower extremity casts are applied with the patient sitting or supine and the foot supported by a bolster or an assistant. The ankle is usually positioned in neutral to prevent equinus contracture. The diameter of a limb changes from proximal to distal, as it is not cylindrical; therefore the padding should be torn on the side of the larger diameter (i.e., proximal part of the padding) to conform the padding material to the limb. The padding is overlapped 50%. The cast material is then applied from the metatarsal heads to the upper limit of the cast.

Short leg casts extend to the tibial tubercle. Patellar tendon-bearing casts are molded over the patellar tendon and patella but allow knee flexion. **Long leg casts** extend to the proximal thigh. Trimming of the leg cast should allow toe flexion and avoid pressure against the fifth toe. To prevent the cast from slipping on wood and linoleum floors, a cast shoe or rubber walking heel is applied. The rubber walking heel is advantageous when a limited axis of loading the lower extremity is desired (e.g., to avoid force transmission through fractured metatarsals). The rubber heel is placed proximal to the fracture.

Tucks in the cast material are taken on the side of the limb with the smaller diameter to conform the material to the limb. **Additional longitudinal splints** (i.e., a posterior splint at the ankle and medial and lateral splints at the knee) provide additional strength to the casts. **Molding** the cast material over bony prominences while it is being applied increases stability. The **cast is trimmed** by removing excess material with scissors or a cast saw, pulling the stockinette over the edge of the cast, and wrapping it with additional cast material.

A Gore-Tex cast liner is currently available to allow bathing, pool swimming, and hydrotherapy to a person with a fiberglass cast. Because the exposure to water does not wet the liner but only the skin, rapid drying by evaporation prevents skin maceration. Use of this material in casts covering damaged skin or surgical wounds would not be appropriate.

Techniques of Splinting

The technique of splinting usually involves the use of a casting material that hardens after it is applied. However, there are other types of splints that are preformed. These are often used at the site of an accident (e.g., aluminum universal arm and leg splints, ladder splints, and inflatable splints) and are seldom left in place after the initial evaluation is completed. Preformed splints used for definitive management are the cervical collar, figure-of-eight clavicle splint, knee immobilizer, and ankle stirrup (air cast). A functional fracture brace can also be used for the definitive management of diaphyseal fractures of the humerus and tibia. The brace must fit adequately and the soft tissue damage must be minimal.

The **upper extremity** is splinted while the arm is in fingertrap traction or held by an assistant. Plaster or synthetic material 4 to 5 in. wide and 10 to 15 layers (sheets) thick is used. When plaster is used, the splint is conformed to the extremity with a gauze wrap and Ace bandage. The material is applied from the metacarpal heads to the proximal extent of the splint. A short arm splint is applied to the dorsal, volar, or lateral surface of the forearm and extends to the elbow. The sugar-tongs splint starts on the volar surface of the hand and forearm and wraps around the elbow, extending to the dorsal surface of the hand. The thumb spica splint extends from the tip of the thumb along the radial aspect of the forearm to just below the flexion crease of the elbow. The radial styloid is padded to prevent injury to the superficial branch of the radial nerve.

The **lower extremity** is splinted with the patient sitting and the ankle in neutral. The ankle is splinted with a sugar-tongs splint. The splint extends down the medial aspect of the leg under the foot and then back up the lateral aspect of the leg. When a posterior splint is applied, it must be thicker than the sugar-tongs splint, and additional splints are used medially or laterally at the ankle to provide strength. To prevent thermal injury, cold water is used; excessively thick splints and heavy wrapping are avoided.

Complications of Splinting and Casting

Complications include pressure sores, burns, and skin irritation.

Pressure sores occur when sensation is reduced (e.g., diabetic peripheral neuropathy); decreased sensation is a major concern in splinting and casting. To minimize the incidence of skin breakdown, bony prominences are padded, and the splint or cast is changed frequently. Pain underneath a splint or cast is a complaint to be taken seriously; it is managed by windowing of the cast over the involved area or by cast removal and inspection of the skin.

Burns after the application of a splint or cast occur most commonly when plaster is used with warm water and the material is excessively thick or wrapped with a bandage that does not allow heat dissipation. To minimize the incidence of burns, the use of cold water and adequate padding are essential.

Itching beneath the splint or cast can often be controlled with the use of mild analgesics such as aspirin and a hair dryer set on room temperature to blow cool air underneath the cast. Powders and ointments should not be applied to the skin under the cast in hopes of drying or lubricating the skin.

TRACTION

Traction is used temporarily to splint or definitively manage fractures. Traction is applied through the skin (skin traction) or a pin inserted into a long bone (skeletal traction).

Skin Traction

The advantage of skin traction is that it does not require insertion of a pin. The disadvantage is that it can result in skin breakdown. The danger of skin breakdown limits the length of time it can be used and the amount of weight applied (10 lb). Skin traction is applied through adhesive strips applied to the skin.

Buck's traction uses a "Buck's" boot to apply traction temporarily before surgery to the lower extremity with a fractured hip. It employs a prefabricated soft synthetic boot held in place with Velcro straps through which 7 to 10 lb of weight is applied. A pillow is placed beneath the knee, slightly flexing it. The most common error occurs when the patient slides down in bed and the weights rest on the floor or the boot lies against the end of the bed. A push box between the end of the bed and the opposite foot prevents the patient from sliding down in bed.

Recent investigations indicate that a pillow placed beneath the patient's knee and distal thigh is just as effective by itself in reducing pain, suggesting that the addition of traction is not necessary.

Skeletal Traction

Skeletal traction is used most frequently to manage acetabular and femoral fractures temporarily and occasionally fractures of the distal humerus and distal tibia. More weight can be applied for a longer period of time through skeletal traction than through skin traction.

Basic rules of skeletal traction are as follows: (1) the pin should be inserted at 90 degrees to the long axis of the bone; (2) skeletal traction is contraindicated where there is damage to the ligaments of the joint proximal to the pin site; (3) radiographs in traction are obtained immediately after application and as required for adjustments; and (4) the neurologic and vascular status of the extremity is examined daily.

The technique of pin insertion is as follows: the area is shaved and scrubbed; local infiltration anesthesia (taking care to infiltrate the periosteum and skin on both sides) and parenteral sedation are used; pins are inserted from the side most vulnerable to neurovascular damage so that the point is accurately applied to the bone (e.g., lateral to medial in the distal femur and ulnar to radial in the proximal ulna); the skin is incised with a no. 11 blade; the pin is drilled by hand or power through the bone; the skin on the opposite side is incised as it is tented by the point of the pin; and stability of the pin is evaluated by pushing proximally and distally on one end of the pin to see if the bone moves with the pin—the "toggle test." Oblique placement of femoral traction pins for femoral fractures has been associated with an increased incidence of varus or valgus malalignment.

Pin selection is based on the following considerations: threads prevent the pin from loosening and sliding in the bone; threaded pins must have a larger caliber than smooth pins because the threads weaken the pin; smooth pins that are threaded in their midportions are especially useful; and threaded pins are not used when the pin will pass near a neurovascular bundle (e.g., through-and-

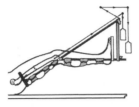

FIG. 3-1 Skeletal traction using a Thomas splint and Pierson attachment.

through olecranon pin), for fear of wrapping the soft tissues around the pin and causing a neurovascular injury.

Traction maintenance consists of supporting the part distal to the pin; twice-daily cleaning of the pin sites with sterile saline or peroxide; sterile dressings, and release of skin under tension to prevent skin irritation, with resulting pain and local infection.

For acetabular and femoral fractures, the pins are inserted through the distal femur at the flare of the condyles or through the proximal tibia 2 cm posterior and 1 cm inferior to the tibial tubercle. As longitudinal traction is applied through the pin, the leg is supported with slings or in a frame. The frame used most frequently is the Thomas frame with a Pierson attachment. The Pierson attachment is an outrigger that slides up and down the Thomas frame to compensate for the length of the femur and allow knee flexion (Fig. 3-1). Depending on the size of the patient, 15 to 30 lb of longitudinal traction is appropriate initially.

The safest type of **olecranon pin** is a screw with an eyelet, inserted at 90 degrees to the long axis of the ulna. A through-and-through pin can be used in the proximal ulnar metaphysis just distal to the olecranon fossa, but the ulnar nerve must be protected. When olecranon traction is used, it must be supplemented by supporting the hand and forearm with a sling or skin traction. Initially, 5 to 10 lb of longitudinal traction is applied (Fig. 3-2). The calcaneal pin is inserted 2 cm distal and 2 cm posterior to the medial malleolus. The leg is supported on a frame, and 5 to 10 lb of weight is applied initially.

ARTHROCENTESIS

Arthrocentesis, or aspiration, of a swollen, painful joint is both therapeutic and diagnostic. The traumatic hemarthroses most frequently aspirated are those

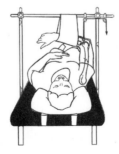

FIG. 3-2 Overhead olecranon traction with a forearm support.

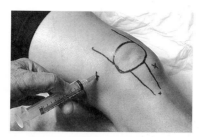

FIG. 3-3   Aspiration of the knee.

of the knee and elbow. The shoulder joint can be injected with local anesthetic to obtain anesthesia while a traumatic dislocation is being reduced.

Strict adherence to aseptic technique is essential: the area through which the joint is aspirated is shaved and scrubbed and sterile gloves are used. Local infiltration anesthesia is recommended. Large joints are aspirated with a 19-gauge needle. Smaller joints of the fingers and toes are aspirated with a 22-gauge needle, but its smaller diameter makes obtaining fluid difficult. The larger the syringe, the more negative pressure is generated, which tends to draw obstructive particles into the needle opening. A 10-mL syringe seems ideal.

The **contraindications to arthrocentesis** are periarticular sepsis and uncorrected coagulopathy. Tubes for synovial fluid cell count, microscopic examination, and culture should be available in the event that an effusion suggestive of an acute inflammatory arthritis is found.

Techniques of Arthrocentesis

The **knee** is aspirated with the patient supine and the joint extended. The needle is directed posterior to the quadriceps tendon at the superior lateral pole of the patella. Alternatively, the knee can be aspirated with the knee flexed. The needle is directed toward the center of the joint, starting just below and just medial or lateral to the inferior pole of the patella (Fig. 3-3).

Aspiration of the hip is done with the aid of fluoroscopy. The patient is supine and the hip is extended. A spinal needle is inserted lateral to the

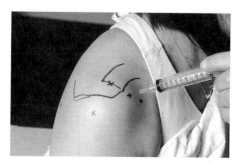

FIG. 3-4   Aspiration of the shoulder.

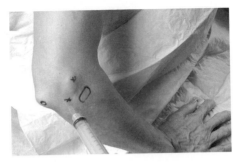

FIG. 3-5 Aspiration of the elbow.

femoral artery and 2 cm distal to the inguinal ligament. It is directed toward the inferior aspect of the femoral head and neck. The resistance of the hip capsule is apparent as the needle enters the joint.

Shoulder aspiration is performed with the patient sitting and the humerus in neutral or slight external rotation. Unless the patient is unusually large, a 1.5-in. needle is used. The needle is inserted lateral to the coracoid process and below the acromioclavicular joint. It is directed posteriorly into the interval just medial to the biceps tendon and near the junction of the supraspinatous and subscapularis tendon (Fig. 3-4).

Intraarticular lidocaine can be used to assist in obtaining analgesia during reduction of uncomplicated shoulder dislocations. In this technique, 20 mL of 1% lidocaine is injected with a 1.5-in. 20-gauge needle 2 cm inferior and lateral to the acromion in the sulcus formed by the absent humeral head. The needle is directed slightly caudad, and care must be taken to avoid the axillary nerve.

The **elbow** is aspirated with the patient sitting and the elbow in 80 degrees of flexion. A tense hemarthrosis can often be palpated in the interval between the lateral epicondyle, radial head, and olecranon. The needle is directed medially through the center of this triangular area (Fig. 3-5).

The **ankle** is aspirated through the interval between the tibialis anterior tendon and the medial malleolus at the joint line or just proximal and medial to the flare of the lateral malleolus at the level of the joint line (Fig. 3-6).

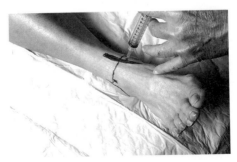

FIG. 3-6 Aspiration or injection of the ankle.

SELECTED READINGS

Davids JR, Frick SL, Skewes E, et al. Skin surface pressure beneath an above-the-knee cast: plaster casts compared with fiberglass casts. *J Bone Joint Surg* 79A:565–569, 1997.

Marson BM, Keenan MAE. Skin surface pressures under short leg casts. *J Orthop Trauma* 7:275–278, 1993.

4 | Anesthetic Techniques

Carl H. Nielsen

Physicians without specialty training in anesthesiology may safely employ the technique of minimal sedation and regional anesthesia for short surgical procedures provided that a few basic rules are followed. Drugs must never be administered to a patient without a plan for establishment of an airway, administration of oxygen, and immediate management of an overdose or side effect of the administered drug. The following recommendations apply only to healthy, nonpregnant patients without allergy to the drugs.

MODERATE AND DEEP SEDATION

Moderate sedation, frequently called conscious sedation, may allow the patient to tolerate unpleasant procedures by relieving anxiety, discomfort, and pain. Because it is not always possible to predict how a specific patient will respond to sedative and analgesic medication, both moderate and deep sedation may result in cardiac or respiratory depression. These adverse effects must be rapidly recognized and appropriately managed to avoid the risk of hypoxic brain damage, cardiac arrest, or death. "Practice Guidelines for Sedation and Analgesia by Non-Anesthesiologists" (see "Selected Readings" at the end of this chapter) gives an overview of this complex issue. Drug recommendations and dosages, monitoring, and recovery are beyond the scope of this handbook.

MINIMAL SEDATION

Midazolam (Versed) has a wide margin of safety, but it may cause respiratory depression with rapid injection and/or overdose. Dosage must be reduced for geriatric patients. Midazolam is administered intravenously, and 0.03 mg/kg is used as a single dose. The dose may be repeated after 5 min if the patient needs additional sedation. Midazolam has no analgesic properties. Mental function may be impaired for hours after midazolam administration.

ANALGESIA

Opioids rarely provide complete analgesia for even minor procedures, but they add to patient comfort when used as adjuncts to sedation and/or regional anesthesia. All opioids are potent dose-dependent respiratory depressants. Intramuscular injection is to be avoided because absorption may be slow and time to onset variable. An intravenous bolus of 2.5 mg morphine, 25 mg meperidine, or 50 m g fentanyl is used. The bolus dose may be repeated to a total of 10 mg morphine, 100 mg meperidine, or 100 m g fentanyl.

REGIONAL ANESTHESIA

Infiltration techniques inhibit excitation of sensory nerve endings and provide sensory anesthesia. Intravenous regional anesthesia is usually classified as an infiltration block, although the exact mechanism of action is unclear. Peripheral nerve block involves reversible block of nerve action potentials along all types of nerve fiber and is called *conduction anesthesia*.

Bier Block

Bier block, or intravenous regional anesthesia (IVR), is a suitable technique for operative procedures on the hand and forearm, with a duration of less than 1 h. This technique may also be used for foot and lower leg anesthesia, but the quality of anesthesia is not as good for the lower extremity as for the upper extremity. The following diseases of the limb are contraindications for the use of IVR: infection, malignant tumor, and vascular insufficiency.

A 20- or 22-gauge cannula is placed and secured in a distal vein on the limb to be anesthetized. A tourniquet is placed as proximally on the limb as possible; for longer-lasting procedures, two tourniquets or a double tourniquet must be used. The limb below the tourniquet is exsanguinated by compression with an elastic Esmarch bandage. The tourniquet is inflated to a pressure 100 mmHg above the systolic blood pressure. The source of the pressure must be calibrated and must continuously maintain the desired preset pressure. A regular cuff, sphygmomanometer, and bulb with release valve are inadequate as a tourniquet for IVR. Immediately after exsanguination, tourniquet inflation, and removal of the Esmarch bandage, a single dose of 50 mL 0.5% (250 mg) lidocaine (Xylocaine) is injected into the indwelling cannula. Complete IVR of the leg requires about 75 mL of local anesthetic. Use lidocaine only from a sealed single-dose vial without epinephrine. The cannula may be removed after the injection, and satisfactory anesthesia is obtained within 10 min. When two tourniquets are used, the distal one is deflated at this point. Should the patient complain about tourniquet pain before completion of the operation, the distal cuff is reinflated and about 20 s later the proximal cuff is deflated (Fig. 4-1). At completion of the operation, the tourniquet is deflated. This is not

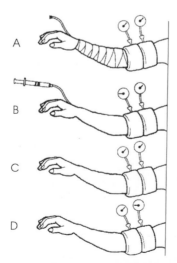

FIG. 4-1   Bier block. (*A*) The limb is exsanguinated and the tourniquets inflated. (*B*) The distal tourniquet is deflated and anesthetic injected. If there is tourniquet pain, the distal tourniquet is inflated (*C*) and the proximal tourniquet is deflated (*D*).

done until at least 15 min has elapsed after injection. Early release of the tourniquet may bring about a systemic reaction to the lidocaine.

Nerve Block

The following nerve blocks are all performed with 1 to 1.5% lidocaine, 1 to 1.5% mepivacaine (Carbocaine), or 0.5% bupivacaine (Marcaine). Distal blocks (i.e., of fingers and toes, wrist and ankle) must never be performed with local anesthetics containing epinephrine because of the risk of prolonged vasospasms. When epinephrine is used to prolong peripheral nerve blocks, the optimal concentration is 1:200,000, which is equivalent to 5 m g epinephrine per milliliter of local anesthetic. When small amounts of local anesthetics are injected, multiple-dose vials are appropriate. When larger amounts of local anesthetics are injected, the single-dose vial is used. The difference is that single-dose vials contain no preservatives, whereas multiple-dose vials do.

Digital Nerve Block

Four nerves innervate each finger and toe: two are palmar/plantar and two are dorsal. Block of these four nerves provides adequate anesthesia for minor operations. The injection may be performed at the base of the digit, but an injection about 1 cm farther proximal is less painful. Despite anesthesia of half of the two digits next to the anesthetized digit, it is the preferred method (Fig. 4-2).

A 23-gauge 1-in. needle is advanced from the dorsal side to the palmar/plantar fascia so that the needle tip can be palpated. It is retracted 2 mm, and 3 mL of local anesthetic is injected. The needle is retracted so that the tip is just below the subcutaneous tissue, and another 2 mL is injected. The procedure is repeated on the other side of the digit.

Wrist Block

Blocks of one, two, or all three nerves at the wrist will provide adequate anesthesia of the part of the hand innervated by the blocked nerve or nerves.

The **median nerve** runs in the wrist between the palmaris longus and flexor carpi radialis tendons. It is blocked approximately 2 cm proximal to the proximal wrist crease. With the hand slightly dorsiflexed, a 23-gauge 1-in. needle is advanced perpendicular to the skin between these two tendons, and the area is infiltrated with 5 to 8 mL of local anesthetic (Fig. 4-3). If there is paresthe-

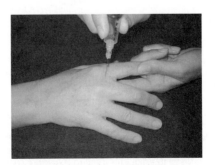

FIG. 4-2 Digital nerve block.

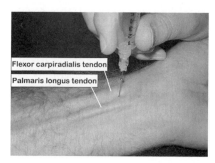

Flexor carpiradialis tendon

Palmaris longus tendon

FIG. 4-3 Median nerve block at the wrist.

sia, the needle is stopped and the entire volume is injected. If there is no paresthesia, the local anesthetic is deposited with a fanwise injection. This block is not used in patients with carpal tunnel syndrome and is not performed distally at the level of the carpal tunnel.

The **ulnar nerve** is blocked approximately 6 cm proximal to the proximal wrist crease, just to the radial side of the tendon of the flexor carpi ulnaris. The nerve is on the ulnar side of the ulnar artery. A 23-gauge 1-in. needle is inserted perpendicular to the skin, and 8 to 10 mL of local anesthetic is injected. If the block is performed less than 6 cm proximal to the wrist, it will not include the dorsal branch of the ulnar nerve; a block of this branch must be performed with a subcutaneous ring of anesthesia around the ulnar aspect of the wrist, starting from the flexor carpi ulnaris tendon. For this block, 5 mL of local anesthetic is used.

The **radial nerve** is blocked with infiltration under the brachioradialis tendon 8 cm proximal to the proximal wrist crease. Alternatively, the radial nerve is blocked with a subcutaneous ring of anesthesia. The ring starts at the radial aspect of the wrist at the flexor carpi radialis and continues around the wrist dorsally to the styloid process of the ulna. Both methods require approximately 5 to 8 mL of local anesthetic.

Elbow Block

The **ulnar nerve** is blocked 3 cm proximal to its course in the groove behind the medial epicondyle. A 23-gauge 1-in. needle, pointed either distally or proximally, is advanced at a 45-degree angle to the course of the nerve; 5 to 8 mL of local anesthetic is injected around the nerve.

The median nerve lies on a line drawn on the anterior elbow between the two epicondyles on the medial side of the brachial artery and is easily palpated in thin individuals. The block is performed at this level with a 23-gauge 1-in. needle. When paresthesia is encountered, 5 to 8 mL local anesthetic is injected (Fig. 4-4). A subcutaneous infiltration is required to block the cutaneous branches to the forearm.

To find the **radial nerve**, a line is drawn from the most prominent point of the humeral head to the lateral epicondyle. The nerve crosses the humerus one-third of the way up from the lateral epicondyle. It can be palpated on the bone; the block is performed with a 23-gauge 1-in. needle and 5 to 8 mL of local anesthetic. Alternatively, the radial nerve is blocked with the lateral cutaneous nerve of the forearm, as described next.

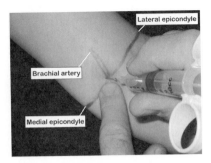

FIG. 4-4   Median nerve block at the elbow.

The **lateral cutaneous nerve** of the forearm is a continuation of the musculocutaneous nerve and perforates the deep fascia on the lateral side of the biceps muscle just proximal to the elbow. The lateral cutaneous nerve and the radial nerve can both be blocked with a 23-gauge 1.5-in. needle inserted between the brachioradialis muscle and the biceps tendon (Fig. 4-5). The needle is directed proximally toward the anterolateral surface of the lateral epicondyle, and 3 mL of local anesthetic is injected just above the periosteum. Bone contact is made two more times, and 3 mL is injected each time above the periosteum. An additional 5 mL of local anesthetic is injected as the needle is withdrawn. If paresthesia is elicited, 5 to 8 mL of local anesthetic is injected and no further bone contact is necessary. A subcutaneous ring of 5 mL of local anesthetic from the biceps tendon to the brachioradialis muscle will provide anesthesia of the superficial branches of the musculocutaneous nerve.

Ankle Block

Foot operations lasting less than 2 h can be done with an ankle block. The block provides anesthesia for a tourniquet at the level of the malleoli. A common mistake is to block the ankle too distally. Injections 1 to 2 cm above the malleoli provide a more complete block. The block is a conduction block of the five nerves that innervate the foot: three on the dorsal side and two on the plantar side. The block is performed with a 23-gauge 1-in. needle, and 5 to

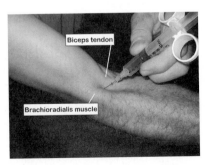

FIG. 4-5   Block of the lateral cutaneous and radial nerves at the elbow.

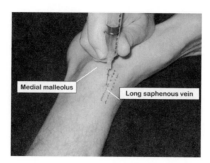

FIG. 4-6   Saphenous nerve block.

10 mL local anesthetic is infiltrated around each of the nerves, as described in the following section.

The **saphenous nerve** is blocked at the greater saphenous vein 1 to 2 cm above the medial malleolus (Fig. 4-6).

The **deep peroneal nerve** is blocked around and deep to the dorsalis pedis artery. Alternatively, the infiltration is performed between the tibialis anterior and the extensor hallus longus tendons; flexion of the first and second toes improves visualization of the two tendons (Fig. 4-7).

The **superficial peroneal nerve** is blocked with subcutaneous ring infiltration from the anterior edge of the tibia to the anterior edge of the fibula (Fig. 4-8).

The **sural nerve** is blocked with subcutaneous fanwise infiltration between the Achilles tendon and fibula (Fig. 4-9).

The **tibial nerve** is blocked with a needle advanced just lateral to the posterior tibial artery toward the posterior surface of the tibia. The needle is retracted 1 cm after contact with the tibia, and the anesthetic is injected (Fig. 4-10).

Hematoma Block

Spread of local anesthetic to the nerve fibers supplying soft tissue and periosteum around a fracture is obtained with a hematoma block. This technique is contraindicated if there is any risk of contamination of the fracture site from the skin puncture.

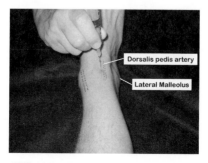

FIG. 4-7   Deep peroneal nerve block.

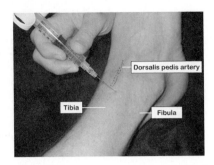

FIG. 4-8   Superficial peroneal nerve block.

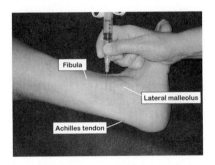

FIG. 4-9   Sural nerve block.

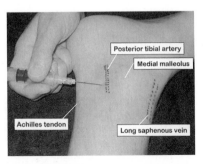

FIG. 4-10   Tibial nerve block.

A large-bore needle, (e.g., 19 gauge, 1.5 in.) is used for this block because it is important to withdraw blood from the fracture hematoma and replace it with local anesthetic. This method provides better anesthesia and reduces the risk of a high compartment pressure. After aspiration of the hematoma, 10 to 15 mL of 1% lidocaine is injected. When there is an associated distal radioulnar joint injury, 5 to 8 mL of 1% lidocaine is injected into the radioulnar joint in addition to the hematoma block.

SELECTED READINGS

American Society of Anesthesiologists Task Force on Sedation and Analgesia by Non-Anesthesiologists. Practice guidelines for sedation and analgesia by non-anesthesiologists. *Anesthesiology* 84:459–471, 1996.

5 | Radiologic Evaluation

Ron C. Gaba   Margaret A. Stull

This chapter provides an overview of radiography and diagnostic imaging as it applies to the evaluation of fractures.

IMAGING MODALITIES

Imaging modalities employed in the investigation of musculoskeletal trauma include **radiography**, **computed tomography** (**CT**), **magnetic resonance imaging** (**MRI**), **radionuclide bone scan** (**scintigraphy**), **ultrasound**, and **fluoroscopy**. Clinical information is needed to appropriately direct an evaluation by diagnostic imaging.

Radiography

Radiographs (analog or digital), commonly referred to as x-rays, are the primary imaging modality used to evaluate musculoskeletal injuries. Radiographic examination of a fracture requires at least two orthogonal views, the AP (anteroposterior) and lateral. Frequently, extremity radiographs include the proximal and distal joints in order to assess for concomitant joint injury. Oblique projections and joint-specific special views improve sensitivity and help visualize complex anatomy (Fig. 5-1). Careful image inspection is crucial, as nondisplaced fractures may be seen on only a single view or with magnification. Weight-bearing and stress views provide functional information about joint stability and ligament integrity. Radiographs of contralateral structures are often obtained for comparison in children and with injuries of the wrist and foot.

Computed Tomography (CT)

CT is generally performed to further analyze a known or suspected abnormality. The excellent anatomic detail and contrast resolution of CT helps define the extent of complex fractures, identify articular involvement, and delineate soft tissue injury. CT images are reviewed using soft tissue and bone window settings. Multiplanar two- (2D) and three-dimensional (3D) image reformations aid in fracture assessment (Fig. 5-2) and in preoperative planning. Advances such as 16-slice multidetector (M-D) CT permit isotropic image reconstruction (i.e., image reconstruction in any plane). Intravenous iodinated contrast is usually unnecessary for fracture evaluation. Contrast-enhanced studies are obtained in patients with suspected vascular, abdominal, or pelvic trauma. Metallic objects, such as orthopedic hardware and bullet fragments (Fig. 5-3), produce streak artifacts that can degrade image quality.

CT is commonly necessary to detect and characterize wrist, foot, skull, spine, and pelvic fractures (Fig. 5-4 *A* to *C*). Occasionally, nondisplaced fractures are not readily apparent on CT. MRI is more sensitive in the identification of these radiographically occult fractures. Nuclear medicine is also employed in this regard, particularly in osteoporotic patients.

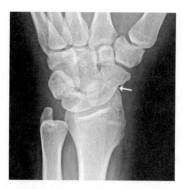

FIG. 5-1   Scaphoid fracture. An oblique view of the wrist best displays the fracture through the waist of the scaphoid.

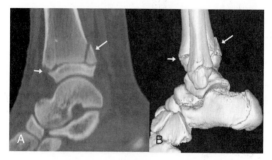

FIG. 5-2   Distal tibial fracture in 8-year-old girl. Reformatted 2D sagittal (*A*) and 3D (*B*) CT images reveal the Salter-Harris type 2 injury of the distal tibia. The distal metaphyseal fracture fragment is minimally displaced posteriorly (*long arrow*) and the physis is widened anteriorly (*short arrow*).

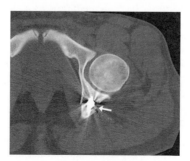

FIG. 5-3   Open fracture secondary to a gunshot wound to the buttock. Artifact from bullet fragments embedded in the posterior column of the acetabulum limits visualization of the pelvic fracture (*arrow*) on this axial CT image.

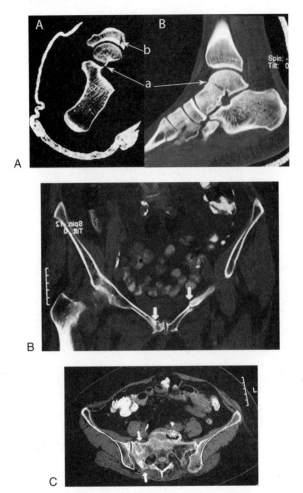

FIG. 5-4 *A.* This CT image of the foot after a crush injury shows an occult navicular fracture in addition to the talar fracture. Fractures of the second metatarsal base and middle cuneiform were also evident only on CT. *B* and *C*. Fractures of the pubis and sacral ala in a patient with groin pain after a fall. The pelvic radiograph was unremarkable.

Magnetic Resonance Imaging

MRI is the method of choice for the detection of radiographically occult, clinically significant acute fractures, such as hip fractures in osteoporotic patients (Fig. 5-5). Stress fractures are easily recognized on MRI, and bone edema is immediately apparent. MRI provides excellent resolution of soft tissue structures and is invaluable in the detection of soft tissue injuries, particularly involving joints (Fig. 5-6).

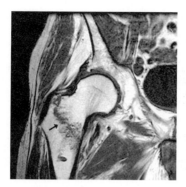

FIG. 5-5 Radiographically occult hip fracture in an elderly osteoporotic man. Coronal T1 MR image demonstrates a nondisplaced intertrochanteric femoral fracture and surrounding bone edema (*arrow*).

MRI pulse sequences used in the setting of acute musculoskeletal trauma include T1, proton density (PD) or T2 with fat suppression, and inversion recovery (IR) techniques. Lengthy scan acquisition time (compared to CT) and high cost are disadvantages of MRI. Contraindications to MRI include certain metallic implants, such as cardiac pacemakers and some cerebral aneurysm clips. Metal workers require screening orbital CT before MRI.

Radionuclide Bone Scan (Scintigraphy)

Bone scans evaluate skeletal metabolic activity. In the realm of musculoskeletal injury, bone scans are most valuable in the detection of stress fractures

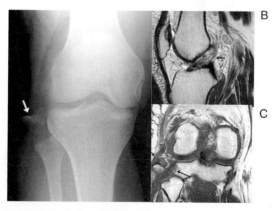

FIG. 5-6 Extensive soft tissue injury of the knee. AP radiograph (*A*) shows proximal retraction of an avulsed fracture fragment (*arrow*) of the fibular head. Sagittal T2 (*B*) and coronal T1 (*C*) MR images reveal rupture of the anterior cruciate ligament (*arrow*), grade 3 sprain of the lateral collateral ligament (LCL) (*short arrow*), and Segond fracture (tibial avulsion of the midcapsular ligament of LCL) (*long arrow*).

and radiographically occult fractures. Although they are not visible on radiographic or tomographic studies, these fractures may be detected in their early stages using bone scanning (Fig. 5-7). Radiographically occult fractures in osteoporotic patients may require 48 h to demonstrate increased osseous activity. The inherent low specificity and limited spatial resolution of bone scanning may preclude precise anatomic localization of an injury.

Ultrasound

The role of ultrasound in the evaluation of musculoskeletal injuries is broadening. While useful in the investigation of some radiographically occult fractures, including sternal and rib injuries, this modality is primarily used to diagnose soft tissue injuries. Muscular trauma is well demonstrated. Tendon and ligament tears in superficial structures are visible on ultrasound. Sonography is capable of identifying callus prior to its appearance on radiographs. Disadvantages of ultrasound include the inability to penetrate cortical bone, operator dependence, and lack of standard documentation and labeling of sonographic images.

Fluoroscopy

Fluoroscopy, or real-time radiography, may aid in the detection of radiographically unapparent fractures by allowing the radiologist to evaluate osseous structures in numerous projections under direct observation. Joint kinematics may also be assessed. Fluoroscopy is used to guide diagnostic and therapeutic interventional musculoskeletal procedures, such as arthrography and joint injections or aspirations (especially in the spine). Orthopedic surgeons often utilize fluoroscopy during operative reduction and fixation of fractures and dislocations. The ability to reduce a fracture and pass a guide pin across the fracture site from the end of a long bone using real-time imaging has made possible the entire science of closed, locked intramedullary fixation as well as facilitating other procedures involving closed reduction and placement of pin (or screw) fixation.

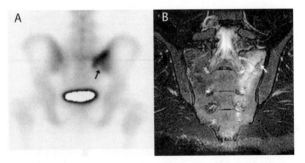

FIG. 5-7 Sacral stress fracture in marathon runner with left gluteal pain. Bone scan (*A*) shows abnormal uptake in the region of the left sacroiliac joint (*arrow*). Oblique coronal fat-suppressed T2 MR image of the sacrum (*B*) displays the stress fracture and edema in the left sacral ala (*arrow*).

TERMINOLOGY

Precise terminology must be used to convey an accurate description of a fracture to the treating orthopedic surgeon.

Location

A detailed description of the anatomic location of the fracture is essential. Long bone fractures may involve the **diaphysis** (shaft), **metadiaphysis**, **metaphysis**, **physis** (growth plate), or **epiphysis**. Division of the long bone diaphysis into thirds (proximal, middle, and distal) assists in injury localization. Involvement of an articular surface must be determined if a fracture is located near a joint. In these cases, fractures are described as **intraarticular** (Fig. 5-8*A* and *B*) or **extraarticular**.

Extent or Type

Complete fractures extend across a bone and interrupt both cortices, whereas **incomplete** fractures display a single cortical break. Incomplete fractures in adults are termed **fissures**. Incomplete fractures frequently occur in children due to bone flexibility. **Bowing** as well as **torus** and **greenstick** fractures are incomplete fractures that are unique to the immature skeleton. Bowing refers to plastic bending of soft, incompletely mineralized bone. Torus fractures result in a localized cortical buckle caused by longitudinal compression of soft bone (Fig. 5-9). Greenstick fractures are unilateral cortical breaks along the convex margin of a bowed bone (Fig. 5-10).

Avulsion injuries occur at tendon and ligament insertions. A bone fragment is avulsed, or sheared, from its original position by forceful pulling (Fig. 5-11).

Closed (**simple**) fractures are injuries in which the overlying skin is intact. **Open** (**compound**) fractures communicate with the outside environment through a skin wound. A fractured bone may extend through the skin or an external force may penetrate the skin. Designation of closed or open fractures is more readily determined on physical examination.

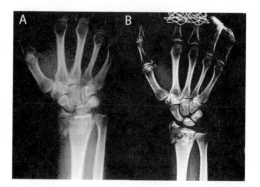

FIG. 5-8   Distal radial fracture. The radiograph shows a comminuted, displaced, angulated fracture of the distal radius with intraarticular extension. Before (*A*) and after (*B*) traction has been applied.

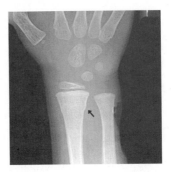

FIG. 5-9   Torus fracture. This PA radiograph displays cortical buckle (*arrow*) in the distal radial metaphysis.

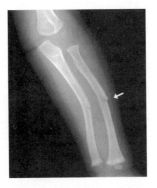

FIG. 5-10   Greenstick fractures of the left radius and ulna. This AP radiograph demonstrates bowing deformities of the radius and ulna, with fractures along the convex surfaces (*arrow*).

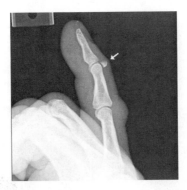

FIG. 5-11   Avulsion fracture of the distal phalanx. This lateral radiograph shows proximal retraction of the dorsal plate fracture fragment from the base of the distal phalanx (*arrow*). The avulsion occurs at the insertion of the extensor tendon and is referred to as a baseball or mallet finger.

Plane

The plane of a fracture is best described in relation to the long axis of the broken bone. **Transverse** fractures lie perpendicular to the long axis of a bone, whereas **longitudinal** (or **vertical**) fractures are parallel to the long axis. **Oblique** fractures form oblique angles with the cortical long axis, and **spiral** fractures rotate along the long axis of a bone.

A fracture that results in the formation of more than two fragments is termed **comminuted. Additional fracture lines indicating comminution may not be initially apparent on routine radiographs. Segmental** fractures are comminuted fractures in which a long bone is divided into successive pieces by consecutive transverse fractures. **Butterfly** fractures result in the formation of a wedge-shaped fragment that is split from the major fracture fragments.

Alignment

Fracture alignment refers to the position of adjacent major fracture fragments and is described in terms of **displacement**, **length discrepancy**, **angulation**, and **rotation**.

Displacement refers to loss of cortical continuity in the transverse plane. By convention, displacement of the distal fracture fragment is specified as anterior, posterior, medial, or lateral. *Partial continuity* implies that fracture ends maintain contact, but with offset cortices. An accurate description of displacement is important, as fractures that maintain some continuity may be amenable to closed reduction in the emergency room, while fractures that have lost end-to-end continuity may require operative intervention.

Length discrepancy describes the longitudinal continuity of osseous fragments. **Distraction** indicates longitudinal separation of fracture fragments. **Apposition** (or **bayonet** apposition) refers to fragment overlap, which results in shortening.

Angulation indicates the angular relationship of the longitudinal axis of adjacent fracture fragments and is typically described according to the orientation of the distal fragment. Angulation may occur in the anterior, posterior, medial, and lateral directions. A laterally oriented distal fracture fragment is reported as having **valgus** angulation (Fig. 5-12), whereas a medially oriented

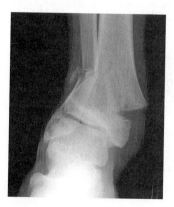

FIG. 5-12   Ankle fractures. This AP radiograph displays valgus angulation of the major distal fracture fragments of distal tibial and fibular fractures.

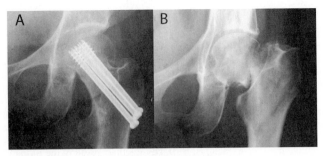

FIG. 5-13   *A.* An impacted fracture of the femoral neck that was pinned in situ. The femoral neck has moved under the femoral head in a valgus configuration. *B.* A fracture of the femoral neck in which the femoral neck has moved superiorly in relation to the femoral head. This varus displacement is unstable and is frequently treated with prosthetic replacement.

distal fracture fragment has **varus** angulation (Fig. 5-13*A* and *B*). The fracture apex is less commonly used to designate the direction of angulation.

Relative rotation of fracture fragments is defined by the distal fracture fragment and may be **internal** (medial) or **external** (lateral).

Special Features

Impaction occurs when osseous bodies are forcibly driven into one another (Fig. 5-14). *Depression* is the inward displacement of bone and results when the hard surface of one bone presses into a relatively softer bone (Fig. 5-15). This usually involves articular surfaces and results in loss of joint congruence. Compression deformities commonly involve vertebral bodies.

Joint dislocation refers to total loss of congruence of opposing articular surfaces and often occurs in conjunction with fractures (Fig. 5-16). Subtotal loss of articular surface contact is termed **subluxation**. The direction of a dislocation or subluxation is described in reference to the distal structure. **Diastasis** is the widening of a slightly movable articulation, such as the symphysis pubis or sacroiliac joint (see Chap. 16).

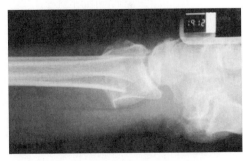

FIG. 5-14   Distal radial fracture. Impaction of the transverse extraarticular fracture is seen as overlapping bony trabeculae.

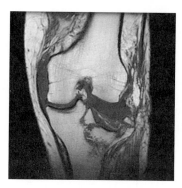

FIG. 5-15 Fracture of the tibial plateau. Coronal T1 MR image reveals a comminuted, depressed fracture of the lateral tibial plateau associated with soft tissue injury.

Special Fractures

Stress fractures are subdivided into **fatigue** and **insufficiency** fractures. These injuries result from persistent trauma that overwhelms the healing mechanisms of bone. Fatigue fractures result when normal bone suffers repeated microtrauma and most commonly occur in the weight-bearing bones of the lower extremities (see Fig. 5-7). Insufficiency fractures are a consequence of normal stresses placed on abnormally weakened bone. Metabolic disorders—such as osteoporosis, osteomalacia, and osteopetrosis—predispose to insufficiency fractures (Fig. 5-17).

   Pathologic fractures occur in locations where bone has been affected by a disease process (Fig. 5-18), such as neoplasm or infection. Detection of a pathologic fracture will affect therapy. A lytic bone lesion that is larger than 2 cm or involves more than 50% of the cortex of a weight-bearing bone is termed an **impending** fracture. This designation indicates a high risk of future fracture.

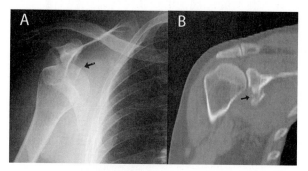

FIG. 5-16 Anterior dislocation of the right shoulder. AP radiograph (*A*) demonstrates anterior dislocation of the shoulder. A small triangular bone fragment is superimposed over the dislocated humeral head (*arrow*). Postreduction coronal 2D reformatted CT image (*B*) confirms fracture of the inferior glenoid (Bankart lesion) (*arrow*).

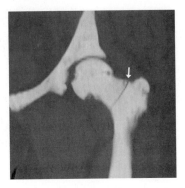

FIG. 5-17   Insufficiency fracture in man with osteopetrosis (marble bone disease). Coronal 2D reformatted CT image of the hip demonstrates a nondisplaced fracture through the left femoral neck.

Indirect Signs

Subtle fractures may not be readily apparent on radiographs, and indirect signs may provide a clue to their presence. **Soft tissue swelling** helps localize the site of injury. Displacement of adjacent fat stripes and loss of soft tissue planes are associated with bone trauma. **Joint effusions** accompany fractures with intraarticular extension (Fig. 5-19). **Hemarthroses**, or bloody effusions, may contain fat-fluid levels. These fat- and blood-containing effusions are termed **lipohemarthroses**. *Periosteal reaction* indicates early fracture healing (or in some instances a response to a neoplastic process).

Fracture Healing

Bone healing is affected by fracture location and type, patient age, associated abnormalities, and therapeutic intervention. The healing fracture demonstrates the formation of callus, which is a bridging tissue composed of fibrous mate-

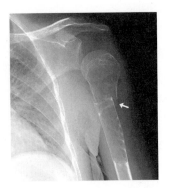

FIG. 5-18   Pathologic fracture in a patient with polyostotic fibrous dysplasia. A comminuted, minimally displaced, angulated fracture of the proximal humeral diaphysis (*arrow*) has occurred through the expansile osteolytic lesion.

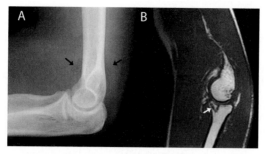

FIG. 5-19   Radiographically occult elbow fracture. Lateral radiograph (*A*) demonstrates displacement of elbow fat pads (*arrows*), which indicates elbow joint effusion. No fracture is identified. Sagittal T1 MR image (*B*) reveals nondisplaced fracture through the radial head (*arrow*).

rial, blood vessels, cartilage, and bone. Normal healing results in osseous bridging, or **union**, between fracture fragments. **Delayed osseous union** is fracture healing retarded beyond the usual time frame of 2 to 4 months and is manifest by persistent visualization of the fracture line and lack of adequate callus bridging the fracture fragments. **Fibrous union** may be present despite the lack of bony bridging.

Complications

Nonunion occurs when bone fragments have not united and healing has ceased (Fig. 5-20). Nonunion may result in the formation of a **pseudarthrosis**, which represents a false "articulation," between the fracture fragments. Nonunion may be **reactive (hypertrophic)**, **nonreactive (atrophic)**, or **infected**. Reactive nonunion is characterized by bone formation and sclerosis at the fracture margins, while nonreactive nonunion demonstrates a lack of bone formation (osteopenia) at the fracture site. Infected nonunions can be associated with osteomyelitis.

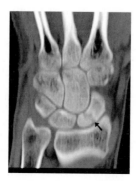

FIG. 5-20   Nonunited scaphoid fracture. Coronal 2D reformatted CT image reveals nonunited fracture of the scaphoid bone (*arrow*). Sclerosis of the proximal pole is compatible with avascular necrosis.

Malunion refers to fractures that have not healed in clinically acceptable alignment.

Other fracture complications include **avascular necrosis (osteonecrosis)**, **secondary osteoarthritis (degenerative joint disease)**, **myositis ossificans**, **disuse osteoporosis**, and **reflex sympathetic dystrophy (regional pain syndrome)**. Avascular necrosis (osteonecrosis) is bone death secondary to vascular insufficiency (Fig. 5-20). Posttraumatic osteoarthritis occurs following injury to the articular surface. Myositis ossificans is potentially painful posttraumatic heterotopic bone formation within a muscle. Immobilization or pain may produce decreased bone density secondary to disuse, which is termed *disuse osteoporosis*. Reflex sympathetic dystrophy is a complex, often posttraumatic regional pain process associated with loss of motion, tissue atrophy, and functional loss of an extremity.

SELECTED READINGS

Berquist TH (ed). *Imaging of Orthopedic Trauma and Surgery.* Philadelphia: Saunders, 1986.

Bohndorf K, Imhof H, Pope TL Jr (eds). *Musculoskeletal Imaging: A Concise Multimodality Approach.* New York: Thieme, 2001.

El-Khoury GY (ed). *Imaging of Orthopedic Trauma, The Radiologic Clinics of North America,* Vol. 35, No. 3. Philadelphia: Saunders, 1997.

Greenspan A. *Orthopedic Radiology: A Practical Approach,* 3d ed. Philadelphia: Lippincott, Williams & Wilkins, 2000.

Rogers LF (ed). *Radiology of Skeletal Trauma,* 3d ed. Philadelphia: Churchill Livingstone, 2002.

Schultz RJ. *The Language of Fractures,* 2d ed. Baltimore, Lippincott, Williams & Wilkins, 1990.

6 | Fracture Healing and Bone Grafting

Eleftherios Tsiridis   Sanjeev Kakar
Thomas A. Einhorn

FRACTURE HEALING BIOLOGY

Clinical Anatomy of Fracture Healing

Fracture healing is a complex biological process involving four distinct responses: those that take place in the bone marrow, the cortex, the periosteum, and the external soft tissues.

1. **Bone marrow:** Within a few hours after a fracture is sustained, normal bone marrow architecture is lost, blood vessels in the region adjacent to the fracture clot, and the cellular components of the bone marrow reorganize into regions of high and low cellular density. In the high-density region, endothelial cells appear to transform to polymorphic cells, which express an osteoblastic phenotype and begin to form bone 24 h after the fracture occurs.

2. **Cortex:** In terms of histology, *primary healing* refers to a direct attempt by the cortex to reestablish continuity. The bone ends at the fracture site, deprived of their blood supply, become necrotic and are resorbed, thus creating a radiographically apparent gap at the fracture site several weeks after fracture. Primary healing (healing without callus formation) occurs when there is anatomic restoration of the fracture fragments and rigid fixation can be achieved with internal fixation devices. Osteoclasts on either side of the fracture initiate a tunneling resorptive response and develop discrete remodeling units known as "cutting cones." These units reestablish new haversian systems, thus providing pathways for the penetration of blood vessels and bone formation. These processes convert the resorption cavities in fully formed osteons.

3. **Periosteum:** The most important response in secondary fracture healing (healing with callus formation) is that of the periosteum. Committed osteoprogenitor cells and uncommitted, undifferentiated mesenchymal cells recapitulate embryonic intramembranous ossification and endochondral bone formation in this tissue. Unlike primary healing, secondary fracture healing is enhanced by motion and inhibited by rigid fixation. Bone formed by intramembranous ossification is found in the periphery of the fracture site, forming the so-called hard callus, which results in bone formation directly without the prior formation of cartilage. Consequently, structural proteins associated with bone matrix appear very early. On the other hand, callus that forms by endochondral ossification is found adjacent to the fracture site and involves the development of a cartilage archetype that becomes calcified and is then replaced by bone (Fig. 6-1).

4. **External soft tissues:** The response of the soft tissues is mainly complementary to the secondary healing of fracture. A rapid cellular activity and the development of an early bridging callus immobilize the fragments and evolve into the process of endochondral ossification along with the periosteal reaction.

49

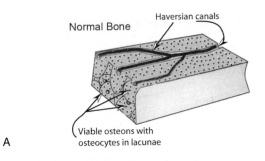

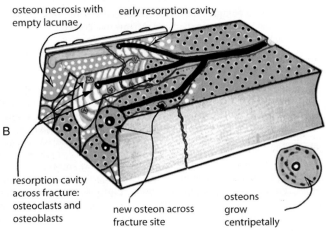

FIG. 6-1 *A.* Normal cortical bone: Lacunae are filled with viable osteocytes and the osteonal pattern is preserved. *B.* Primary cortical healing by haversian remodeling.

Histologic Types of Fracture Healing

Two types of healing processes take place following a fracture and are dependent on the type of bone in which a fracture occurs (cancellous vs. cortical) and the type of fixation achieved (rigid vs. nonrigid); thus:

1. Primary bone healing occurs in cortical and cancellous (metaphyseal) bone (healing by primary intention), following rigid fixation (compression and buttress plating, screw fixation) or after impaction in cancellous bone.
2. Secondary bone healing occurs in cortical bone, following intramedullary fixation (controlled dynamic motion) or casting (uncontrolled motion).

Primary Fracture Healing

Fracture healing can occur without callus formation in either cancellous or cortical bone when the fragments are rigidly held in contact. Many impacted epiphyseal, metaphyseal, and vertebral fractures, due to the interlocking of fragments, present sufficient stability to permit primary bone healing. There are two types of primary bone healing: "contact healing" (or haversian healing), when the fragments are in absolute contact, and "gap healing," when a small gap occurs between fragments without compromising rigid fixation.

Rigid fixation is a prerequisite of primary healing. It means that there is no micromovement at the fracture site.

Primary Cortical Healing

In the cortex of a fracture, haversian remodeling begins with the formation of resorption cavities that penetrate longitudinally from the viable bone through the necrotic fragment ends. Resorption cavities are formed by groups of osteoclasts that have formed a cutting cone. This cone advances longitudinally, leaving behind a resorption cavity. A thin-walled capillary loop that runs in the center of the resorption cavity follows the osteoclasts. These vessels are accompanied by mesenchymal cells and osteoblast precursors. Newly formed osteoblasts eventually line the resorption cavity and begin producing osteoid in a centripetal direction. Eventually the resorption cavity fills entirely with concentric layers of new bone, thus becoming an osteon across the fracture line (Fig. 6-1) and in the process healing the fracture.

When small gaps (200 to 500 m m) are present at the fracture site, the healing process is called "gap healing." During the first stage of this process, the fracture gap is filled with primary or woven bone without the prior interference of a fibrocartilaginous stage. The pattern of the newly formed bone does not correspond with its original structure, as it lies perpendicular to its neighbor fragments. Furthermore, necrotic areas are present on both sides of the fracture as a consequence of the interruption of the vascular circulation in the haversian canals. The second stage of gap healing, which finally leads to the healing of a fracture, is characterized by the longitudinal reconstruction of the fracture site by haversian remodeling through the woven bone in the gap, as described above.

Primary Cancellous Healing

Primary healing is healing in the areas of the cancellous bone where the fracture fragments are in direct tight apposition, without gaps, held together by rigid fixation or after impaction. In this type of healing, remodeling of the fracture site begins immediately, without the primary deposition of woven bone. Osteoclastic cutting cones advance across the fracture line, followed by capillaries and osteoprogenitor cells, which become the source of osteoblasts. Osteoblasts lay osteoid and form bone spicules/trabeculae. This process leads to the simultaneous union and reconstruction of the fracture ends (Fig. 6-2).

Secondary Fracture Healing

There are six identifiable stages in this type of fracture repair (Fig. 6-3).

Stage 1: Hematoma and Inflammation

Blood clots provide signaling molecules able to initiate the cascade of cellular events essential for fracture healing. Inflammatory cells secrete cytokines, such as interleukins-1 and -6 (IL-1 and IL-6), which may be important in regulating the early stages of healing, while degranulating platelets in the clot may release transforming growth factor beta (TGF-b) and platelet-derived growth factor (PDGF), which may be important in regulating cell proliferation, differentiation, and chemotaxis of committed mesenchymal stem cells.

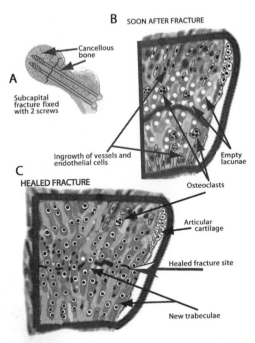

FIG. 6-2 Primary cancellous healing: *A*. Subcapital fracture with cancellous bone in the head and neck is fixed with two cancellous screws; no periosteum is found in the adult. *B*. Healing a block of cancellous bone at the fracture site where it reaches the articular surface. *C*. A block of bone at the healed fracture site.

Stage 2: Cartilage Formation and Angiogenesis

In a rat fracture model, intramembranous and endochondral bone formation is initiated during the first 7 to 10 days after fracture. By the middle of the second week, abundant cartilage overlies the fracture site, and it is this chondroid tissue that initiates the biochemical events leading to calcification of the callus. At this time, the callus may be divided histologically into hard callus, where intramembranous ossification is taking place, and soft callus, where endochondral ossification is proceeding. Neoangiogenesis occurs simultaneously with those events, and new blood vessels, originating from the periosteum, penetrate both hard and soft callus.

Stage 3: Cartilage Calcification

Fracture callus calcification occurs by a mechanism similar to that which takes place during physeal growth. A large number of elongated and proliferative chondrocytes appear 9 days after the fracture occurs and dominate the fracture callus. Chondrocytes produce vesicularized bodies, known as matrix vesicles, from their cellular membrane; these migrate to the extracellular matrix. The matrix vesicles contain the enzyme complements needed for proteolytic modification of the matrix, a necessary step in the preparation of the cells for cal-

FRACTURE HEALING RESPONSES

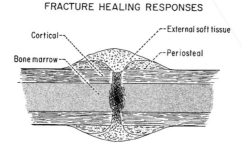

FIG. 6-3 Secondary healing. This type of healing occurs with callus formation. Hard callus is formed at the periphery (intramembranous ossification) and soft callus is formed adjacent to the fracture site (endochondral ossification).

cification. Matrix vesicles also contain phosphatases needed for the degradation of matrix phosphodiesters, resulting in phosphate ion release for precipitation with calcium. Proteases hydrolyze large proteins and proteoglycans in the extracellular matrix approximately 14 days after a fracture takes place, thus preventing inhibition of calcification. Alkaline phosphatase (ALP) levels increase approximately 3 days later.

Stage 4: Cartilage Removal

Once the cartilage is calcified, neoangiogenesis occurs. New vessels carry perivascular osteoprogenitor cells and the calcified cartilage is then resorbed by chondroclasts. New woven bone is then laid down to replace calcified cartilage.

Stage 5: Bone Formation

Formation of intramembranous bone by periosteum begins immediately after a fracture but stops 2 weeks later. At the same time, adjacent to the fracture site, the endochondral ossification process reaches the stage of woven bone formation. By the third week, the fracture is united by woven bone, bridging the gap within the callus.

Stage 6: Bone Remodeling

This is a chronic process of gradually replacing the woven bone with lamellar bone. With time, the healing fracture recovers its biomechanical properties, while it modulates its shape under the influence of environmental mechanical stimuli.

Expression of Extracellular Matrix Proteins during Fracture Healing

During endochondral ossification, two main proteoglycans are expressed in the extracellular matrix: dermatan sulfate, produced by fibroblasts during early callus formation, and chondroitin 4-sulfate, produced by chondroblasts during the second week of fracture healing. Proteoglycan degradation is essential for callus calcification, as is the presence of ALP, IL-1, and IL-6.

Collagens (types I, II, III, V, IX, X, and XI) are essential throughout the healing process, as are noncollagenous extracellular matrix proteins (osteonectin, osteocalcin, osteopontin, and fibronectin).

Regulation of Fracture Healing

The transforming growth factor beta (TGF-b) superfamily of morphogenetic proteins has a prominent role in fracture repair (Table 6-1). Bone morphogenetic proteins 2 and 4 (BMP-2 and BMP-4) have been shown to be expressed during the first 4 weeks of fracture healing. BMP-1 to BMP-8; growth and differentiation factors (GDFs) 1, 5, 8, and 10; and TGF-b 1 to 3 act in combination to promote the various stages of intramembranous and endochondral bone formation during fracture healing. It is now well established that the signals which initiate and establish the symmetry of repair around the fracture line are part of the initial inflammatory process. Tumor necrosis factor alpha (TNF-a) signaling may facilitate the repair process by promoting the chemotaxis and differentiation of the mesenchymal stem cells, while bone remodeling appears to be regulated by IL-1, IL-6, and TNF-a. Furthermore, the final stages of endochondral ossification and bone remodeling are dependent on the action of specific matrix metalloproteinases that degrade cartilage and bone, allowing for the invasion of blood vessels. Angiogenesis is regulated mainly by the vascular endothelial growth factor (VEGF), a promoter of neoangiogenesis, and an endothelial cell-specific mitogen. Moreover, fibroblast growth factor (FGF) and platelet-derived growth factor (PDGF) are mitogenic for mesenchymal stem cells, chondrocytes and osteoblasts, and insulin-like growth factor (IGF); promote the proliferation and differentiation of osteoprogenitor cells; and mediate the anabolic action of parathyroid hormone (PTH) on the skeleton. Several systemic and local factors, related to the patient or attributed to the nature and impact of the original injury, tissue quality, and the surgical technique, may enhance or inhibit fracture healing. (Table 6-2).

Failure of Fracture Healing

Failure of bone healing is attributed to mechanical and biological factors as well as apposition of fragments and interposition of soft tissue or muscle, complete interruption, and subsequent retraction of the periosteum. Failure of bone healing may result from inadequate stability of the fragments, leading to the formation of a large volume of callus without bridging of the fracture gap (**hypertrophic nonunion**). Second, it may be due to deficient biological substrate, resulting in the arrest of the healing process, with little or

---

TABLE 6-1 Members of the TGF-b Superfamily

BMPs	BMP-1(procollagen C-proteinase), BMP-2, BMP-3 (osteogenin), BMP-3b(GDF 10), BMP-4 (BMP-2b), BMP-5, BMP-6, BMP-7(OP-1), BMP-8a(OP-2), BMP-8b(OP-3), BMP-9, BMP-10, BMP-11, BMP-12(GDF-7), BMP-13 (GDF-6, CDMP-2), BMP-15(GDF-9b)
GDFs	GDF-1, GDF-3, GDF-5(CDMP-1), GDF-8, GDF-9
TGF-b isoforms	TGF b1, TGF b2, TGF b3
MIF	
Activins	
Inhibins	

BMPs = bone morphogenetic proteins; CDMP = cartilage-derived morphogenetic protein; GDF = growth and differentiation factors; MIF = mullerian inhibition factor; OP = osteogenic protein; TGF = transforming growth factors.

TABLE 6-2 Factors Influencing Fracture Healing

Systemic factors	Promote healing	Inhibit healing
Age	Childhood	
Nutrition		Malnutrition
Hormones	Growth hormone (GH), PTH, calcitonin, androgen, estrogen	Corticosteroids
Diseases		Diabetes, anemia
Vitamin deficiencies		A, C, D, K
Substances		Nicotine, alcohol
Medication		Nonsteroidal anti-inflammatories, anticoagulants, phenytoin

Local factors	Promote healing	Inhibit healing
Tissue-related factors		Bone necrosis (radiation, avascular necrosis), bone disease (osteoporosis, osteomalacia, osteogenesis imperfecta, fibrous dysplasia), tumors, infection
Injury-related factors		Fracture comminution, velocity of injury, vascular and neurologic trauma, bone loss
Treatment-related factors	Bone graft, bone morphogenetic proteins, electrical stimulation	Inadequate fracture stabilization, surgical trauma, implant-related periosteal and vascular impairment, soft tissue interposition between fragments

no callus formation (**atrophic nonunion**). In some nonunions, cartilaginous tissue is formed over the fracture surface and the cavity between the surfaces fills with clear fluid, which resembles synovial joint fluid, creating the so-called **pseudoarthrosis**. A variation of nonunion, **fibrous nonunion**, presents with dense fibrous tissue between the fragments and union is not restored.

BONE GRAFTING

Clinical Need

Each year, more than 2.2 million bone-grafting procedures are performed worldwide, 450,000 of them in the United States. These grafts provide osteo-inductive, osteoconductive, and osteogenic activity to enhance the local bone-healing response. *Osteoinduction* refers to the process by which pluripotent mesenchymal stem cells are recruited from the surrounding host tissues and differentiate into bone-forming osteoprogenitor cells. An osteoconductive material is one that acts as a scaffold, supporting the ingrowth of capillaries, perivascular tissue, and osteoprogenitor cells from the recipient bed. Although current interest has focused on bone-graft substitutes to provide this property, human cancellous bone is the best example of an osteoconductive material. *Osteogenesis* refers to the process of local bone formation. In terms of bone grafting, an osteogenic material is one that contains living cells capable of differentiating into bone.

AUTOLOGOUS BONE

Bone graft incorporation follows a similar sequence of events to those seen in fracture repair.

Cancellous bone graft is mainly harvested in fragments from sites such as the iliac crest, distal radius, or greater trochanter. It is an excellent choice for the treatment of nonunion with small defects that do not require structural integrity from the graft.

Cortical bone graft is usually harvested from the ribs, fibula, or shell of the ilium and can be transplanted with or without its vascular pedicle. It is mostly osteoconductive, with little or no osteoinductive property. The thickness of the matrix of cortical bone limits the diffusion of nutrients to support the survival of any useful fraction of osteocytes after transplantation, thereby limiting its osteogenic properties.

Autologous bone marrow contains osteogenic precursor cells and has been used in the management of tibial fractures.

ALLOGENEIC BONE

This is an attractive alternative to autogenous bone, as it avoids donor-site morbidity; moreover, its relative abundance allows for tailoring to fit the defect size. It is available in many preparations, including morcellized and cancellous chips, corticocancellous and cortical grafts, osteochondral segments, and de-mineralized bone matrix.

Cortical allografts are available as whole bone segments for limb-salvage procedures or may be cut longitudinally to yield struts that can be used to fill bone defects or reconstitute cortical bone after periprosthetic fractures.

Allogeneic osteochondral grafts are composed of cortical bone, metaphys-eal cancellous bone, and articular cartilage. Once implanted, the graft is incor-porated by similar processes to those observed for cortical allografts. Despite this, nonunion is a common complication at the host-graft interface. Osteochondral allografts are immunogenic, increasing vulnerability to direct injury by cytotoxic antibodies or lymphocytes and indirect injury by inflammatory mediators and enzymes.

Demineralized bone matrix (DBM) is an osteoconductive scaffold produced by acid extraction of banked allograft. It contains noncollagenous proteins, osteoinductive growth factors, and type I collagen but provides little structural support. DBM has greater osteoinductive potential than allografts due to the bioavailability of these growth factors. DBM is available in various forms: as a freeze-dried powder, granules, gel, putty, or strip (i.e., Grafton DBM, Dynagraft, DBX, Osteofil, etc.). At this time, however, there are no data from well-designed, appropriately powered, randomized controlled trials to support the use of DBM in patients.

BONE GRAFT SUBSTITUTES

An ideal bone graft substitute must provide three elements necessary to maximize its bone-forming ability: the scaffolding for osteoconduction, growth factors for osteoinduction, and progenitor cells for osteogenesis.

Calcium Phosphate Ceramics

Calcium phosphate (CaP) ceramics are synthetic scaffolds that have a stoichiometry similar to that of bone. Their mechanical properties resemble those of ceramics, as their manufacturing process involves sintering, for thermal consolidation of the inorganic compounds, at temperatures above 1000°C. When they are implanted next to healthy bone, osteoid is secreted directly onto their surfaces; this subsequently mineralizes, and the resulting bone undergoes remodeling. CaP ceramics are highly biocompatible and differ only in their resorbability. The mechanical properties of CaP scaffolds are not suited to withstand the torsional and tensile forces imposed on the skeleton; thus their use is limited to non-weight-bearing sites and in conjunction with internal or external fixation devices.

1. **Hydroxyapatite (HA) of natural origin.** Commercial HA of natural origin is derived from sea coral (genus *Gonipora,* genus *Porites)* and is prepared by hydrothermal conversion (*Replamineform*) to HA (ProOsteon Interpore International, Inc., Irvine, CA) or from bovine bone (Bio-Oss Geistlich Biomaterials, Geistlich, Switzerland; Osteograf-N CeraMed Co., Denver, CO; and Endobon Merck Co., Darmstadt, Germany).
2. **Synthetic CaP biomaterials.** Synthetic HA [$Ca_{10}(PO_4)_6(OH)_2$] is used as bone-graft material and for the coating of orthopedic and dental implants (Calcitite Sulzer Calcitek, Carlsbad, CA), while b-TCP is used mainly as a bone-graft substitute in non-weight-bearing applications (Vitoss Orthovita, Inc., Philadelphia). Biphasic CaP has better resorbability than HA and is mechanically sounder than b-TCP (Triosite, Zimmer, Warsaw, IN; BCP, Sofamor Danek, Roissy Cdg Cedex, France).

Calcium Phosphate/Collagen Composites

A composite of porous calcium phosphate granules and purified bovine-derived fibrillar collagen, to which autogenous bone marrow aspirate is added during implantation, is called Collagraft (Zimmer Corporation, Warsaw, IN). It can be used as a paste or in strips and serves as a carrier for the porous ceramic and the autogenous marrow.

Calcium Sulfate

Calcium sulfate or plaster of Paris has been used since the early 1900s as void filler (Osteoset, Wright Medical Technology, Inc., Arlington, TN) or mixed with bone marrow aspirate, demineralized bone, or autograft. A mixture of $CaSO_4$ putty with demineralized bone matrix (Allomatrix, Wright Medical, Arlington, TN) has recently been investigated in an effort to improve the osteoinductive properties of calcium sulfate.

Bioactive Glasses

A family of glasses in the form of beads, identified under the trade name Bioglass (U.S. Biomaterials Corporation, Alachua, FL), represents a further approach to bone substitutes. The beads range in size from 90 to 710 m m and are composed of silica (SiO_2, 45%), calcium oxide (CaO, 24.5%), disodium oxide (Na_2O, 24.5%), and pyrophosphate (P_2O_5, 6%). Bioactive glasses stimulate osteoprogenitor cell function and possess controlled resorbability and proven biocompatibility.

Polyglycolic Acid Polymers and Composites

Polymeric membranes have been investigated for bone graft substitution. The most prominent types are the polytetrafluoroethylene (PTFE) and degradable polyesters poly-a-hydroxy acids (PHAs), such as polylactic acid (PLA) and polyglycolic acid (PGA). PLA/PGA/PLGA has been successfully combined with rhBMP-2 in animal models, and the results were biomechanically comparable to those obtained with autogenous cancellous bone grafts.

Calcium Phosphate Cements (CPCs)

CPCs were introduced in the early 1990s. Currently, two CPC categories are available, based on their end product: the apatite CPCs (the end product being precipitated HA) and the brushite CPCs (the end product being dicalcium phosphate dehydrate). CPCs can be used only in combination with metal implants (osteoporotic intertrochanteric femoral fractures) or in certain weight-bearing skeletal sites (comminuted tibial plateau fractures). Some CPCs are injectable, such as the Norian Skeletal Repair System (SRS) (Norian-Synthes, Oberdorf, Switzerland), the a-BSM (Etex, Cambridge, MA), and the Callos (Skeletal Kinetics, Cupertino, CA), as they maintain their cohesion in an aqueous environment without disintegrating. Others are not injectable, such as the BoneSource (Leibinger, Mülheim-Stettin, Germany) and the Cementek (Teknimed, Bigorre, France), as blood must be kept away from the implanting site until the material has set.

Future Technologies

A more adaptive "biomimetic" scaffold may be achieved by making it responsive to the mechanical environment in which it is placed. For example, peptides of the arginine-glycine-aspartic acid range-gated Doppler (RGD) sequence have been incorporated onto scaffold surfaces in an effort to increase cell adhesion, proliferation, and biocompatibility. The use of supercritical fluid technology in the development of porous biodegradable scaffolds represents another promising approach. This technology is involved in the development of biodegradable scaffolds and does not employ solvents or thermal processing, thus allowing for the incorporation of growth factors into the scaffold at construction.

SYSTEMIC ENHANCEMENT OF FRACTURE HEALING

Parathyroid Hormone (PTH)

Contrary to the assumption that PTH is a bone-resorbing hormone with catabolic effects on the skeleton, the response of the osteoclasts to PTH is more likely to be mediated by osteoblastic activity, as PTH receptors are found on osteoblast membranes. Indeed, while continuous exposure to PTH leads to an increase of osteoclast numbers and activity, intermittent exposure stimulates osteoblasts and results in increased bone formation in rats and humans.

Growth Hormone (GH)

IGF-1 is known as somatomedin-C and seems to be mediating the effect of GH on the skeleton. IGF-1 promotes the formation of bone matrix (type I collagen and noncollagenous matrix proteins) by the fully differentiated osteoblasts. In animal models of distraction osteogenesis, biomechanical testing, quantitative computed tomography (qCT), histomorphometric analysis, and serum levels of IGF-1 showed that administration of recombinant GH leads to increased stimulation of IGF-1 in serum during fracture healing and accelerates ossification of the regenerated bone.

The Effect of Head Injury on Fracture Healing

Perkins and Skirving (1987) and Spencer (1987) were the first to examine the volume of fracture callus and time to union in patients with traumatic brain injury (TBI). They found that the volume of callus was greater and the average time to union shorter in patients with TBI. Bidner et al. (1990) examined the hypothesis that sera from TBI patients displayed increased cell proliferation, attributed to a circulating growth factor released following TBI. The relation between TBI and enhanced fracture healing represents an important field of research, as it reveals the autocrine and/or paracrine effects of circulating factors that take part in fracture healing under the possible influence of the central nervous system.

TISSUE ENGINEERING OF FRACTURE HEALING

Current Technologies

Since the discovery of the osteoinductive properties of DBM, attention has focused on the role of bone morphogenetic proteins (BMPs) in embryologic bone formation and bone repair in the postnatal skeleton. BMPs are a group of noncollagenous glycoproteins that belong to the transforming growth factor beta (TGF-b) superfamily. Over 15 different BMPs have been identified and their genes cloned. The best-studied examples are BMP-2, BMP-3, and BMP-7 (osteogenic protein 1, or OP-1), as these are known to play important roles in bone repair by stimulating MSC differentiation. Riedel and Valentin-Opran (1999) were the first to report preliminary results from the use of BMP-2 to augment the treatment of open tibial fractures. Govender et al. (2002) conducted a large prospective, randomized, controlled multicenter trial evaluating the effects of recombinant (rh) BMP-2 on the treatment of open tibial fractures.

In a larger prospective randomized controlled and partially blinded multi-center study, Friedlaender et al. (2001) assessed the efficacy of rhBMP-7 over iliac crest bone graft in the treatment of 122 patients with 124 tibial nonunions. Recombinant human BMP-2 and BMP-7 appeared equally osteoinductive to autograft in these studies.

Peptide-Signaling Molecules

Transforming growth factor beta (TGF-β) influences a number of cell processes, such as the stimulation of MSC growth and differentiation; it also enhances collagen and the secretion of other extracellular matrix products and acts as a chemotactic factor for fibroblast and macrophage recruitment.

Fibroblast growth factors (FGF) are a group of structurally related compounds that share between 30 and 50% sequence homology. Acidic FGF (aFGF, FGF 1) and basic FGF (bFGF, FGF 2) are the best-studied members of this family, with bFGF considered to be most potent. It stimulates angiogenesis and endothelial cell migration and is mitogenic for fibroblasts, chondrocytes, and osteoblasts.

Insulin-like growth factors (IGF) exert an anabolic effect on bone metabolism. Two types have been described: IGF 1 and IGF 2, which stimulate osteoblast and osteoclast cell proliferation and matrix synthesis.

Platelet-derived growth factor (PDGF) is synthesized by numerous cell types, including platelets, macrophages, and endothelial cells. It consists of two polypeptide chains, A and B, which share 60% amino acid sequence homology. PDGFs possess strong mitogenic properties and stimulate the proliferation of osteoblasts.

Gene Therapy

Gene therapy is an emerging field in bone tissue engineering, involving the transfer of genetic material into the genome and thereby altering cellular synthetic function. For this process, the selected gene's messenger ribonucleic acid (mRNA) is reversely transcribed into complementary deoxyribonucleic acid (cDNA). It is then inserted into a plasmid and placed into a vector (viral or nonviral) carrier that facilitates gene transfer into the targeted cell lines. Successful gene transfer using nonviral vectors is termed *transfection*, whereas gene transfer using viral carriers is known as *transduction*. The two main approaches to gene therapy involve in vivo and ex vivo gene transfer. The in vivo technique involves the direct transfer of genetic material into the host. It is technically an easier method to perform but is limited by the inability to perform in vitro safety testing on transfected cells. In vivo gene therapy has been used to promote fracture repair through the expression of BMP-2. Using the principles of ex vivo gene transfer, Lieberman et al. (1999) generated BMP-2–producing bone marrow cells and investigated their ability to heal critically sized femoral segmental defects in syngeneic rats.

CONCLUSION

Molecular biology is now offering new tools for the investigation and understanding of the spatial and temporal gene expression of the skeletal repair cascade, but fracture healing remains highly challenging. Our ability to influence skeletal repair events pharmacologically is appearing to improve, and new biomaterials possessing osteoconductive and osteoinductive properties to facilitate the healing process are being produced.

Molecular biotechnologies have been emerging in the field of skeletal tissue engineering, involving manipulation of the genetic material of targeted cells. Issues of biosafety and efficacy, however, need to be answered before human trials take place.

SUGGESTED READINGS

Bidner SM, Rubins IM, Desjardins JV, et al. Evidence for a humoral mechanism for enhanced osteogenesis after head injury. *J Bone Joint Surg Am* 72:1144, 1990.

Brighton CT, Hunt RM. Early histological and ultrastructural changes in medullary fracture callus. *J Bone Joint Surg Am* 73:832, 1991.

Einhorn TA. The cell and molecular biology of fracture healing. *Clin Orthop* 355(suppl): S7, 1998.

Einhorn TA, Hirschman A, Kaplan C, et al. Neutral protein-degrading enzymes in experimental fracture callus: a preliminary report. *J Orthop Res* 7:792, 1989.

Einhorn TA, Majeska RJ, Rush EB, et al. The expression of cytokine activity by fracture callus. *J Bone Miner Res* 10:1272, 1995.

Friedlaender GE, Perry CR, Cole JD, et al. Osteogenic protein-1 (bone morphogenetic protein-7) in the treatment of tibial nonunions. *J Bone Joint Surg Am* 83(suppl 1, pt 2):S151, 2001.

Geesink RG, Hoefnagels NH, Bulstra SK. Osteogenic activity of OP-1 bone morphogenetic protein (BMP-7) in a human fibular defect. *J Bone Joint Surg Br* 81:710, 1999.

Gerstenfeld LC, Cho TJ, Kon T, et al. Impaired intramembranous bone formation during bone repair in the absence of tumor necrosis factor-alpha signaling. *Cells Tissues Organs* 169:285, 2001.

Govender S, Csimma C, Genant HK, et al. BMP-2 Evaluation in Surgery for Tibial Trauma (BESTT) Study Group. Recombinant human bone morphogenetic protein-2 for treatment of open tibial fractures: a prospective, controlled, randomized study of four hundred and fifty patients. *J Bone Joint Surg Am* 84:2123, 2002.

LeGeros RZ. Properties of osteoconductive biomaterials: calcium phosphates. *Clin Orthop* 395:81, 2002.

Lieberman JR, Daluiski A, Stevenson S, et al. The effect of regional gene therapy with bone morphogenetic protein-2-producing bone-marrow cells on the repair of segmental femoral defects in rats. *J Bone Joint Surg Am* 81:905, 1999.

Perkins R, Skirving AP. Callus formation and the rate of healing of femoral fractures in patients with head injuries. *J Bone Joint Surg Br* 69:521, 1987.

Riedel GE, Valentin-Opran A. Clinical evaluation of rhBMP-2/ACS in orthopedic trauma: a progress report. *Orthopedics* 22:663, 1999.

Urist MR, Silverman BF, Buring K, et al. The bone induction principle. *Clin Orthop* 53:243, 1967.

Urist MR. Bone: formation by autoinduction. *Science* 150:893, 1965.

7 | Injuries of the Glenohumeral Joint

Charles M. Court-Brown   *C. M. Robinson*

This chapter reviews fractures of the proximal humerus and dislocations of the humeral head from the glenoid fossa.

PART I. PROXIMAL HUMERAL FRACTURES

Proximal humeral fractures are relatively common, comprising about 5 to 6% of all fractures. They occur mainly in elderly patients with osteopenic bone. Despite this, many of the studies of proximal humeral fractures have examined the treatment of younger patients, and the results are difficult to extrapolate to an older population with different functional requirements and expectations. This chapter discusses the treatment of both patient groups.

ANATOMY

The basic anatomy of the proximal humerus is shown in Fig. 7-1. The anatomic neck lies behind the articular surface and the greater and lesser tuberosities lie between the anatomic and surgical necks. The surgical neck connects the humerus to the shaft. It is the displacement of the anatomic and surgical necks and the two tuberosities that define the different proximal humeral fractures.

The rotator cuff muscles insert into the proximal humerus behind the insertion of the joint capsule. Teres minor inserts onto the back of the greater tuberosity and the proximal humeral shaft. Infraspinatus runs above teres minor and inserts onto the greater tuberosity behind supraspinatus, which runs under the acromion and inserts into the tip of the greater tuberosity. Subscapularis runs anteriorly from the scapula and inserts into the lesser tuberosity and the proximal humeral shaft.

The main approach to the proximal humerus is the deltopectoral approach, which separates deltoid and pectoralis major. The deltoid arises from the lateral clavicle, acromion, and spine of the scapula and inserts into the deltoid tuberosity on the humeral diaphysis. Pectoralis major arises from the chest wall and the clavicle and inserts into the proximal humeral diaphysis. The cephalic vein lies between the muscles and serves as a marker for the space between the two muscles. The short head of biceps and coracobrachialis lie between the deltoid and pectoralis major and the anterior rotator cuff. They originate from the coracoid process. The musculocutaneous nerve pierces coracobrachialis about 4 cm below the coracoid and is at risk in anterior shoulder surgery. The axillary nerve runs behind the proximal humerus and can also be damaged by a proximal humeral fracture or during surgery. The main arterial supply to the area is the axillary artery, which gives rise to the anterior and posterior circumflex humeral arteries; these anastomose around the surgical neck of the humerus and supply ascending branches to the humeral head. Damage to the vascular supply by fracture may cause avascular necrosis; this is of particular importance in four-part proximal humeral fractures and fracture-dislocations.

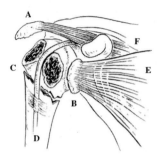

FIG. 7-1   The anatomy of the proximal humerus as it relates to fractures. *A.* Greater tuberosity. *B.* Lesser tuberosity. *C.* Surgical neck. *D.* Long head of biceps. *E.* Infraspinatus. *F.* Supraspinatus.

CLASSIFICATIONS

There are two classifications, which, to an extent, are complementary, and both are used in this chapter. Neer (1970) introduced a classification that subdivided proximal humeral fractures. It was based on the degree of displacement of the tuberosities and the anatomic and surgical neck and the presence of an associated dislocation. He defined a displaced fragment as one with more than 1 cm displacement or more than 45 degrees of angulation. Using these criteria, he defined proximal humeral fractures as minimally displaced, displaced two-part anatomic neck, surgical neck, and greater and lesser tuberosity fractures. He also defined three- and four-part displaced fractures as those that had displacement of either one or both of the tuberosities together with a surgical neck fracture. In addition he recognized two-, three-, and four-part fracture-dislocations and head-splitting fractures. Table 7-1*A* lists the types of proximal humeral fracture defined by Neer.

The Orthopaedic Trauma Association (OTA) classification (1997) has 27 subtypes and therefore better defines the different fractures (Fig. 7-2). Type

TABLE 7-1A The Neer Classification of Proximal Humeral Fractures[a]

Neer type	Percent
Minimally displaced	49
Two-part anatomic neck	0.3
Two-part surgical neck	28
Two-part greater tuberosity	4
Two-part lesser tuberosity	0
Three-part fracture	9.3
Four-part fracture	2
Two-part fracture-dislocation	5.2
Three-part fracture-dislocation	0.2
Four-part fracture-dislocation	1.1
Head-splitting fracture	0.7

[a]The different categories of proximal humeral fracture as defined by the Neer (1970) classification, together with their incidence, according to Court-Brown et al., 2001.

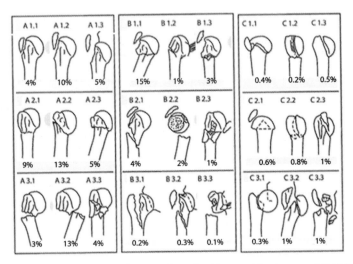

FIG. 7-2 The OTA classification of proximal humeral fractures and their incidence. *From Orthopaedic Trauma Association Committee for Coding and Classification. Fracture and dislocation compendium.* J Orthop Trauma *1996; 10(suppl):2–5.*

A fractures are unifocal fractures, with A1 fractures involving the greater tuberosity. A2 and A3 fractures are surgical neck fractures, with A2 being impacted and A3 nonimpacted. In A1 fractures, the suffixes 0.1 to 0.3 refers to the displacement of the greater tuberosity or glenohumeral dislocation. In A2 and A3 fractures, the suffix 0.1 to 0.3 refer to the different fracture types. Type B fractures are bifocal, with B1 fractures having metaphyseal impaction. B2 fractures are nonimpacted, and B3 fractures are associated with glenohumeral dislocation. The suffixes 0.1 to 0.3 refer to the different fracture patterns. Type C fractures are fractures of the anatomic neck, with C1 fractures showing slight displacement and C2 fractures showing marked displacement. C3 fractures are associated with a dislocation and/or head-splitting fractures. Again the suffixes 0.1 to 0.3 denote different fracture configurations.

The two classification systems should be seen as complementary. The Neer system does not define the different fracture patterns very well and makes no mention of valgus-impacted fractures. The OTA classification is more comprehensive but does not take fracture displacement into account. It is therefore best to combine the OTA classification with Neer's displacement criteria, and that is done in this chapter.

EPIDEMIOLOGY

The incidence of the different fracture types defined by the Neer classification is shown in Table 7-1*A*. Figure 7-2 shows the incidence of the different types of proximal humeral fracture when the OTA classification is used. The data in both Table 7-1*A* and Fig. 7-2 are from Court-Brown et al. (2001). In this study of 1027 consecutive fractures, the average age was 66 years. Some 27%

were male (average age 56 years) and 73% were female (average age 70 years). Age and sex incidence curves show that both males and females have a unimodal distribution, with very few fractures under the age of 40. It is a fracture of the fit elderly, with 90% of patients being independent at the time of fracture.

If the Neer classification is used, 49% of proximal humeral fractures are minimally displaced, 28% are two-part surgical neck fractures, 9% are three-part fractures, and 5% are two-part anterior fracture-dislocations. Only 2% are four-part fractures and only 1.3% are three- or four-part fracture-dislocations. If the OTA classification is used, 66% of fractures are type A unifocal fractures affecting the greater tuberosity or surgical neck. A further 27% are bifocal fractures, and only 6% of fractures are variations of the anatomic neck fracture, including four-part fractures. The most common proximal humeral fracture is the B1.1 impacted valgus fracture (15%), followed by the A3.2 translated two-part fracture (13%), the two-part impacted varus fracture (13%), and the A1.2 displaced greater tuberosity fracture (10%). All together, about 21% of proximal humeral fractures are impacted valgus fractures (A2.3, B1.1, C1.1, and C2.1).

Associated Injuries

About 10% of patients present with associated injuries. As the patients are usually elderly, multiple injuries are rare. Most patients present with either an ipsilateral distal radial fracture or an associated proximal femoral fracture. Vascular injury is very rare, with axillary artery damage having been reported in less than 20 cases. However, neurologic damage is fairly common and may involve the brachial plexus or peripheral nerves. The posterior cord of the brachial plexus is most commonly affected; axillary, suprascapular, and radial nerve involvement is not infrequent.

CLINICAL HISTORY AND EXAMINATION

Patients who have proximal humeral fractures tend to be elderly and to have isolated injuries. They present with a painful shoulder and a very restricted range of motion. Nerve damage is not uncommon; therefore a neurologic examination of the arm should be undertaken and the results recorded. In view of the patient's age, a thorough social history is important, as the fracture may well prevent an independent existence, at least on a temporary basis. If the patient is multiply injured, a complete clinical examination according to the Americal College of Surgeons' Advanced Trauma Life Support (ATLS) guidelines is mandatory.

Radiologic Examination

Adequate information to diagnose and classify the fracture should be obtained from anteroposterior and axial radiographs (Fig. 7-3). An axillary view can also be useful. A lateral scapular view is often suggested, but it does not add much information. Computed tomography (CT) scans will show the extent of the fracture but are rarely required. Magnetic resonance imaging (MRI) may help to delineate the extent of associated soft tissue damage in fracture-dislocations.

The essential information to be gained from the radiographs is listed in Table 7-1*B*.

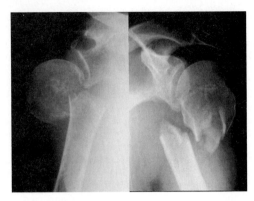

FIG. 7-3 Anteroposterior and lateral radiographs of an A3.2 translated surgical neck fracture.

TREATMENT

Minimally Displaced Fractures

Table 7-1A shows that about 50% of proximal humeral fractures are minimally displaced (Fig. 7-4). Analysis shows that about 56% of type A, 41% of type B, and 15% of type C fractures are minimally displaced (Court-Brown et al, 2003). There is universal acceptance that these fractures should be managed nonoperatively and that the results of such management are generally good. The literature indicates that about 85% of patients have excellent or good results with nonoperative treatment. About 70% of these patients are pain-free; on average, patients regain about 85% of normal shoulder function. Analysis shows that the results are age-dependent, with most patients below age 50 achieving normal shoulder function. Poor results tend to occur in older patients who have coexisting medical morbidities. Nonoperative management consists of 2 weeks in a sling followed by a course of physical therapy. There is no evidence that other types of nonoperative treatment or a longer duration of immobilization gives better results.

TABLE 7-1B Important Radiographic Features of Proximal Humeral Fractures

1. Is there a proximal humeral fracture?
2. How extensive is the fracture? Does it involve either or both of the tuberosities, the surgical neck, or the anatomic neck?
3. How displaced are the fragments (>1 cm displacement or >45 degrees of angulation)?
4. Is an isolated fracture of the greater tuberosity displaced by >0.5 cm?
5. Is it a valgus impaction fracture?
6. Is there an anterior or posterior dislocation?
7. Is there an impaction fracture of the head associated with a dislocation?
8. Is there a glenoid rim fracture?
9. Is there high-riding of the humeral head, suggesting a chronic rotator cuff tear?
10. What is the state of the bone? Is it osteopenic?

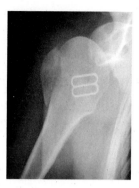

FIG. 7-4   An A1.2 minimally displaced fracture.

Displaced Fractures

Two-Part Fractures

Greater tuberosity fractures.   Greater tuberosity fractures (Fig. 7-5) account for about 19% of proximal humeral fractures. About 4% are undisplaced (A1.1), 5% are associated with glenohumeral dislocation (A1.3), and the remaining 10% are displaced (A1.2). These fractures occur in younger patients with an average age of about 55 years. All greater tuberosity fractures should be regarded as possible rotator cuff tears. The true incidence of rotator cuff tears associated with greater tuberosity fractures is unknown, but it seems likely that they are more common in older patients, in high-energy injuries, and where there is significant tuberosity displacement. It is accepted that displacement of more than 5 mm is an indication for surgical reconstruction of the greater tuberosity.

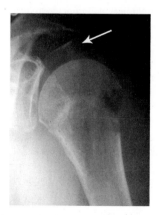

FIG. 7-5   An A1.3 fracture showing marked displacement of the greater tuberosity (*arrow*).

If there is evidence of significant shoulder dysfunction with 2 or 3 weeks of the fracture, all greater tuberosity fractures should have an ultrasound examination or an MRI scan to check the integrity of the rotator cuff. If there is more than 5 mm of displacement of the tuberosity or imaging shows a cuff tear, operative treatment is indicated. Surgery is best undertaken through a lateral deltoid splitting approach. The tuberosity can be fixed by an intrafragmentary screw if the bone fragment is large enough or with interosseous sutures or suture anchors if screw fixation is impossible. Care must be exercised in using screw fixation, as large tuberosity fragments tend to occur in older patients with osteopenic bone. Any rotator cuff tear must be repaired.

Surgical neck fractures. About 47% of proximal humeral fractures are in the surgical neck, although about only 28% are significantly displaced. The majority of surgical neck fractures are translated fractures (A3.2) and impacted varus fractures (A2.2).

TRANSLATED SURGICAL NECK FRACTURE. This fracture (Fig. 7-3) has received considerable attention in the literature. Suggested methods of treatment include nonoperative management, percutaneous Kirschner wires (K wires), plating, antegrade intramedullary nailing, and retrograde intramedullary fixation with flexible pins. Table 7-2 presents an analysis of the results of the literature dealing with these techniques.

Nonoperative management. Most surgeons would treat A3.2 fractures associated with less than 50 to 60% translation nonoperatively. The debate about treatment concerns more severely displaced fractures. Table 7-2 shows that nonoperative management is associated with better results than percutaneous K-wire fixation or plating despite the much higher average age of the patients in published series. As with all treatment methods, the results of nonoperative management are age-dependent. Table 7-2 suggests that nonoperative management remains the treatment of choice for older patients with displaced A3.2 fractures. The treatment involves using a sling for 2 weeks and then instituting a physical therapy program.

Percutaneous K-wire fixation. This technique is widely talked about, but there is little evidence to justify its use. After fracture reduction, K wires are inserted, using either an antegrade or retrograde technique under fluoroscopic control. The technique is much more difficult than it appears and the difficulty of transfixing the fracture combined with pin loosening in osteopenic bone leads to high pin-failure and infection rates. It is a useful technique in proximal humeral epiphyseal fractures in young adolescents, where bone quality is good and union is rapid. It should not be used in older patients.

TABLE 7-2 Excellent and Good Results Associated with the Different Methods of Treating A3.2 Translated Two-Part Fractures of the Surgical Neck

Treatment method	Age	Excellent/good (%)
Nonoperative	72	69
Kirschner wires	56	50
Plates	56	67
Antegrade nailing	63	78
Retrograde flexible nails	60	82

Plating. Many surgeons have utilized T- or L-shaped neutralization plates or blade plates to treat displaced two-part surgical neck fractures. As with percutaneous K-wire fixation, the results for patients below age 50 are much better than those in older patients, but fractures are rare in this age group. It is probable that the new generation of locking plates will improve the results shown in Table 7-2, but this is as yet unknown.

Antegrade intramedullary nailing. The results of both antegrade nailing (Fig. 7-6) and retrograde pinning of two-part surgical neck fractures are shown in Table 7-2. The average age of the series dealing with this technique lies between those with K wires and plating and nonoperative management, but it is clear that the results are better than those associated with K wires and plating. The problem associated with antegrade nailing is rotator cuff damage. Antegrade nailing is usually undertaken through a deltoid splitting approach under fluoroscopic control. A locked short intramedullary nail is usually used.

As with all methods of treatment, better results are gained in younger patients; but unlike the case with K wiring and plating, the difference between the results in the young and older groups is less marked. The results of retrograde nailing using two or more flexible intramedullary pins are similar to those of antegrade nailing and, indeed, to those of nonoperative management in patients of a similar age. Retrograde nailing is undertaken using thin, flexible nails inserted from above the olecranon fossa. The drawback is that the nails tend to back out, causing loss of elbow extension, usually of less than 20 degrees. This technique is less popular than the other techniques listed in Table 7-2, but it can give good results.

TWO-PART VARUS IMPACTED FRACTURES. These are extremely common, accounting for 13% of all proximal humeral fractures, and it is surprising that there has been only one study of their treatment (Court-Brown and McQueen, 2004). In a series of 133 consecutive fractures, the average age of the patients was 68 years, and 89% were above 50 years of age. Nonoperative management was used, and 78% of patients had excellent or good results. There is understandable concern that increasing varus angulation causes increased impingement between the greater tuberosity and the acromion and therefore

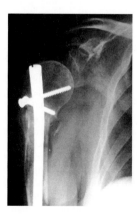

FIG. 7-6   Intramedullary nailing of a surgical neck fracture.

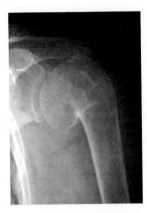

FIG. 7-7 An A2.2 impacted varus fracture.

increased pain and decreased function. However analysis shows that while the outcome of A2.2 fractures is age-dependent, it is independent of the degree of varus of the humeral head. Nonoperative management is therefore indicated in these fractures (Fig. 7-7).

Lesser tuberosity fractures. These are extremely rare and are treated in the same way as fractures of the greater tuberosity. If displaced, they should be internally fixed; if undisplaced, they can be treated nonoperatively. As with greater tuberosity fractures, imaging of the rotator cuff is indicated, with repair being undertaken as required.

Anatomic Neck Fractures

Isolated two-part anatomic neck fractures are very rare. If undisplaced, they should be treated nonoperatively; but if they are significantly displaced, the vascular supply of the humeral head will be compromised and a hemiarthroplasty prosthesis will usually be used in older patients. Screw fixation is advised in younger patients.

Three- and Four-Part Fractures

Three and four-part fractures are uncommon. In three-part fractures, the surgical neck and greater tuberosity are usually involved; very rarely, the fracture may involve the surgical neck and the lesser tuberosity. In four-part fractures, both tuberosities and the surgical neck are fractured, thus compromising the vascularity of the humeral head. The original Neer classification assumed that three- and four-part fractures were always associated with rotation of the humeral head; but surgeons have now realized that most three- and four-part fractures involve a valgus malposition of the head (Fig. 7-8), which is impacted onto the humeral metaphysis. These fractures are not associated with the same degree of vascular damage, and internal fixation rather than joint replacement is often used to treat valgus impaction fractures. Three- and four-part fractures can be treated nonoperatively or operatively using plates, percutaneous screws, cerclage wire fixation, or hemiarthroplasty. The results of these treatment methods are given in Table 7-3.

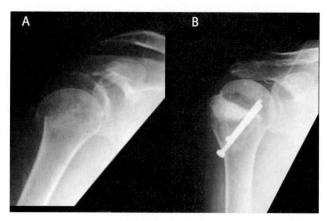

FIG. 7-8   A three-part impacted valgus fracture showing significant valgus of the head (*A*) and treatment with calcium phosphate cement and screw fixation. (*Courtesy of C. M. Robinson, M.D.*)

Treatment Methods

Nonoperative

Table 7-3 shows the results of nonoperative treatment in the management of three- and four-part fractures. As with two-part fractures (Table 7-2), the patients tend to be older, and a poorer prognosis can therefore be expected. The results for nonoperative management of three-part fractures are at least equivalent to those of plating and are only slightly worse than those of two-part fractures. However, the results of the use of nonoperative management in four-part fractures are poor.

Plating

The results of plating of three- and four-part fractures are poor. Table 7-3 shows that the technique is no better than nonoperative management in three-part fractures. In four-part fractures, it is better than nonoperative management but worse than percutaneous screw fixation or the use of sutures or cerclage wires. There is

TABLE 7-3   Results Associated with the Treatment of Three- and Four-Part Fractures[a]

	Three-part fractures		Four-part fractures	
	Age	Excellent/good (%)	Age	Excellent/good (%)
Nonoperative	73	63	73	29
Plating	67	63	66	48
Percutaneous screws	52	87	52	74
Cerclage wire/suture	51	93	51	77
Hemiarthroplasty	—	—	68	53

[a]The average age and excellent and good results associated with the different treatments of three- and four-part fractures. The results for hemiarthroplasty include both three- and four-part fractures.

no evidence that the technique should be used, although, as with two-part fractures, the new locking compression plates may improve results.

Percutaneous Screw Fixation

This technique is designed for valgus impacted fractures (Fig. 7-8). Under fluoroscopic control, minimal dissection techniques are used to reduce the fragments into an anatomic position and percutaneous screws are used to fix the fracture. Calcium phosphate cement may be used to fill the void in the humeral head. Table 7-3 shows good results in both three- and four-part fractures, although the average age of the patients in these series is much younger than that of the population who sustain these injuries. There is no good information about the use of this technique in older patients, but the osteopenic nature of the bone will make the procedure difficult.

Suture/Cerclage Wire

It is possible to reduce and hold the tuberosities with nonabsorbable sutures or use a cerclage wire or tension band to hold the reduced tuberosities to the humeral shafts. The soft tissue dissection is less than with plating, but again, Tables 7-2 and 7-3 show that while good results can be obtained, it is the younger patients who have been treated; there are no results for older patients.

K Wires and Tension Banding

This technique is not appropriate in the treatment of three- and four-part fractures. The osteopenic nature of the bone in the majority of patients means that results are poor.

Intramedullary Nailing

Good results have been published, but there are very few good studies, and up to 71% fixation failure has been reported. Both antegrade and retrograde nailing provides good results in two-part fractures, but these techniques are not appropriate for more complex fractures.

Hemiarthroplasty

The results of the use of hemiarthroplasty prostheses (Fig. 7-9) to treat three- and four-part fractures are given in Table 7-3. A number of different implants

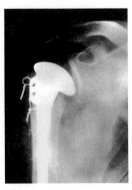

FIG. 7-9   A hemiarthroplasty prosthesis.

have been used, but the literature suggests that there is little difference between them. They are inserted through an anterior deltopectoral approach, with the tuberosities being reconstructed after the prosthesis has been inserted. The literature clearly shows that their use is associated with good pain relief but relatively poor shoulder function, particularly in the elderly. A number of factors have been shown to affect outcome. These are listed in Table 7-4.

Table 7-3 shows that these prostheses are usually used in older patients and that only about 50% of patients will get excellent or good results. As with other techniques, the success of the technique correlates with age. However, over 85% of patients have little or no pain and regain functional movement. Patient satisfaction is high and the operation is better than nonoperative management in the fit elderly. There has only been one prospective study comparing hemiarthroplasty with nonoperative management in elderly patients. This showed that function was relatively poor in both groups, but the patients who had arthroplasties had better pain relief. There has been no prospective study comparing hemiarthroplasty with operative reconstruction.

Fracture-Dislocations and Head-Splitting Fractures

Three- and four-part fracture-dislocations and head-splitting fractures are very rare, all together accounting for 2% of proximal humeral fractures. The prognosis is worse than for three- and four-part fractures, with very high rates of avascular necrosis and shoulder dysfunction often being recorded. Hemiarthroplasty is the best treatment method.

Valgus Impacted Fractures

These fractures (Fig. 7-8) have assumed greater importance in the last 20 years. They represent about 21% of proximal humeral fractures. About 48% are minimally displaced, 31% are two-part, 18% are three-part, and 3% are four-part fractures. The average age of patients with a valgus impacted fracture is 72 years. The incidence of avascular necrosis is less than in fractures associated with rotation of the head. Minimally displaced and two-part valgus impacted fractures will usually be treated nonoperatively, with 90 and 72% excellent and good results being obtained. Nonoperative treatment of three-part surgical neck and greater tuberosity fractures results in 66% excellent and good results. Four-part impacted valgus fractures are best treated by percutaneous screw fixation or hemiarthroplasty, depending on the age of the patient.

Operative treatment of three-part valgus impaction fractures is indicated if there is excessive valgus. These fractures have been treated successfully with reduction, the insertion of calcium phosphate cement to fill the void in the

---

TABLE 7-4 Factors Affecting the Outcome of Shoulder Hemiarthroplasty Performed for Fracture

Increasing age
Neurologic deficit
Timing of surgery (early surgery produces better results)
Displacement of the prosthesis in relation to the glenoid
Nonunion of the tuberosities
Displacement of the tuberosities
Alcohol consumption
Tobacco usage
Experience of the surgeon

humeral head, and either screw or plate fixation (Fig. 7-8). Unfortunately there is as yet no definition as to what constitutes the extreme valgus of the humeral head, but consideration should be given to operative treatment of three-part impacted valgus fractures that show significant valgus of the head, particularly if they occur in younger patients.

COMPLICATIONS

Nonunion

The inference in some texts is that proximal humeral nonunion is common, but this is not the case. In a study of 1027 consecutive proximal humeral fractures, only 11 (1.1%) occurred (Court-Brown, 2001). Five (45.4%) were OTA type A2 fractures and three (27.3%) were B2 fractures. The highest incidence of nonunion is in the rare B2.3 fracture, with 33% nonunions being recorded. This is followed by the B2.2 fracture (4.2%) and the A3.2 fracture (2.3%).

Nonunion can be extremely disabling. The humeral head becomes stuck and all movement is at the site of the nonunion. Treatment depends on the age and degree of infirmity of the patient, but symptomatic nonunion is best treated by internal fixation and bone grafting in younger patients and by hemiarthroplasty in older patients, in whom pain relief is the most important outcome. Good results have been reported with locked antegrade nails and bone grafting. The results of hemiarthroplasty are also encouraging, but function is not as good as for primary hemiarthroplasty.

Malunion

Malunion is relatively common after proximal humeral fractures but rarely requires surgery. However, in younger patients, repositioning of displaced tuberosities may improve shoulder function and a proximal humeral osteotomy and refixation can be carried out. More commonly, however, hemiarthroplasty is the treatment of choice for symptomatic proximal humeral malunion.

Avascular Necrosis

Avascular necrosis has been reported in up to 3% of three-part fractures and 20% of four-part fractures. If this condition is causing symptoms, it should be treated by hemiarthroplasty.

Heterotopic Ossification

Heterotopic ossification has been reported to occur in up to 56% of hemiarthroplasty procedures. However, in 50 to 65% of cases, it is minor. Rarely, it is more severe and symptomatic. Under these conditions, excision can be carried out with indomethacin or with radiation therapy to minimize the risk of recurrence.

Axillary Artery Damage

This is extremely rare. It occurs in high-energy injuries, usually in younger patients. The head of the humerus is forced into the axilla, damaging the artery. Vascular reconstruction is usually required.

Neurologic Damage

Neurologic damage is surprisingly common after proximal humeral fractures. The brachial plexus, suprascapular nerve, or axillary nerve are most commonly involved. The lesion is usually a neuropraxia and treatment is expectant, although physical therapy may be required. Recovery is usually complete.

SUGGESTED TREATMENT

Guidelines for the treatment of proximal humeral fractures are given in Table 7-5. These are based on the results detailed in the literature and are not followed by every surgeon. The interpretation of age is particularly difficult. Surgeons should assess the patient's general health, degree of dependence, and functional requirements before making a decision regarding treatment. They should also remember that fracture treatment is constantly evolving.

PART II. DISLOCATIONS OF THE GLENOHUMERAL JOINT

FUNCTIONAL ANATOMY

The **proximal humerus** consists of the head, greater and lesser tuberosities, and anatomic and surgical necks. The **greater tuberosity** carries the insertion of the supraspinatus superiorly and the infraspinatus and teres minor posteriorly. The **lesser tuberosity** is the site of insertion of the subscapularis. The long head of the biceps takes origin from the superior glenoid and lies in the intertubercular groove between the two tuberosities. The **anatomic neck** of the humerus is delineated by the area of the head covered by articular cartilage, whereas the **surgical neck** is the narrowest portion of the proximal humeral metaphysis. The anterior and posterior circumflex humeral arteries and the axillary nerve circle the proximal humerus at the level of the surgical neck. The vascular supply of the humeral head is through the anterior lateral ascending (arcuate) artery, which originates from the anterior humeral circumflex artery. The arcuate artery runs proximally along the lateral aspect of the intertubercular groove and enters the humeral head through foramina along its course.

The **glenoid** serves as a fulcrum against which the muscles of the shoulder work to move the humerus. The bony glenoid is a shallow socket that has an articular surface area of only one-third that of the humeral head.

Although both the humeral head and the glenoid are typically retroverted with respect to their long axes, the scapula is protracted forward on the chest wall (Fig. 7-10). Excessive posterior translation of the humeral head is therefore prevented by the strong buttressing action of the posterior glenoid.

The **glenohumeral articulation** functions as a multiaxial ball-and-socket joint and is the most mobile joint in the body, at the expense, however, of intrinsic stability. The stability of the articulation is dependent on passive and active mechanisms. Passive mechanisms of stability include the glenoid labrum, negative intraarticular pressure, the coracoacromial ligament, the capsule, and the glenohumeral ligaments. The **glenoid labrum** deepens the glenoid fossa and consists of dense fibrocartilage. The anteroinferior labrum is usually detached from the rim of the glenoid during anterior dislocations of the shoulder **(Bankart lesion).** The supraspinatus tendon, coracoacromial ligament, and acromion form the roof of the glenohumeral articulation and, with other components of the rotator cuff, prevent proximal migration of the humeral head. The capsule of the glenohumeral articulation is large and baggy, allowing the extensive range of motion of the shoulder. The three **glenohumeral ligaments (superior, middle, and inferior)** are thickenings of the capsule and are major passive stabilizers of the joint. The superior and middle ligaments vary widely in size and shape, but the inferior glenohumeral ligament is a constant

TABLE 7-5 Guidelines for the Treatment of Proximal Humeral Fractures

Fracture type	Suggested treatment
Proximal physis	Closed reduction and K wiring
Minimally displaced	Nonoperative
Two-part surgical neck (<65 years)	Antegrade nailing
(>65 years)	Nonoperative
Two-part greater tuberosity (<5 mm displacement)	Nonoperative
(>5 mm displacement)	Screw or suture fixation. Cuff repair
Three-part fracture (<65 years)	Percutaneous screw fixation
(>65 years)	Nonoperative
Four-part fracture (<65 years)	Percutaneous screw fixation
(>65 years)	Hemiarthroplasty
Two-part fracture-dislocation	Reduce and as for two-part fracture
Three- and four-part fracture-dislocation	Hemiarthroplasty
Head-splitting fracture	Hemiarthroplasty

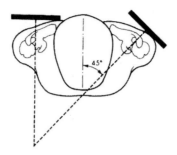

FIG. 7-10   Techniques of shoulder imaging show the ventral inclination of the scapula on the chest wall, creating a buttressing effect by the glenoid surface.

"hammock," which suspends the humeral head and prevents anteroinferior subluxation. The anterosuperior aspect of the shoulder capsule and the subscapularis tendon limit posterior glenohumeral translation, even when the entire posterior capsule has been divided. An intact rotator interval is felt to be a major stabilizer, opposing posterior and inferior humeral displacement on the glenoid. The coracohumeral ligament is a fold in the anterosuperior glenohumeral capsule that becomes prominent with inferior translation of the humeral head.

The muscles of the rotator cuff and the long head of the biceps contribute to active glenohumeral stability. The **rotator cuff muscles** function to maintain the humeral head against the glenoid and also serve to tension the capsulolabral complex during movement of the shoulder. The other, larger shoulder girdle muscles either produce the major shoulder movements in the three planes (deltoid, pectorals, teres major, and latissimus dorsi) or coordinate and stabilize movements of the scapula on the chest wall (serratus anterior and the rhomboids).

DISLOCATIONS OF THE GLENOHUMERAL ARTICULATION

Dislocations of the glenohumeral articulation are classified according to their direction (anterior, posterior, inferior, multidirectional), degree (subluxation or dislocation and "microinstability"), chronicity (acute, recurrent, or chronic), volition (voluntary or involuntary), and cause (traumatic or atraumatic). In addition, all acute dislocations may be associated with neurovascular or soft tissue injuries and fractures.

The majority of glenohumeral dislocations are **anterior** (Fig. 7-11) and occur in the young following sporting injuries and in the middle-aged and elderly following low-energy falls. **Posterior dislocations** (Fig.7-12A to C) are uncommon but are difficult to diagnose and may be overlooked without a careful physical examination and adequate radiograph or CT scan of the involved shoulder. These injuries occur in all age groups and occur following either high-energy injury or during seizures, which may be triggered either by epilepsy, diabetic hypoglycemia, electrocution, or alcohol or drug withdrawal. **Inferior dislocations** are extremely uncommon and are known as traumatic **luxatio erecta** (Fig. 7-13). *Multidirectional instability* refers to instability of the shoulder in more than one direction (characteristically anterior, posterior, and inferior instability) and is usually associated with constitutional ligamentous laxity.

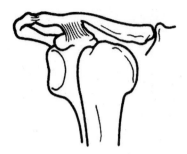

FIG. 7-11   Anterior glenohumeral dislocation.

Glenohumeral dislocations are further classified as acute, chronic, or recurrent. **Acute dislocations** are diagnosed within the first 2 weeks after injury. **Chronic dislocations** are diagnosed after 2 weeks, either because the dislocation was missed by the physician initially or due to delayed presentation by the patient. The elderly and patients with posterior dislocations are at risk of substantial delay before the diagnosis is made. Instability may become **recurrent** if the shoulder repeatedly resubluxates or redislocates following an initial episode of instability. Anterior dislocations in the young are particularly at risk of this complication.

Instability may be classified according to its degree into **dislocation** (complete dissociation of the humeral head from the glenoid), **subluxation** (excessive symptomatic translation of the humeral head on the glenoid), and

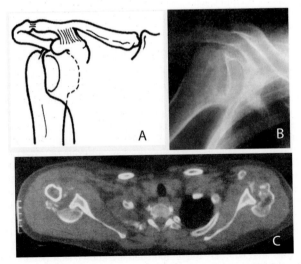

FIG. 7-12   *A.* Posterior glenohumeral dislocation. *B.* Superimposition of humeral head on glenoid indicates posterior dislocation. *C.* Computed tomography indicates bilateral posterior fracture dislocations of the shoulder.

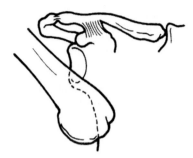

FIG. 7-13   Luxatio erecta, or an inferior glenohumeral dislocation.

microinstability (instability produced by acquired laxity of the shoulder, caused by repetitive movements, particularly in the throwing athlete; this form of instability often presents with pain rather than instability when the arm is in the provocative position for instability).

Instability may also be classified according to whether or not it is under voluntary control. **Voluntary dislocation** is produced willfully, usually by emotionally disturbed individuals who dislocate a shoulder for the sake of secondary gain. In the majority of patients, dislocation is not under voluntary control and occurs accidentally (**involuntary instability**).

Glenohumeral dislocations are classified according to their etiology as being traumatic or atraumatic. A **traumatic** dislocation occurs following injury to the shoulder, whereas **atraumatic** instability develops more insidiously and is usually associated with a degree of constitutional ligamentous laxity. In these patients there is often evidence of instability in other joints, and the shoulder instability is often bilateral and multidirectional.

Associated Injuries

Injuries associated with traumatic dislocations include fractures, rotator cuff tears, nerve injuries, and, rarely, arterial disruption. Fractures commonly associated with glenohumeral dislocations include tuberosity fractures and fractures of the glenoid rim. Fractures of the surgical or anatomic neck of the humerus may occur in association with a dislocation, but they are best considered with other proximal humeral fractures (see Part I of this chapter). All of these associated injuries are more common in middle-aged and elderly patients.

Careful review of the radiographs is required to determine the presence of fractures. It is important to be aware of the possibility of an undisplaced fracture of the humeral neck, which may displace during attempted reduction of the dislocation. In this situation, to minimize the probability of displacement, reduction is performed under general anesthesia with muscle relaxation and is monitored fluoroscopically.

Fracture of more than 25% of the anteroinferior glenoid rim may result in acute recurrent instability and may require acute open reduction and internal fixation. The **Hill-Sachs lesion** is an osteochondral fracture of the posterior surface of the humeral head produced by its impaction on the glenoid during an anterior dislocation. With recurrence, this lesion progressively enlarges and is pathognomonic of recurrent traumatic instability. A reverse Hill-Sachs lesion is the corresponding lesion of the anterior part of the humeral head, associated with a posterior dislocation.

Both displaced fractures of the tuberosities and rotator cuff tears undermine the function of the rotator cuff muscles; they may lead to chronic pain and shoulder weakness if neglected. Suspicion of a rotator cuff tear is raised by positive findings on physical examination (inability to initiate abduction of the glenohumeral joint and specific weakness on selective testing of each muscle). The diagnosis is confirmed by arthrography, ultrasound, or MRI scanning. All significantly displaced tuberosity fractures and confirmed rotator cuff tears occurring after a traumatic dislocation should be treated by surgical repair in medically fit patients.

The neurologic injury most frequently associated with glenohumeral dislocation involves the **axillary nerve**, although injury to the entire brachial plexus or other individual nerves, trunks, or divisions may occur. Injury to the axillary nerve is confirmed by the presence of hypoesthesia in the cutaneous distribution of the nerve (the "sergeant's badge area") and lack of voluntary contractions of the anterior and middle portions of the deltoid muscle. It is a mistake to assume that weakness of the shoulder following a dislocation is due entirely to an axillary nerve palsy; a concomitant rotator cuff injury must always be suspected and treated if present. Most dislocations with closed nerve injuries will be treated expectantly; the prognosis for recovery following an isolated nerve injury is usually better than when a more proximal plexus lesion is present.

Axillary artery injury is very uncommon and more likely to occur following a high-energy injury, in older patients, and in association with a brachial plexus injury. Physical signs include an expanding hematoma in the axilla and absent pulses at the elbow and wrist. Rupture of the axillary artery is an absolute surgical emergency.

Diagnosis and Management

Acute (first-time) dislocations. HISTORY AND PHYSICAL EXAMINATION. A clear history of when the injury occurred and whether there have been previous problems with instability must be determined. Traumatic anterior dislocation typically results from a contact sports injury or simple fall, whereas acute posterior dislocations result from either high-energy injury, an epileptic or hypoglycemic fit, alcohol or drug withdrawal, or electrocution. Any patient with shoulder pain following a "blackout" should have a posterior shoulder dislocation specifically excluded.

Acute traumatic dislocations are typically painful and the patient is usually reluctant to move the arm. Anterior dislocations are recognized by "squaring off" of the normal deltoid profile, while posterior dislocations are associated with a fixed mechanical block to external rotational movements of the arm. The physical examination of the patient with luxatio erecta is dramatic, with the humerus locked in greater than 90 degrees of abduction.

RADIOGRAPHIC EXAMINATION. Radiographic examination of the injured shoulder confirms the direction of the dislocation and delineates any associated fractures. The patient with a glenohumeral dislocation is unable to move the arm so that a true axial view of the shoulder may be obtained. Therefore, in addition to the standard anteroposterior radiograph in the transscapular plane, a "modified" axial or Velpeau view, taken with the arm in a sling, is essential to confirm the diagnosis (Fig. 7-14).

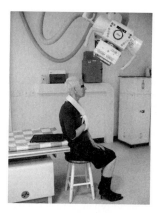

FIG. 7-14   Modified radiographic axial view (Velpeau view).

Specialized imaging, in the form of CT, MRI, or ultrasound, may be useful to delineate the nature and extent of associated soft tissue injuries.

Initial management.   Acute dislocations should be reduced under sedation. It is important to document the presence of any neurovascular injury prior to any attempted manipulation. Prior to reduction, venous access is established, the patient is sedated, and intravenous analgesics are administered. The reduction maneuver used is determined by the type of dislocation. Anterior dislocations are reduced with straight traction in line with the humerus. Gentle internal and external rotation of the arm will relocate the humeral head. Countertraction is applied by an assistant using a sheet wrapped around the patient's chest. The traction is firm and consistent. It is important not to attempt to force the humeral head back into place, because this will result in muscle spasm, making reduction more difficult and traumatic. Other methods of reduction of anterior dislocations that bear mention include Stimson's method and the Hippocratic method. **Stimson's method** involves hanging 5 to 10 lb of weight from the arm of the prone patient. After 10 to 20 min, gentle internal and external rotation of the arm will relocate the humeral head. Stimson's method is useful as a last resort for dislocations that are difficult to reduce by other methods. The **Hippocratic method** involves applying lateral traction through the arm and countertraction by placing the foot in the axilla.

Posterior dislocations are reduced with gentle traction, with pressure over the front of the humeral head, to disengage the engaged reverse Hill-Sachs lesion. Following disengagement, the shoulder can usually be reduced by gentle external rotation of the arm. **Luxatio erecta** is reduced with traction along the line of the arm, bringing it down to the side from its fixed abducted position.

Following reduction of the shoulder, a focused reexamination is performed to assess the integrity of the axillary nerve and rotator cuff. Repeat radiographs are obtained to ensure the adequacy of reduction. The shoulder is immobilized in a sling, with the arm internally rotated and in neutral flexion/abduction. Uncomplicated anterior dislocations are usually stable in this position, although rarely acute instability may be caused by a large glenoid rim fracture. In these circumstances, the fracture should be treated by acute open reduction and internal fixation to stabilize the shoulder. Posterior dislocations are often unstable after reduction due to reengagement of the reverse Hill-Sachs lesion in the sling with the arm in internal rotation. The treatment options in this situation include either immobilization of the shoulder in a position of external rotation or an acute stabilization procedure to address the reverse Hill-Sachs lesion. This may include either transplantation of the subscapularis tendon into the defect (**McLaughlin procedure**) or bone grafting of the defect with an allograft. These procedures should be performed by an experienced shoulder surgeon.

Most acute shoulder dislocations are treated by immobilization for the first 3 to 4 weeks in the sling, followed by a program of active physiotherapy to reestablish range of motion and strengthen the musculature of the shoulder girdle and rotator cuff.

ADJUNCTIVE TREATMENT. Associated fractures and rotator cuff lesions, typically in the middle-aged and elderly patient, should be treated on their merits as described above. Recurrent instability of the shoulder may be prevented by an acute arthroscopic Bankart repair to reattach the anteroinferior glenoid labrum within the first few weeks following an acute first-time anterior dislocation. The evidence suggests that this may reduce the risk of recurrent instability from approximately 75% down to 15% in individuals below 30 years of age. This procedure requires considerable expertise.

Recurrent instability. Recurrent instability, in the form of recurrent subluxation or dislocation, is usually a complication of an initial traumatic anterior dislocation, though recurrent posterior instability is being increasingly diagnosed and treated.

HISTORY AND PHYSICAL EXAMINATION. The clinical assessment of the patient presenting with symptoms of recurrent shoulder instability is primarily directed toward identifying those individuals with predominantly traumatic instability, who would benefit from surgical treatment. The acronym TUBS— for traumatic, typically unilateral, with a Bankart lesion, and usually requiring surgery to stabilize the shoulder—can serve to identify such cases. These patients must be distinguished from those with predominantly atraumatic or voluntary instability, who are best treated nonoperatively in the first instance. The acronym AMBRI—for atraumatic, multidirectional, commonly bilateral, treatment by rehabilitation, and inferior capsular shift in some refractory patients—may be useful here.

Details about the onset, duration, and frequency of the symptoms should be sought in the history. Physical examination should include screening for evidence of generalized ligamentous laxity and the use of provocative tests to define the direction and extent of instability.

RADIOGRAPHIC EXAMINATION. A plain radiographic series is useful in delineating any associated bony pathology, including glenoid rim and humeral head defects. Further specialist radiologic investigation, examination under anesthesia, or diagnostic arthroscopy may be used for patients in whom the precise diagnosis is in doubt. MRI of the shoulder is superior to CT in the assessment of shoulder instability owing to the better definition of soft tissue provided by MRI.

MANAGEMENT. Patients with atraumatic shoulder instability should be treated by an intensive 6-month course of physiotherapy, concentrating on proprioceptive exercises and rotator cuff strengthening. A small minority of these individuals who fail to adequately stabilize their shoulders on this regimen are treated with a Neer inferior capsular shift procedure to retension the antero-inferior capsule and reduce the overall joint volume.

Emotionally disturbed patients may learn to dislocate a shoulder at will for secondary gain; it is important not to make the mistake of treating these patients by way of a surgical stabilization procedure. Psychological counseling is the mainstay of treatment for these individuals.

Most patients with recurrent anterior traumatic instability are best treated by a surgical stabilization procedure to repair the Bankart lesion to the decorticated glenoid rim (Bankart repair), combined with a procedure to retension the redundant, stretched anteroinferior capsule-ligamentous complex, by advancing it superiorly in a capsular shift procedure. These procedures have traditionally been performed at open surgery, through a deltopectoral approach, with a high degree of success (typically with a less than 5% failure rate). Increasingly nowadays, these procedures can be carried out arthroscopically, although the expected failure rate by that technique is slightly higher.

Recurrent posterior shoulder instability is commonly associated with concomitant inferior or multidirectional instability. The results of surgical stabilization have previously been poor for this condition. However, there is evidence that targeted "lesion-specific" surgery, along similar lines to the treatment of anterior instability, particularly when performed arthroscopically, may be associated with a higher success rate.

Chronic dislocations. Most dislocations that present late occur in elderly patients and many of these are posterior in direction. The management of these injuries depends on the activity and health of the patient, length of time that the glenohumeral joint has been dislocated, and size of associated humeral head defect. Nonoperative treatment is usually preferred if the patient is inactive or a poor surgical candidate. Despite the chronic dislocation, the patient will regain a surprisingly functional, pain-free shoulder within the limited expectations in these circumstances.

Operative treatment is indicated for all younger patients with chronic dislocations, especially when the dislocation is less than 6 weeks old and the humeral head defect involves less than 50% of the articular surface of the humeral head. In these circumstances, closed reduction may be attempted, but often an open reduction is required to disengage the humeral head defect from the glenoid rim. Ancillary stabilizing techniques, including soft tissue rebalancing and bone grafting of the humeral head defect, are often required to stabilize the shoulder following open reduction.

When the dislocation is more chronic and the defect involves more than 50% of the articular surface of the humeral head, a total shoulder arthroplasty or hemiarthroplasty is usually the best surgical option.

SELECTED READINGS—PART I

Bhandari M, Matthys G, McKee MD. Four part fractures of the proximal humerus. *J Orthop Trauma* 18:126–127, 2004.

Court-Brown CM. The epidemiology of proximal humeral fractures. *Acta Orthop Scand* 72:365–371, 2001.

Court-Brown CM, Garg A, McQueen MM. The translated two-part fracture of the proximal humerus. Epidemiology and outcome in the older patient. *J Bone Joint Surg* 83B:799–804, 2001.

Court-Brown CM, McQueen MM. The impacted varus (A2.2) proximal humeral fracture: prediction of outcome and results of nonoperative treatment in 99 patients. *Acta Orthop Scand* 75:736–740, 2004.

Frankle MA, Mighell MA. Techniques and principles of tuberosity fixation for proximal humeral fractures treated with hemiarthroplasty. *J Shoulder Elbow Surg* 13:191–195, 2004.

Gaebler C, McQueen MM, Court-Brown CM. Minimally displaced proximal humeral fractures: epidemiology and outcome in 507 cases. *Acta Orthop Scand* 74:580–585, 2003.

Green A, Izzi J. Isolated fractures of the greater tuberosity of the proximal humerus. *J Shoulder Elbow Surg* 12:641–649, 2003.

Jakob RP, Miniaci A, Anson PS, et al. Four-part impacted valgus fractures of the proximal humerus. *J Bone Joint Surg* 73:295–298, 1991.

Kralinger F, Schwaiger R, Wambacher M, et al. Outcome after primary hemiarthroplasty for fracture of the head of the humerus. A retrospective multicentre study of 167 patients. *J Bone Joint Surg Br* 86B:217–219, 2004.

Neer CS. Displaced proximal humeral fractures. Part 1. Classification and evaluation. *J Bone Joint Surg* 52:1077–1089, 1970.

OTA fracture and dislocation compendium. *J Orthop Trauma* 10(suppl 1):1–5, 1996.

Park MC, Murthi AM, Roth NS, et al. Two-part and three-part fractures of the proximal humerus treated with suture fixation. *J Orthop Trauma* 17:319–325, 2003.

Robinson CM, Page RS. Severely impacted valgus proximal humeral fractures. Results of operative treatment. *J Bone Joint Surg* 85A:1647–1655, 2003.

SELECTED READINGS—PART II

Gonzalez D, Lopez RA. Concurrent rotator cuff tear and brachial plexus palsy associated with anterior dislocation of the shoulder: a report of two cases. *J Bone Joint Surg* 73A:620–621, 1991.

Matthews D, Roberts T. Intraarticular lidocaine versus intravenous analgesic for reductions of acute anterior shoulder dislocations. *AM J Sports Med* 23:5458, 1995.

Rowe CR, Zarins B. Chronic unreduced dislocations of the shoulder. *J Bone Joint Surg* 64A:495–505, 1982.

Wirth MA, Groh GI, Rockwood CA. Capsulorrhaphy through an anterior approach for treatment of atraumatic posterior glenohumeral instability with multidirectional laxity of the shoulder. *J Bone Joint Surg* 80A:1570–1578, 1998.

8 | Fractures and Dislocations of the Clavicle and Scapula

John A. Elstrom

This chapter reviews fractures of the clavicle, injuries of the sternoclavicular and acromioclavicular joints, and fractures of the scapula.

ANATOMY

The clavicle is the strut that connects the upper extremity to the chest. It stabilizes and serves as a fulcrum for the scapula. Without the clavicle, contraction of muscles that cross the glenohumeral joint (e.g., the pectoralis major) would pull the proximal humerus to the chest instead of lifting the arm.

The **clavicle** is S-shaped when viewed from above. The flat acromial end is covered by the deltoid origin anteriorly and the trapezius insertion posteriorly. The round sternal end gives rise to the origin of the pectoralis major anteriorly and the sternocleidomastoid posteriorly.

The **scapula** is a flat, triangular bone located on the posterior aspect of the chest. It has three bony processes: the coracoid process; the spine; and the continuation of the spine, the acromion. It has two articulations: the acromioclavicular joint and the glenohumeral joint. The scapula is buried in muscles. The costal, or anterior, surface is covered by the subscapularis muscle. The posterior surface is covered by the supra- and infraspinatus muscles. The spine is the origin of the posterior deltoid and the insertion of the trapezius. The short head of the biceps, the coracobrachialis, and the pectoralis minor originate from the coracoid process and insert on it. The trapezius and levator scapulae elevate the scapula. The serratus anterior moves the scapula anteriorly, holding it against the chest wall. Paralysis of the serratus anterior results in "winging" of the scapula.

The **acromioclavicular joint** is a diarthrodial plane joint. Its articular surfaces are covered by fibrocartilage and separated by a meniscus. The joint is stabilized by weak acromioclavicular ligaments, the deltoid and trapezius muscles, and the coracoclavicular ligaments (i.e., the trapezoid and conoid ligaments). Disruption of the acromioclavicular capsule increases joint translation in the anteroposterior plane; the coracoclavicular ligaments are more efficient in resisting superior displacement. The range of motion through the acromioclavicular joint is 20 degrees, with most of it occurring in the initial 30 degrees of shoulder abduction.

The **sternoclavicular joint** is a diarthrodial saddle joint. Its surfaces are covered with fibrocartilage, and the joint is completely divided by an articular disc. This disc attaches to the articular border of the clavicle, first rib, and joint capsule. The sternoclavicular joint is strengthened by anterior and posterior sternoclavicular ligaments, the interclavicular ligament running between the clavicles behind the sternum, and by the costoclavicular ligament running between the first rib and the clavicle. The clavicle abducts or elevates about 40 degrees through the sternoclavicular joint. This motion occurs throughout shoulder abduction up to 90 degrees. The medial physis of the clavicle fuses around the age of 25 years; therefore, epiphyseal separations rather than

85

true sternoclavicular dislocations occur in patients below 25 years of age. This is important, because physeal injuries will remodel and joint dislocations will not.

Behind the sternoclavicular joint are the major blood vessels, the trachea, and the esophagus. The brachial plexus and subclavian artery continue laterally, posterior to the clavicle, passing over the first rib, and anterior to the scapula just distal to the coracoid. The costoclavicular space may be decreased by a fracture of the first rib or medial portion of the clavicle, resulting in acute neurovascular injury or late compression. The axillary nerve passes below the neck of the glenoid and is frequently injured in shoulder dislocations. The suprascapular nerve passes through the scapular notch medial to the base of the coracoid under the transverse scapular ligament. It continues distally through a fibroosseous tunnel (spinoglenoid notch) formed by the scapular spine and the spinoglenoid ligament to end in the infraspinatus muscle.

FRACTURES OF THE CLAVICLE

Classification

Clavicular fractures are classified according to location as distal-, middle-, and proximal-third fractures. The mechanism of injury is either a direct blow or an axial load resulting from a fall or blow on the lateral aspect of the shoulder.

Distal-third fractures are further classified into three types (Fig. 8-1). Type I fractures are the most common and occur between intact coracoclavicular and acromioclavicular ligaments. The ligaments hold the fragments in alignment. Type II fractures are characterized by disruption of the coracoclavicular ligaments. The weight of the arm pulls the distal fragment inferiorly, and the trapezius and sternocleidomastoid pull the proximal fragment superiorly. Type III fractures are intraarticular, usually undisplaced, and frequently become symptomatic years later as posttraumatic arthritis.

Middle-third fractures are the most common type of clavicular fracture. The proximal fragment is displaced superiorly by muscle pull; the distal fragment is displaced inferiorly by the weight of the arm.

Fractures of the proximal third of the clavicle, excluding injuries of the sternoclavicular joint, are uncommon and frequently pathologic.

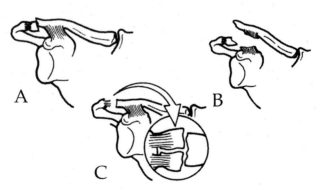

FIG. 8-1   The three types of distal clavicular fracture: (*A*) type I, (*B*) type II, and (*C*) type III.

Diagnosis and Initial Management

History and Physical Examination

The clavicle is subcutaneous; therefore swelling and deformity are obvious, and tenderness on palpation reveals the site of the injury.

Radiographic Examination

Radiographic confirmation and evaluation of fractures of the clavicle are done with anteroposterior and 45-degree cephalic tilt views with the patient upright. Radiographs of proximal-third fractures may occasionally have to be augmented with computed tomography (CT). In fractures of the distal third of the clavicle anteroposterior, radiographs of both acromioclavicular joints with the use of 5- to 10-lb weights are obtained to determine the presence of ligamentous disruption.

Initial Management

Initial management consists of a sling.

Associated Injuries

Associated injuries to the chest, brachial plexus, and major vessels are ruled out by history and physical examination. Visceral injury is associated with high-energy trauma, an open fracture, and fracture of the first rib or scapula. Scapulothoracic dissociation is a devastating injury associated with clavicular fracture or dislocation. The diagnosis is confirmed by lateral displacement of the scapula, with an associated injury of the clavicle, acromioclavicular joint, or sternoclavicular joint. There is frequently an associated injury of the brachial plexus or axillary artery. Complete brachial plexus injury is an indication for primary above-elbow amputation. Axillary artery disruption can be managed by prompt vascular surgical repair.

Ipsilateral fracture of the clavicle (or acromioclavicular separation) associated with an extraarticular fracture of the glenoid neck results in a "floating shoulder" (Fig. 8-2).

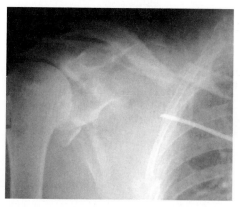

FIG. 8-2   Floating shoulder. (*Courtesy of Dr. Enes Kanlic.*)

Definitive Management

Open reduction and internal fixation of **fractures of the distal third of the clavicle** is indicated if there is superior displacement of the proximal fragment due to disruption of the coracoclavicular ligaments or there is intraarticular displacement. Type I and undisplaced type III distal clavicular fractures are managed symptomatically with a sling. The figure-of-eight splint has no value for fractures of the distal third. Type II distal clavicular fractures and the rare displaced type III fractures are managed with open reduction and internal fixation. The distal clavicle is exposed through an incision over its anterior subcutaneous border. The fracture is stabilized with a T (or one-third tubular) plate. Type II fractures of the distal third of the clavicle treated nonoperatively are associated with a high rate of symptomatic nonunion (Fig. 8-3A and B).

Fractures of the middle and proximal third of the clavicle are treated with manipulative reduction and immobilization with a figure-of-eight splint that holds the shoulders dorsally. The splint is applied and tightened with the shoulders retracted. It will stretch and loosen; therefore it must be tightened every morning for the first few days. A sling supports the arm the first week. After 4 or 5 weeks, fracture healing has usually progressed to the point where immobilization is no longer required.

Indications for primary open reduction of middle- and proximal-third clavicular fractures include the threat of skin penetration by fracture fragments, initial fracture shortening of 2 cm or more, irreducible displacement (e.g., buttonholing of the proximal fragment), neurovascular compromise, open fractures, and frequently fractures associated with other injuries of the shoulder girdle (e.g., displaced extraarticular fractures of the glenoid neck and scapulothoracic dissociation). Exposure of the clavicle is through an incision along

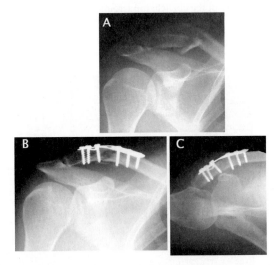

FIG. 8-3   Type II fracture of the distal clavicle treated by open reduction and internal fixation.

the superior surface of the clavicle. A 3.5-mm limited-contact dynamic compression plate with a minimum of six holes is contoured and placed on the flat superior surface of the clavicle. Autogenous cancellous grafting is required with extensive comminution, devitalized bone fragments, or loss of continuity. Postoperatively, the arm is supported in a sling until callus formation becomes evident at about 4 weeks.

Complications

Complications consist of nonunion, malunion, and neurovascular compromise.

Nonunion of fractures of the middle third of the clavicle occurs more frequently following high-energy injuries. Atrophic nonunions are radiographically obvious. Tomography or fluoroscopic examination may be required to demonstrate the more common hypertrophic nonunion. Management of symptomatic nonunions includes open reduction, internal fixation, and bone grafting (Fig. 8-4).

Malunion of middle-third clavicular fractures is frequent and usually a cosmetic problem associated with shortening of the shoulder girdle and inferior displacement of the shoulder. Shoulder pain and weakness are frequently associated. Symptomatic shortening or angulation resulting in tenting of the skin is managed with osteotomy, with internal fixation to restore clavicular length and bone grafting.

Neurovascular complications result from displacement of the fracture fragments at the time of injury, from associated injuries (e.g., first rib fracture), and from late sequelae associated with hypertrophic callus or shortening of the clavicle. Dysesthesias on the ulnar side of the hand and forearm as well as weakness and pain in the involved shoulder brought on by prolonged activity suggest a thoracic outlet syndrome and must be differentiated from symptoms associated with a hypertrophic nonunion. Provocative testing, angiography, electromyography, and CT are useful in determining the presence of neurovascular compromise. Corrective osteotomy to restore clavicular length and resect hypertrophic callus may be required.

Subclavian vein obstruction between the clavicle and first rib is characterized by prominence of the veins in the ipsilateral upper extremity.

FRACTURES OF THE SCAPULA

Fractures of the scapula are rare and often associated with other severe injuries. As a result, nearly 50% of injuries are overlooked initially. The most common associated injury is fracture of the ipsilateral ribs, with hemopneumothorax occurring in approximately one-third of high-energy injuries.

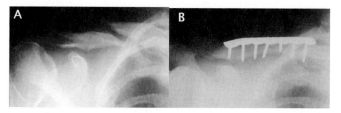

FIG. 8-4   Nonunion of the clavicle.

Classification

The most important factor in classifying a scapular fracture is whether it was caused by high-energy (e.g., an automobile accident) or low-energy (e.g., avulsion of a muscle insertion) trauma. Comminution and displacement, the "burst fracture," indicate high-energy trauma. Scapular fractures are further classified according to the location: fractures of the body and spine, the glenoid neck (extraarticular), the acromion, the coracoid process, and the glenoid (intraarticular). Intraarticular fractures of the glenoid are subdivided into undisplaced and displaced fractures. Displaced fractures are simple (i.e., part of the glenoid is intact) or complex (i.e., the entire articular surface of the glenoid is fractured) (Fig. 8-5).

Diagnosis and Initial Management

History and Physical Examination

Pain is localized in the shoulder and back. The arm is adducted and protected against motion. Ecchymosis and swelling are minimal due to the location of the scapula beneath layers of muscle. Loss of active abduction and forward elevation of the arm, known as **pseudoparalysis of the rotator cuff**, is often associated with scapular fracture and is the result of intramuscular hemorrhage and pain.

Radiographic Examination

Radiographic evaluation of the scapula includes true anteroposterior and lateral views of the scapula and an axillary view. The anteroposterior view of the scapula will show fractures of the glenoid and glenoid neck. Lateral scapular views show fractures of the scapular body and acromion. The axillary view will show fractures of the coracoid and glenoid. Magnetic resonance imaging (MRI), CT, and anteroposterior and lateral chest radiographs provide additional information.

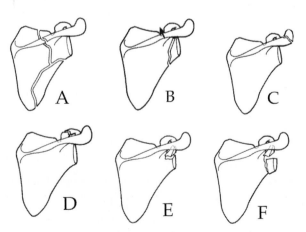

FIG. 8-5 The six types of scapular fractures: (*A*) fracture of the body, (*B*) extraarticular fracture of the neck of the glenoid, (*C*) fracture of the acromion, (*D*) fracture of the coracoid, (*E*) simple fracture of the glenoid, and (*F*) complex fracture of the glenoid.

Initial Management

The initial management consists of a sling.

Associated Injuries

The most important factor in the initial management of scapular fractures is their frequent association with life-threatening visceral injuries. The most common associated visceral injuries include hemopneumothorax, pulmonary or cardiac contusion, aortic tear, brachial plexus injury, axillary artery injury, and closed head injury. The most common associated osseous injuries are fractures of the ribs and clavicle. Fracture of the first rib is frequently associated with injury of the brachial plexus and subclavian vessels.

Definitive Management

Management of **fractures of the body and spine** is usually nonoperative. The muscles surrounding the scapula prevent further displacement. A sling and ice are used for the first few days to control pain. As the pain subsides, pendulum exercises in the sling are initiated. Healing is rapid; usually, active motion can be initiated after 4 weeks. Burst fractures with proximal displacement of the lateral margin of the body may impinge on the glenohumeral joint capsule. When this occurs, the fracture is reduced and stabilized or the offending bony spike is osteotomized.

Extraarticular fractures of the glenoid neck are the second most common type of scapular fracture and occur when the humeral head is driven into the glenoid fossa. A CT scan may be necessary to confirm that the fracture does not involve the joint. Reduction is not attempted. The arm is supported in a sling, and management is as described for fracture of the body and spine. The prognosis is good for near full return of function.

Fractures through the neck of the glenoid with an associated clavicular fracture (floating shoulder) are unstable because of loss of the suspensory function of the clavicle. The weight of the arm pulls the glenoid fragment distally, resulting in deformity and ultimate loss of function. Open reduction and internal fixation of the fractured clavicle has been recommended but is controversial. Open reduction and internal fixation of the glenoid neck fracture through a posterior approach, as described by Brodsky et al. (1987), with the patient in the lateral decubitus position, may also be required (Fig. 8-6). Postoperative radiographs of such a patient are shown in Fig. 8-2.

The **acromion** is fractured by a direct blow from the superior aspect or by superior displacement of the humeral head. Stress fracture results from superior migration of the humeral head due to a long-standing rotator cuff tear. A stress fracture, therefore, may be an indication for MRI with intraarticular contrast to evaluate the rotator cuff. Depression of the acromion is associated with traction injury of the brachial plexus. Care should be taken not to mistake a bipartite acromion (os acromiale) for a fracture.

Minimally displaced fractures of the acromion are treated conservatively. These are followed closely for the first 3 weeks because they may displace. Significant displacement impairs glenohumeral motion because of impingement on the rotator cuff. Displaced fractures are managed with open reduction and internal fixation with a screw or tension-band wire.

Isolated **fracture of the coracoid process** results from a direct blow, avulsion by muscle pull, or stress (i.e., "trap shooter's shoulder"). Fractures occur through the base or the tip. When minimally displaced, they heal uneventfully.

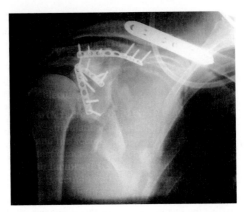

FIG. 8-6   Postoperative radiograph of the patient shown in Fig. 8-2. (*Courtesy of Dr. Enes Kanlic.*)

Displaced coracoid fractures occur in combination with an acromioclavicular dislocation. The coracoid is avulsed from the scapula by the coracoclavicular ligaments. Management is open reduction and fixation of the coracoid with a single screw and temporary transarticular fixation of the acromioclavicular dislocation. Displacement of the coracoid can cause compression of the suprascapular nerve and paralysis of the external rotators of the shoulder (i.e., the supraspinatus and infraspinatus). When this occurs, open reduction and fixation of the coracoid and decompression of the nerve are indicated.

The management of **intraarticular fractures of the glenoid** is based on the amount of displacement, the type of fracture, and the presence of glenohumeral instability.

Undisplaced fractures are managed with a sling and immobilization as described for fractures of the body of the scapula. Displaced simple fractures (3 mm or more) are managed with open reduction and internal fixation. The degree of congruity of the articular surface is determined by anteroposterior, glenoid tangential, and axillary radiographs and CT. Instability of the glenohumeral articulation is expected when the fragment is displaced 1 cm and when the fragment comprises one-fourth of the articular surface. Frequently, subluxation will be evident on the initial radiographs. An anterior approach through the deltopectoral interval is used to expose fractures of the anterior glenoid rim only. Transverse, vertical, and minimally comminuted fractures where reduction and fixation can be obtained should be approached posteriorly, as described by Brodsky et al. (1987) and Kavanagh et al. (1993). Posterior exposure is accomplished with the patient prone or in the lateral decubitus position. Through a vertical incision, the posterior deltoid is mobilized either by abducting the arm or by a limited release from the scapular spine, and the interval between the infraspinatus and teres minor is developed to expose the fracture and posterior capsule. The axillary nerve and posterior circumflex humeral vessels are identified and protected, as is the suprascapular nerve. Additional exposure may be obtained with a vertical incision through the tendinous portion of the infraspinatus muscle. Large fragments are reduced and stabilized with screws or plates. Kirschner wires and cerclage wires may break or migrate and are not used. In severely comminuted fractures, the fragments are excised and replaced with an iliac crest bone graft contoured to the shape of the osseous defect and fixed to the glenoid with screws. Alternatively, if the fracture involves the anterior rim, the coracoid process is osteotomized and transferred to the defect.

Complex fractures of the glenoid pose special problems. The surgeon must decide whether an extensive surgical procedure will result in a reduced stable glenoid; if not, closed management is indicated. These fractures can be difficult to manage surgically because the necessary exposure is extensive. Postoperative management depends on the stability of fixation and the surgical approach. Ideally, early passive motion becomes possible.

Closed management consists of an initial period of immobilization followed by early range of motion to mold the articular fragments into as normal a position as possible. The optimal position and type of immobilization are determined by comparing anteroposterior and axillary radiographs of the glenohumeral joint with the arm at the side and in various positions of elevation and rotation. Immobilization may be in the form of a sling and swathe, traction, or an airplane splint. At 3 to 4 weeks, healing has progressed to the point that immobilization can be discontinued. Range of motion is continued in a sling for an additional 3 to 6 weeks. Between 6 and 9 weeks, the sling is discontinued and active range of motion is initiated.

Complications

Complications of scapular fractures include chronic glenohumeral instability, posttraumatic glenohumeral arthrosis, rotator cuff injury, and impingement. When these complications occur, conservative management with nonsteroidal anti-inflammatory drugs, physical therapy, intraarticular steroid injection, or a surgical procedure to address the most important pathology can be considered.

MRI with intraarticular contrast and CT can be used to substantiate a clinical diagnosis of rotator cuff tear, impingement syndrome, or glenohumeral arthrosis. Rotator cuff repair, decompression of impingement on the rotator cuff, and replacement arthroplasty would be the major surgical options for usual complications. Arthrodesis would be indicated rarely in those instances when posttraumatic glenohumeral arthrosis is associated with neurologic deficit from axillary nerve or brachial plexus injury.

STERNOCLAVICULAR JOINT INJURIES

Classification

Injuries of the sternoclavicular joint are classified as sprains or dislocations. Sprains are undisplaced. Dislocations are anterior or retrosternal.

Diagnosis and Initial Management

History and Physical Examination

A history of injury, pain, and asymmetry of the sternoclavicular joints are the cardinal signs of this injury. The patient supports the injured extremity and tilts his or her head toward the affected side. Pain and swelling without injury may be signs of osteoarthritis or septic arthritis of the proximal end of the clavicle. Spontaneous atraumatic anterior subluxation occurs in young patients with ligamentous laxity and is managed conservatively. In patients below 25 years of age, epiphyseal separation must be differentiated from dislocation.

Radiographic Examination

Routine anteroposterior radiographs of the sternoclavicular joint are not diagnostic. Two projections designed to show sternoclavicular joint dislocation are the Hobbs view and the Rockwood view. In the Hobbs view, the seated patient leans forward over a cassette so that the back of the neck is parallel to the table. The beam is directed through the neck onto the cassette. In the Rockwood view, the patient is supine. The beam is tilted 40 degrees cephalad and aimed at the sternum. A cassette is placed on the table so that the beam will project both clavicles onto the plate. In an anterior sternoclavicular dislocation, the clavicle appears to be anterior and riding higher than that on the uninjured side (Fig. 8-7). In a retrosternal dislocation, the clavicle appears to be posterior and is lower than that on the uninjured side. CT scans provide a more accurate assessment of the injury (differentiating sternoclavicular dislocation from fracture of the medial end of the clavicle) and the adequacy of reduction (Fig. 8-8).

Initial Management

Initial management consists of a sling. The patient is observed for respiratory and circulatory problems.

Associated Injuries

Compression of the structures of the superior mediastinium may occur with posterior dislocation and should be specifically ruled out. Acutely, this may become life-threatening; subacutely, it is an indication for surgery. Symptoms of compression of these structures include shortness of breath and hoarseness, dysphagia, paresthesia, or weakness of the upper extremity. Chronic thoracic outlet syndrome with symptoms of dysesthesias and ischemia is associated with pallor and venous prominence of the involved extremity when placed in a position of 90 degrees of abduction and external rotation.

Definitive Management

Sprains of the sternoclavicular joint are treated symptomatically. Anterior dislocations become asymptomatic, and reduction (which is usually unstable) is rarely indicated. When reduction is attempted, it is performed in the fol-

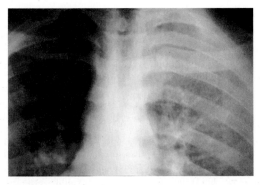

FIG. 8-7   Rockwood view of a right anterior sternoclavicular dislocation.

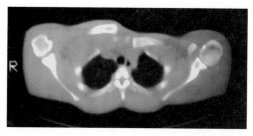

FIG. 8-8   CT scan showing anterior displacement of the right clavicle in relationship to the sternum and the left sternoclavicular joint.

lowing fashion. The patient is supine with a bolster between the shoulder blades. A posteriorly directed force is placed on the anterior aspect of both shoulders, and the medial end of the clavicle is pressed inferiorly and posteriorly. The shoulders are then held retracted with a figure-of-eight clavicular strap.

Treatment of a retrosternal dislocation of the clavicle is more important. A thoracic surgeon is consulted if the patient has compression of the structures of the superior mediastinum. The technique of manipulative reduction has been described by Buckerfield and Castle (1984). A bolster is placed between the shoulders. The bolster should be thick enough to elevate both shoulders from the table. With the arm adducted to the trunk, caudal traction is applied to the arm while both shoulders are forced posteriorly by direct pressure. Percutaneous manipulation with a towel clip may be required. Reduction is confirmed by lordotic radiographs and CT imaging. Once reduced, the retrosternal dislocation is usually stable. A figure-of-eight clavicular strap is used to hold the shoulders retracted for 4 to 6 weeks.

If closed reduction fails, open reduction is indicated when there are symptoms of mediastinal compression or to prevent subsequent damage to retrosternal structures on the medial end of the clavicle. Metallic internal fixation is dangerous and should not be used.

Complications

The incidence of complications from retrosternal dislocation of the clavicle is 25%. The symptoms associated with these complications are usually corrected with reduction; however, pneumothorax, laceration of the great vessels, and rupture of the trachea and esophagus require emergency intervention. The most serious long-term complications are the result of migration of metallic fixation devices.

Most patients with persistent traumatic anterior displacement of the medial end of the clavicle do not require operative treatment. Resection arthroplasty of the sternoclavicular joint with reconstruction using the subclavius tendon or the intraarticular sternoclavicular ligament and repair of the costoclavicular ligament to stabilize the medial portion of the clavicle to the first rib may be indicated for severe pain in chronic traumatic anterior dislocations and to treat thoracic outlet syndrome or to prevent damage to retrosternal structures with chronic unreduced posterior dislocation. Transaxial resection of the first rib might also be considered.

ACROMIOCLAVICULAR JOINT INJURIES

Classification

Acromioclavicular joint injuries are classified according to the amount and direction of displacement into seven groups (Fig. 8-9). In type I injuries, the acromioclavicular capsule is stretched, but the coracoclavicular ligaments remain intact. The clavicle is undisplaced. In type II injuries, the acromioclavicular capsule is torn and the coracoclavicular ligaments are stretched or partly torn. The clavicle is displaced less than one-half of its width. In type III injuries, both the acromioclavicular capsule and coracoclavicular ligaments are torn, the coracoclavicular distance is increased, and the clavicle is completely dislocated from the acromioclavicular joint. The deltoid and trapezius muscles are intact and remain attached to the clavicle. In type IV injuries, the clavicle is displaced posteriorly and is buttonholed through the trapezius, blocking closed reduction. In type V injuries, the trapezius and deltoid are torn, and the distal clavicle is displaced superiorly and is covered only by skin and subcutaneous tissue. In type VI injuries, the distal clavicle is dislocated inferiorly and locked below the coracoid and conjoined tendon. Type VII injuries are panclavicular dislocations.

Diagnosis and Initial Management

History and Physical Examination

There is a history of an axial-loading injury to the lateral aspect of the shoulder, with pain, swelling, and tenderness increasing around the acromioclavicular

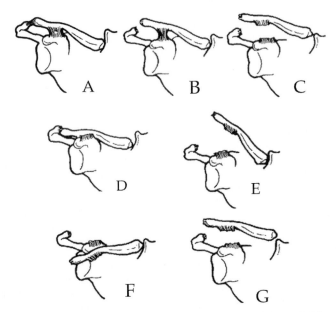

FIG. 8-9   The seven types of acromioclavicular injuries: (*A*) type I, (*B*) type II, (*C*) type III, (*D*) type IV, (*E*) type V, (*F*) type VI, and (*G*) type VII.

joint. Prominence of the distal end of the clavicle is present on inspection (especially when observed from behind), with the patient sitting and the weight of the arm unsupported, in type III injuries. When the amount of displacement is in question, the integrity of the coracoclavicular ligaments is determined by having the patient flex the elbow against resistance, with the arm at the side. When the coracoclavicular ligaments are disrupted, the distal end of the clavicle will seem to rise superiorly as the acromion is pulled distally.

Radiographic Examination

Radiographic confirmation of the acromioclavicular injury and the degree of displacement is obtained with the patient upright and the weight of the arm unsupported. Radiographs taken with the patient supine or with techniques that overpenetrate the acromioclavicular joint obscure displacement. Stress films with the patient holding 5 to 10 lb and comparison films with the opposite side are helpful. An axillary view of the shoulder is obtained to assess displacement in the anteroposterior plane. In type I injuries, there is no displacement of the distal end of the clavicle. In type II injuries, the distal end of the clavicle is slightly elevated but not completely displaced from its articulation with the acromion. In type III injuries, the distal end of the clavicle is displaced superiorly and the coracoclavicular distance is increased. The distance between the coracoid process and the clavicle differs; therefore it is important to obtain comparison views of the other shoulder. In type IV injuries, the distal end of the clavicle is displaced posteriorly. Displacement is best visualized on the axillary view. In type V, VI, and VII injuries, the amount and direction of displacement are indicated by the type of injury.

Initial Management

Initial management is a sling.

Definitive Management

Type I and II injuries are treated symptomatically with a sling and ice. The sling is removed daily for range-of-motion exercises of the shoulder and elbow.

The treatment of type III injuries is controversial. The natural history of unreduced type III dislocations is that the pain diminishes and disappears and the deformity persists but improves. Nonoperative management is recommended. This consists of the use of a sling and early range-of-motion exercises. The use of a shoulder harness to maintain reduction of the acromioclavicular joint is not recommended because it is poorly tolerated and has no effect on ultimate displacement.

If open reduction and internal fixation is attempted, the distal clavicle, acromion, and coracoid are exposed. The joint is debrided, reduced, and stabilized with a large smooth Steinmann pin. The pin is left protruding through the skin laterally and bent to prevent migration. The capsule of acromioclavicular joint is repaired with the coracoclavicular ligaments. Postoperatively, the arm is maintained in a sling. The pins are removed at 6 weeks. Physical therapy is not started until the pins have been removed, so as to prevent breakage. Another surgical option in the acute dislocation is resection of the distal 2 cm of the clavicle and transfer of the coracoacromial ligament along with a piece of bone from its acromial attachment into the distal end of the clavicle, modified from a description by Weaver and Dunn (1972). Procedures that use a Bosworth screw passed through the clavicle into the coracoid and heavy

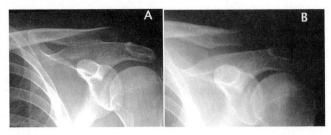

FIG. 8-10   Grade III acromioclavicular separation treated by a modified Weaver-Dunn procedure.

nonabsorbable suture looped under the coracoid process and around the clavicle to tether the clavicle to the coracoid are associated with frequent material complications.

Type IV, V, and VI injuries are treated with open reduction and internal fixation of the acromioclavicular joint. Type VII injuries are managed with open reduction and stabilization of the acromioclavicular joint and closed reduction of the sternoclavicular joint. Reduction of the sternoclavicular joint is maintained with a figure-of-eight splint.

Complications

Complications include shoulder stiffness, deformity, chronic dislocation, and posttraumatic arthritis. Shoulder stiffness is prevented with early range-of-motion exercises. The deformity diminishes but does not disappear. Symptomatic chronic dislocation and posttraumatic arthritis are managed with resection of the distal 2 cm of the clavicle and transfer of the coracoclavicular ligament with a fragment of bone from its acromial attachment to the distal end of the clavicle (Fig. 8-10).

Complications following open management are more significant. The most frequent is loss of reduction. The most significant is breakage and migration of a pin, which is potentially fatal if the pin migrates into the thoracic cavity.

SELECTED READINGS

Fractures of the Clavicle

Hill JM, McGuire MH, Crosby LA. Closed treatment of displaced middle third fractures of the clavicle gives poor results. *J Bone Joint Surg* 79B:537–539, 1997.

Kona J, Bosse MJ, Staeheli JW, Rosseau RL. Type II distal clavicle fractures: a retrospective review of surgical treatment. *J Orthop Trauma* 4:115–120, 1990.

McKee MD, Wild LM, Schemitsch EH. Midshaft malunions of the clavicle. *J Bone Joint Surg* 85A:790–797, 2003.

Robinson CM, Cairns DA. Primary nonoperative treatment of displaced lateral fractures of the clavicle. *J Bone Joint Surg* 86A:778–782, 2004.

Fractures of the Scapula

Brodsky JW, Tullos HS, Gartsman GM. Simplified posterior approach to the shoulder joint. *J Bone Joint Surg* 69A:773–774, 1987.

Egol KA, Connor PM, Karunakar MA. The floating shoulder: clinical and functional results. *J Bone Joint Surg* 83A:1188–1194, 2001.

Goss TP. Fractures of the glenoid cavity. Current concepts review. *J Bone Joint Surg* 74A:299–305, 1992.

Hardegger FA, Simpson LA, Weber BG. The operative treatment of scapular fractures. *J Bone Joint Surg* 66B:725–731, 1984.

Harris RD, Harris JH Jr. The prevalence and significance of missed scapular fractures in blunt chest trauma. *Am J Rheum* 151:747–750, 1988.

Herscovici D Jr, Fiennes AG, Allgower M, Ruedi TP. The floating shoulder: ipsilateral, clavicle and scapular neck fractures. *J Bone Joint Surg* 74B:362–364, 1992.

Kavanagh BR, Bradway JK, Cofield RH. Open reduction and internal fixation of displaced intra-articular fractures of the glenoid fossa. *J Bone Joint Surg* 75A:479–484, 1993.

Leung KS, Lam TP. Open reduction and internal fixation of ipsilateral fractures of the scapular neck and clavicle. *J Bone Joint Surg* 75A:1015–1018, 1993.

Zelle BA, Pape HC, Gerich TG, Garapati R. Functional outcome following scapulothoracic dissociation. *J Bone Joint Surg* 86A:2–8, 2004.

Sternoclavicular Joint Injuries

Buckerfield CT, Castle ME. Acute traumatic retrosternal dislocation of the clavicle. *J Bone Joint Surg* 66A:379–385, 1984.

Eskola A. Sternoclavicular dislocation: a plea for open treatment. *Acta Orthop Scand* 57:227–228, 1986.

Rockwood CA, Groh GI, Wirth MA, Grassi FA. Resection arthroplasty of the sternoclavicular joint. *J Bone Joint Surg* 79A:387–393, 1997.

Spencer EE Jr, Kuhn JE. Biomechanical analysis of reconstructions for sternoclavicular joint instability. *J Bone Joint Surg* 86A:98–105, 2004.

Acromioclavicular Joint Injuries

Bannister GC, Wallace WA, Stableforth PG, Hutson MA. The management of acute acromioclavicular dislocation. A randomised prospective controlled trial. *J Bone Joint Surg* 71B:848–850, 1989.

Tibone J, Sellers R, Tonino P. Strength testing after third degree acromioclavicular dislocations. *Am J Sports Med* 20:328–331, 1992.

Weaver JK, Dunn HK. Treatment of acromioclavicular injuries, especially complete acromioclavicular separation. *J Bone Joint Surg* 54A:1187–1194, 1972.

9 | Fractures of the Humeral Shaft

Prahlad S. Pyati

Fractures of the shaft of the humerus account for 2 to 3% of all fractures treated by orthopedic surgeons. They occur in all age groups and with differing etiology. Most of these fractures heal uneventfully; complications are typically associated with injury to the important neurovascular structures adjacent to the bone.

ANATOMY

Knowledge of the relevant anatomy is essential in the management of humeral fractures. The shaft of the humerus extends from the upper border of the insertion of the pectoralis major tendon proximally to the supracondylar ridge distally. For the most part, the shaft is almost cylindrical; distally, however, it flattens in anteroposterior diameter into a prism shape. The arm is divided into anterior and posterior compartments by the medial and the lateral intermuscular septa, but these compartments are not rigid and compartment syndromes are rare. Several large muscles insert on or originate from the humerus at various levels, and contractions of these muscles exerts predictable deforming forces at different fracture sites. The proximal fragment of the humerus is abducted and externally rotated by the rotator cuff muscles when the fracture occurs above the level of the pectoralis insertion. When the fracture occurs between the deltoid and pectoralis major, the proximal fragment is adducted and the deltoid displaces the distal fragment proximally and laterally. Fractures distal to the deltoid muscle insertion are associated with abduction of the proximal humerus.

Important neurovascular structures surround the entire length of the bone. The nutrient artery to the humeral shaft arises from branches of the brachial artery and enters the shaft near the middle of the medial border. The radial nerve lies in close proximity to the posterior middle third of the humerus and is the most frequently injured structure. The radial nerve courses through the spiral groove, along with the profunda brachii artery in the posterior compartment, and pierces the lateral intermuscular septum approximately 14 cm proximal to the lateral epicondyle, or at the junction of the middle and distal thirds of the humerus, to enter the anterior compartment.

CLASSIFICATION

There is no universally accepted system of classification. However, fractures of the humeral shaft can be classified according to etiology, location, pattern, type, and the AO system.

Etiology

Most fractures are due to low-energy trauma such as falls, minor motor vehicle accidents, gunshot wounds, or birth trauma. More complex fractures usually

100

result from severe vehicular crashes or penetrating injuries. Pathologic fractures are often due to metastatic lesions.

Location

Fractures of the humerus can occur in the proximal, middle, or distal thirds of the shaft (Fig. 9-1). In the proximal half of the humerus, fractures can be above the insertion of the pectoralis major, between the pectoralis major and deltoid insertions, or below the deltoid insertion. The location of the fracture determines the type, extent of angulation, and displacement. Segmental fractures are not uncommon.

Pattern

Most fractures are simple, transverse, oblique, spiral, or comminuted (Fig. 9-1). The Holstein-Lewis fracture is a well-recognized pattern that occurs in the distal portion of the bone (Fig. 9-2).

Type

Most fractures by far are closed. Open fractures are seen occasionally, and these are classified according to the established Gustillo-Anderson system. Complicated fractures are known to be associated with neurovascular injuries, especially injuries involving the radial nerve. The Holstein-Lewis distal-third spiral type of fracture is often associated with radial nerve entrapment.

AO Classification

This classification system, from the Association for the Study of Internal Fixation (AO-ASIF), follows standard ABC groups and represents a spectrum of increasing fracture severity. For humeral diaphyseal fractures, this system is based on the amount of comminution, with type A fractures having no comminution, type B fractures having a butterfly fragment, and type C fractures having comminution.

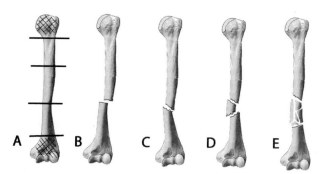

FIG. 9-1   The shaft of the humerus extends from the lesser tuberosity to the supracondylar ridge (*unshaded area*). Fractures may be classified as occurring in the proximal, middle, or distal third (*A*). Types of fractures are described as transverse (*B*), oblique/spiral (*C*), segmental (*D*), or comminuted (*E*).

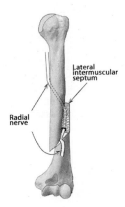

FIG. 9-2   Holstein-Lewis fracture, typically located in the distal third of the humerus. The radial nerve is frequently trapped between the fragments.

DIAGNOSIS

Clinical Features

Fractures of the humeral shaft are fairly easy to diagnose clinically. A history of trauma is followed by severe pain, deformity, and loss of function. Swelling and ecchymosis soon follow. Gradual migration of subcutaneous ecchymosis distally may alarm the patient, who should be reassured.

Physical examination should include an evaluation of the skin to distinguish between closed and open fractures. Neurovascular integrity must be carefully tested and well documented. This should include both motor and sensory examination. Although the most common nerve involved is the radial nerve, injuries to median and ulnar nerves are known to occur. Vascular injuries are well known in fractures secondary to penetrating trauma.

Imaging Studies

Most fractures are diagnosed with routine radiographs to include two orthogonal views. **Care must be taken not to rotate the extremity but to rotate the patient** while obtaining the films. One must insist on visualizing adjacent joints so as not to miss associated injuries to the shoulder and elbow joints. Depending on the clinical evaluation, radiographs of the forearm may be required to exclude floating elbow injuries. Additional studies, such as a computed tomography (CT) and magnetic resonance imaging (MRI) are not necessary unless a pathologic fracture is suspected. If necessary, electrodiagnostic studies for nerve injuries should be performed 3 to 4 weeks after the injury.

Associated Injuries

Radial nerve injury may occur in up to 18% of closed humeral shaft fractures; it is usually of the neuropraxia type owing to fracture displacement at the time of injury. Spontaneous recovery occurs within 4 to 6 months after injury in 90 to 100% of patients. When there is no evidence of spontaneous recovery within 6 to 8 weeks, electromyography should be performed to determine whether exploration is indicated. The Holstein-Lewis fracture is well known to be associated with radial nerve palsy. Radial nerve injuries associated with open fractures and penetrating injuries may involve a laceration of the nerve and are less likely to recover spontaneously; such patients may need surgical exploration. Median and ulnar nerve injuries are rare in closed fractures.

Vascular injuries are less likely to occur in closed fractures. However, they should be suspected in severe open fractures, crush injuries, and penetrating injuries. If such an injury is suspected, angiography may be indicated and an emergency consultation with the vascular service must be obtained.

MANAGEMENT

Initial Management

The goal of initial management is reduction and immobilization of the fracture until plans for definitive treatment are established. In most patients, a simple coaptation splint (Fig. 9-3) or shoulder immobilizer is adequate. However, open fractures need urgent care, as determined by their severity. Patients with fractures associated with simple gunshot wounds, type I open fractures, should receive local wound care and intravenous antibiotics. It is not always necessary to perform extensive debridement unless the soft tissue injury requires it. Vascular injuries demand immediate attention. Nerve injuries do not require special care initially, but one must be mindful of them while manipulating the fracture. Wrist- and finger-drop deformities must be splinted to prevent contracture.

External fixation is often used in the initial care of open fractures with extensive soft tissue injury, severe comminuted fractures, and fractures with vascular injuries (Fig. 9-4A). Most standard external fixation systems can be adapted to the humerus. External fixation is usually applied on the lateral surface of the humerus. In managing fractures in the distal half of the humerus, it is advisable to expose the lateral surface of the bone and insert the pins under direct vision to protect the radial nerve. External fixation systems are often replaced by more definitive methods (Fig. 9-4B) or continued until the fracture is united. Standard protocols for pin-site management must be followed. Complications include loosening of the pins, loss of correction, and pin-tract infection.

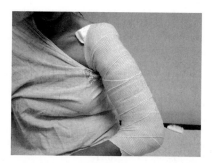

FIG. 9-3   The coaptation splint is a U-shaped, padded plaster splint placed around the medial and lateral aspects of the arm and over the acromion. It works on the principle of soft tissue compression.

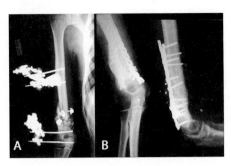

FIG. 9-4   Comminuted fracture of distal shaft of the humerus due to gunshot wound with vascular injury. Initial application of external fixator (*A*). Plate fixation with bone grafting, using a posterior approach, was done after the external fixator was removed (*B*).

Definitive Management

There are two modalities of definitive management of humeral shaft fractures: nonoperative and operative. The goals of treatment are to accomplish solid fracture healing and achieve full functional recovery so that the patient can return to his or her prefracture occupation with the fewest complications.

The key to successful management of a humeral fracture lies in determining the most appropriate of these approaches. Ultimately, the benefits and risks of each procedure must be evaluated, and care must be taken to minimize complications and avoid further injury. The choice of an appropriate method to treat the humeral fracture must be made on an individual basis. Consideration must be given to the fracture pattern, closed or open nature of the injury, associated polytrauma, soft tissue injuries, other associated injuries, and age and body habitus of the patient. The experience of the treating physician will also play a role. Knowledge of the basic mechanism of fracture healing associated with each method is helpful. The biomechanics of fracture healing and fracture stability are described in detail by Sarmiento and discussed in Chap. 6.

Nonoperative Management

For isolated fractures of the humeral shaft, nonoperative treatment methods achieve high union rates of up to 90%, with few complications. Nonoperative treatment should therefore be regarded as the primary option in most patients. Commonly used methods of closed management include the hanging arm cast, coaptation splint, and functional bracing. Other less used methods include the Velpeau dressing, abduction casting or bracing, and skeletal traction.

Unlike the case in long bone fractures of the lower extremities, some minor deformities are acceptable. Klenerman has proposed that as much as 20 degrees of varus angulation, 15 degrees of rotation, and up to 2 cm of shortening are compatible with a good functional outcome. Rotational malalignment is easily compensated by shoulder motion. It is important for the patient to understand and accept these malalignment outcomes.

The **hanging arm cast** (Fig. 9-5) was initially introduced by Caldwell in 1933. A long arm cast is applied from below the axilla with the elbow at 90 degrees of flexion. A loop attached to the forearm is used to suspend the cast from

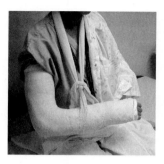

FIG. 9-5   The hanging arm cast is applied with the elbow at 90 degrees of flexion. Gravity maintains alignment. The loop for the sling may be adjusted to correct the alignment.

the neck, helping to maintain correct alignment of the fracture. This method works on the principle of the gentle gravity traction afforded by the cast to maintain alignment of the fracture. Hence the patient must be instructed to remain in an upright or sitting position at all times. Frequent examinations are required to monitor fracture alignment, and the position of the loop may have to be adjusted periodically on the forearm to correct the angulations of the fracture. A hanging arm cast may be used as the definitive treatment option until fracture union is achieved. Alternatively, the cast may be used until satisfactory alignment is obtained and the fracture is "sticky." A coaptation splint or functional brace may then be applied and used until the fracture is fully united. Contraindications for treatment with a hanging arm cast include transverse midshaft fractures and fractures in obese patients and in large-breasted women. In such patients this method is likely to lead to distraction, nonunion, and angulations.

The **coaptation splint** (sugar-tongs or U splint) is fairly simple to use (Fig. 9-3). A padded plaster splint is applied starting in the axilla, going around the elbow, continuing along the lateral aspect of the arm, and ending near or over the acromion. A sling is used to support the arm, and fracture alignment should be closely monitored. To some extent, this method works on the principle of soft tissue compression to maintain fracture alignment. Although the coaptation splint is simple to use, there are some disadvantages, such as minor to moderate swelling of the forearm and hand or stiffness of the shoulder. It may be difficult to maintain acceptable alignment. Again, this method is not well suited for obese patients or female patients with large breasts.

The **functional brace**, introduced by Sarmiento in 1977, is a key advancement in the nonoperative management of humeral shaft fractures and allows many patients to achieve optimal outcomes without surgery (Fig. 9-6). The brace may be used as an initial primary treatment. The functional brace is more often applied 1 to 2 weeks after injury, as a follow-up treatment, once the initial operative or nonoperative treatment has been completed. Because of its simplicity and versatility, this method is widely used. A recent review by Sarmiento and others describes this method in further detail. The functional brace extends from the shoulder to just above the elbow and is usually made of two conforming padded plastic splints, one medial and one lateral, held together with adjustable Velcro straps. The brace (a polypropylene sleeve) is

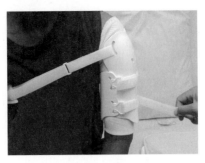

FIG. 9-6   Prefabricated functional brace. An adjustable strap is shown.

either custom-made or obtained as a prefabricated off-the-shelf unit; it works on the principles of gravity and soft tissue compression. Therefore the brace must remain snug around the arm and requires adjustment periodically as the swelling subsides. The brace does not necessarily immobilize the fracture. Some movement does take place at the fracture site, which may be useful in stimulating callus formation. As in other forms of closed management, minimal angulations are acceptable and are compatible with a good functional outcome. One major advantage is that joint stiffness is avoided, as the brace allows for shoulder and elbow motion. For a successful outcome with functional bracing, the patients must be ambulatory, cooperative, and compliant with the rehabilitation programs. This method is not suitable for obese or bedridden patients.

The **Velpeau dressing** requires padding of the axilla and medial sides of the arm with soft pads (to maintain alignment) and suspending the arm with a cuff and collar. The humerus is then immobilized by wrapping an Ace or similar bandage around the entire extremity and the chest. Introduced by Gilchrist, this method is rarely used today for definitive treatment in adults. It can, however, be used as a temporary splint until definitive treatment is selected and has a place in the management of humeral shaft fractures in children.

The following two methods are mentioned only briefly because they have limited indications and are not well tolerated by most patients.

Abduction casting or bracing is similar to a shoulder spica and is applied with varying angles of abduction of the shoulder to maintain alignment. The cast or brace is rarely used today as it makes it awkward for the patient to lead a normal life and there are now better and more effective management options available.

To implement **skeletal traction** at the bedside, a Steinmann pin is inserted in the olecranon process. The patient must remain in bed for this treatment; hence it is used only in very unstable fractures for short periods of time.

Operative Management

Indications for Operative Treatment

As previously mentioned, more than 90% of humeral shaft fractures can be successfully managed by nonoperative methods. Operative treatment of humeral shaft fractures becomes necessary in specific situations, as in patients who cannot tolerate closed management, in those who cannot be placed in a functional brace because of obesity or body habitus, or in those who have multiple injuries. The decision should be based on several factors, including the fracture's characteristics, the surgeon's capability, and the patient's preference. The importance of discussing the pros and cons of the various treatment modalities with the patient cannot be overemphasized.

Specific Indications for Surgery in Acute Fractures

Polytrauma, including head, chest, or multiple system injuries
Bilateral humeral fractures or multiple long bone fractures
Associated ipsilateral fractures of radius and ulna or "floating elbow" injury
Open fractures
Segmental fractures with unacceptable alignment
Nerve injury following manipulation of a fracture
Associated articular injuries
Associated vascular injuries
Obesity
Noncompliant patients
Failed nonoperative treatment
Pathologic fractures
Periprosthetic fractures

Specific Indications for Surgery in Chronic Fractures

Delayed union
Nonunion
Malunion
Infection

Methods of Operative Treatment

Plate osteosynthesis is perhaps the "gold standard" for the fixation of humeral fractures; it offers several advantages, including a high rate of fracture union (Fig. 9-7*A* and *B*). The fracture site is readily exposed, enabling accurate alignment under compression with stable fixation. If necessary, bone grafts can easily be added to enhance fracture healing. The radial nerve can be visualized, freed, and repaired if so indicated. Postoperatively, the adjoining joints can be mobilized early so as to avoid joint stiffness. Functional recovery is fairly rapid,

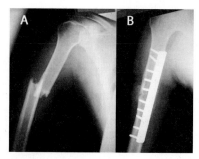

FIG. 9-7 Transverse fracture of middle third of the humeral shaft (*A*). Osteosynthesis achieved by compression plating (*B*). This type of fracture is not suitable for treatment by the hanging cast method.

with the least amount of muscle atrophy. Indications specific to the plating technique include fractures with neurovascular injuries, fractures in the distal part of the humerus, spiral or oblique fractures, and periprosthetic fractures.

However, there are certain drawbacks. The so-called soft tissue envelope is violated, which may prolong fracture healing time. Similarly, the elevation of periosteum and soft tissue necessary to expose the fracture may affect the healing process. It is imperative to keep soft tissue dissection to the minimum. Gentle tissue-handling technique should be followed. Complications such as nonunion, neurovascular injuries, and hardware breakage are well known. Postoperative infection is uncommon, but antibiotic prophylactic measures should nevertheless be used.

Exposure of the fractures is determined by fracture level and pattern. An anterolateral approach along the lateral border of the biceps, which splits the brachialis muscle, is used to expose the the fracture. Alternatively, a modified posterior approach that retracts the entire triceps medially, as described by Gerwin et al. (1996), can be used to obtain more adequate exposure of the humerus than is obtained with the direct posterior triceps-splitting approach. Commonly used plates are 4.5-mm narrow low-contact dynamic compression plates (LCDCPs) with 4.5-mm screws (Fig. 9-7A and B). Preferably the plates should have staggered screw holes. In patients with osteopenic bones, locking plates offer some advantages. Surgeons may choose various combinations of plates and screws, as dictated by the fracture pattern.

Following the successful management of lower extremity fractures with **intramedullary fixation**, a similar approach has been successfully adapted in the management of humeral shaft fractures. Intramedullary nails offer several biomechanical advantages over plate osteosynthesis: the nails are very close to the mechanical axis of the bone and are subject to less mechanical stress. Stress shielding of the cortex is minimized and the soft tissue envelope is not violated. Blood loss is minimal. There is reduced risk infection. However, distraction at the fracture site must be avoided.

Specific indications for intramedullary rod fixation include comminuted fractures, segmental fractures, pathologic fractures, and fractures in patients with osteopenic bones. However, fractures located in the lower fifth of the shaft are not amenable to intramedullary fixation. Though fractures below the lesser tuberosity may be fixed with special intramedullary nails, standard nails are not recommended. Spiral or oblique fractures are better managed by plate osteosynthesis. Fractures with radial nerve palsy and those with vascular injuries are better managed by using plates, as the manipulation needed for the placement of intramedullary nails may aggravate nerve injuries or disrupt the vascular repair.

Antegrade and Retrograde Insertion of Intramedullary Nails

Antegrade insertion. This approach is suitable in the management of fractures of the proximal and middle thirds of the humerus and is easier to implement than distal approach. The nails are introduced from the proximal end of the humerus, near the greater tuberosity. The disadvantage is potential injury to the rotator cuff, with subsequent shoulder problems. However, some systems avoid this problem by inserting the rod slightly distally on the anterolateral surface of the humerus.

Retrograde insertion. An entrance portal is created on the posterior surface of the distal humerus just proximal to the olecranon fossa. This limits the size of the portal. Indications for this approach include fractures of the distal and the middle thirds of the humerus. Shoulder problems are avoided, but minor elbow problems are known to occur. Subsequent fractures of the humerus at the site of the portal have been reported.

Type of nail. Historically, intramedullary nailing systems started out with simple, flexible, nonlocking nails. These were gradually replaced by more advanced, rigid, interlocking nails. Obvious disadvantages of nonlocking systems include suboptimal rigid fixation and lack of torsional control.

Flexible intramedullary nails include Rush pins and Ender's nails. Rush pins are straight rods that are available in various sizes and have a hook at one end for easier removal. They are easy to introduce but lack rigidity and are prone to migration. Hence they are no longer recommended. Ender's nails are flexible and usually two or three are used at a time. These nails offer more rigid fixation than the Rush rods as well as some torsional control. More recently, titanium flexible nails have become available. All types of nails can be inserted using both antegrade and retrograde portals.

Rigid intramedullary nails. The most widely used nails are the rigid interlocking nails. Made by several manufacturers, they follow similar principles and are used in either reamed or nonreamed versions. The standard method of interlocking is by proximal and distal screw fixation (Fig. 9-8*A* and *B*). Seidel nails have a different system of distal locking whereby expansile prongs are deployed to lock into the inner wall of the distal humeral cortex. This type of locking is prone to loosen, leading to complications. Hence, a screw locking mechanism is preferable. For more proximal shaft fractures, special nails with proximal locking screws, which lock into the head of humerus, are available (Figs. 9-8 and 9-9).

Expandable intramedullary nailing systems. More recently, several advanced intramedullary nailing systems have been introduced. Unlike conventional nails that rely on interlocking screws for axial and rotational stability, the walls of the newer nails expand to fill the medullary cavity. Therefore these nails may be better suited for patients with poor bone quality who require humeral stabilization. The nailing system is associated with minimal complications, predictable fracture healing, and excellent functional outcomes in elderly patients.

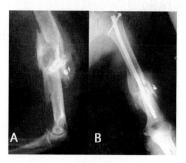

FIG. 9-8 Comminuted fracture of middle third of the shaft of the humerus due to gunshot wound (*A*). Internal fixation by interlocked intramedullary nailing (*B*). The proximal end of the nail is well seated to avoid shoulder impingement.

Flexible locking intramedullary nails. These are articulated flexible nails that allow both antegrade and retrograde implantation and static locking. Nail insertion can be accomplished without violating the rotator cuff or damaging the articular surface of the humeral head. In the antegrade approach, the portal of entry is either the lateral or anterolateral shaft distal to the acromion. After the flexible nail is introduced, it is stiffened by a wire mechanism. Proximal and distal locking screws are also used. This approach avoids the shoulder problems associated with the tuberosity portal. However, this implant should be used with caution in any patient with a medullary canal of 8 mm or less in diameter.

Plating osteosynthesis vs. intramedullary fixation. There is an ongoing controversy regarding the relative benefits of plate osteosynthesis vs. intramedullary fixation with nailing. Valid arguments can be made in support of either method. Two randomized studies are available for review. Results are somewhat comparable; however, each method is associated with different sets of complications. When performed antegrade, nailing is associated with a higher incidence of shoulder pain and dysfunction, whereas plating using the posterior approach is associated with elbow stiffness and pain. Further prospective studies involving large numbers of patients are needed to resolve this issue.

COMPLICATIONS

Initial complications associated with fractures of the humeral shaft have already been mentioned. Complications occurring as a result of treatment methods include nonunion, malunion, infections, radial nerve palsy, vascular injuries, and adjacent joint problems with muscle atrophy.

Nonunion is the most significant complication of humeral shaft fractures (Fig. 9-9). If the fracture shows no evidence of healing by 12 to 16 weeks, it is to be considered a nonunion. Generally speaking, surgical management tends to result in a higher rate of nonunion than closed treatment methods (Fig. 9-9A).

The etiology of nonunion may be patient-, fracture-, or treatment-related. Some of the more common factors include smoking, severe osteopenia, comminution (including segmental fractures), soft tissue interposition, distraction at the fracture site, hardware failure (Fig. 9-9B), and infection.

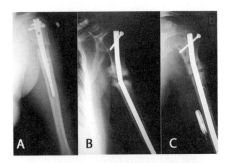

FIG. 9-9   Nonunion of fractures of the proximal third of the shaft of the humerus. This patient had a history of cigarette smoking. *A.* Following interlocked intramedullary nailing. *B.* Hardware failure. *C.* Treatment with reamed nailing, iliac bone grafting, and application of an internal bone stimulator.

Treatment options of nonunion must address the etiologic factors. These must be rectified prior to definitive care. Options for management of nonunion are listed below.

When electrical stimulation using either external or internal stimulators is contemplated, the fractures must be stabilized before this method is applied (Fig. 9-9C).

Reamed intramedullary nailing is less successful in humeral nonunion than in fracture nonunion of the lower extremity. Overreaming must be done with great caution, as it can result in injury to the radial nerve. This technique can be combined with electrical stimulation.

Excision of nonunion with plate osteosynthesis and autogenous bone grafting offers the best chance of success.

Vascularized bone grafting techniques are useful in rare instances where the nonunion is recalcitrant. Even though iliac bone grafting is ideal, it involves an additional surgical procedure, with attendant morbidity. To overcome this problem, synthetic bone graft substitutes may be used. In addition, several biologicals—such as demineralized bone matrix products, bone morphogenetic proteins, and tissue growth factors—are being introduced. These emerging technologies hold great promise and are being widely tested and used.

Malunion can follow any method of treatment. However, it is probably more common after conservative management. Malunion can be angular, rotational, or result in shortening. Fortunately, up to 20 to 25 degrees of angulation, 15 degrees of rotation, and up to 2 to 3 cm of shortening are well tolerated by most patients and compatible with a good functional outcome.

Most cases of **radial nerve palsy** are of the neurapraxia type, and close to 90 percent of patients recover from them within 4 to 6 months of injury. If there is no noticeable recovery within 6 to 8 weeks, it is advisable to obtain electromyography studies; consideration should also be given to exploration and repair of the radial nerve. During the recovery phase, appropriate splinting of the hand and wrist is essential. Early tendon transfers to restore function have been recommended.

Initial vascular injuries should be managed by the vascular service. Vascular injuries as a result of treatment are rare and should be managed accordingly.

Infections following surgical fixation of fractures of the humerus are rare, but when they do occur, they complicate the outcome. Well-established protocols for managing postoperative infections should be followed to secure a healed fracture.

REHABILITATION

Rehabilitation is an important and integral part of managing fractures of the humeral shaft. The ultimate goal of any treatment plan is to regain preinjury functional status. With this goal in mind, a rehabilitation program must be instituted from the onset.

SELECTED READINGS

Amillo S, Barrios RH, Martinez-Peric R, et al. Surgical treatment of the radial nerve lesions associated with fractures of the humerus. *J Orthop Trauma* 7(3):211–215, 1993.

Chapman JR, Henley MB, Agel J, Benca PJ. Randomized prospective study of humeral shaft fracture fixation: intramedullary nails versus plates. *J Orthop Trauma* 14(3): 162–166, 2000.

Fleming P, Lenehan B, Sankar R, et al. One-third, two-thirds: relationship of the radial nerve to the lateral intermuscular septum in the arm. *Clin Anat* 17(1):26–29, 2004.

Franck WM, Olivieri M, Jannasch O, et al. Expandable nail system for osteoporotic humeral shaft fractures: preliminary results. *J Trauma* 54(6):1152–1158, 2003.

Gerwin M, Hotchkiss RN, Weiland AJ. Alternative operative exposures of the posterior aspect of the humeral diaphysis. *J Bone Joint Surg* 78A:1690–1695, 1996.

Lorich DG, Geller DS, Yacoubian SV, et al. Intramedullary fixation of humeral shaft fractures using an inflatable nail. *Orthopedics* 26(10):1011–1014, 2003.

McCormack RG, Brien D, Buckley RE, et al. Fixation of fractures of the shaft of the humerus by dynamic compression plate or intramedullary nail. A prospective, randomized trial. *J Bone Joint Surg* 82B:336–339, 2000.

Sarmiento A, Kinman PB, Galvin EG, et al. Functional bracing of fractures of the shaft of the humerus. *J Bone Joint Surg* 59A:596–601, 1977.

Schemitsch EH, Bhandari M. Fractures of the humeral shaft. In Browner BD, Jupiter JB, Levine AM, Trafton PG (eds): *Skeletal Trauma*, 3d ed. Philadelphia: Saunders, 2003:1481–1511.

Stannard JP, Harris HW, McGwin G Jr, et al. Intramedullary nailing of humeral shaft fractures with a locking flexible nail. *J Bone Joint Surg* 85A:2103–2110, 2003.

10 | Fractures and Dislocations of the Elbow

Edward R. Abraham

This chapter reviews fractures and dislocations of the elbow or cubital articulation. These injuries include fractures of the distal humerus (i.e., isolated medial and lateral condylar fractures, transcondylar fractures, supracondylar fractures, and intercondylar fractures), fractures of the radial head and neck, fractures of the olecranon, and dislocations of the elbow with and without fractures of the proximal ulna (coronoid process) and the radial head and neck.

ANATOMY

The elbow is the articulation of the humerus of the arm to the radius and ulna of the forearm. The distal humerus consists of the extraarticular medial and lateral condyles, which are diverging columns separated by the intraarticular trochlea and capitellum (Fig. 10-1). The distal humerus is angled anteriorly at approximately 30 degrees. The humerus widens and flattens as it angles forward. The trochlea articulates with the trochlear notch of the proximal ulna. The trochlea's articular surface extends from the coronoid fossa anteriorly to the olecranon fossa posteriorly. The anterior and posterior fossae provide space for the coronoid and the olecranon, respectively, at the extremes of motion. The capitellum is a hemispheric termination of the lateral column that articulates with the concave radial head.

The proximal radius consists of a head and neck, which form a 15-degree angle with the radial diaphysis. The radial head is dish-shaped. The outer circumference articulates with the radial (sigmoid) notch of the ulna.

The radial notch of the olecranon forms an arc of 40 to 70 degrees. The trochlear notch forms an arc of 180 degrees.

The prominent medial epicondyle is the origin for the flexor-pronator muscles and the medial collateral ligaments. The epicondyle protects the ulnar nerve, which runs posteriorly in its sulcus. Originating from the smaller lateral epicondyle are the supinator–extensor muscle group and lateral collateral ligament.

The distal articular surface of the humerus is oriented in 7 degrees of valgus in relation to the long axis. The valgus orientation of the distal humerus combines with the ulnar angulation of the olecranon to produce a carrying angle of up to 20 degrees with the elbow in full extension. When viewed from the side, the capitellum and trochlea are anterior to the long axis of the humerus; a line drawn along the anterior cortex of the humeral shaft transects the center of the capitellum.

The medial collateral ligament of the elbow originates on the medial epicondyle and consists of two portions; the anterior portion, which inserts on the medial aspect of the coronoid process, and the posterior portion, which attaches to the medial aspect of the olecranon. The lateral collateral ligament originates on the lateral epicondyle and has insertions on the annular ligament and the olecranon. The annular ligament surrounds the radial neck and stabilizes the radioulnar articulation. Anteriorly, the annular ligament is attached to

113

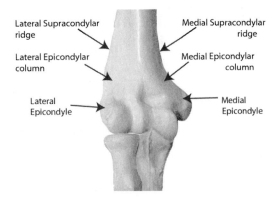

FIG. 10-1 Anterior view of the humerus showing the relation of the lateral and medial columns to the trochlea and capitellum.

the anterior margin of the radial notch. Posteriorly, it is broader and attached to a ridge posterior to the radial notch (Fig. 10-2).

The capsule of the elbow joint attaches to the humerus anteriorly above the coronoid and radial fossae and posteriorly above the olecranon fossa. Distally, it attaches to the base of the coronoid process of the ulna and to the annular ligament; it is continuous with the lateral and medial collateral ligaments.

The principal muscles responsible for active elbow motion are divided into four groups. The extensors are the triceps brachii and anconeus. The triceps muscle inserts into the posterior surface of the olecranon process and along the proximal ulna, where it is referred to as the *extensor expansion*. The flexors comprise the brachialis, biceps, and brachioradialis. Anteriorly, the brachialis muscle attaches to the coronoid process. The biceps tendon attaches to the radial tuberosity. Forearm supination is the function of the biceps and supinator, and forearm pronation is produced by the pronator teres and pronator quadratus.

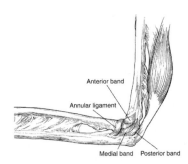

FIG. 10-2 Lateral view of the elbow showing the relation of the lateral collateral ligament to the annular ligament; also shown is the attachment of the anterior band on the annular ligament and the posterior band on the olecranon.

BIOMECHANICS

The humeral ulnar and humeral radial articulations function as a hinge. The joint permits flexion to 160 degrees and extension to 0 degrees. Valgus stability is provided primarily by the anterior fibers of the medial ulnar collateral ligament and secondarily by the radiocapitellar articulation and anterior capsule. The flexor-pronator muscles (especially the flexor carpi ulnaris) provide an important dynamic component.

The lateral collateral ligament provides varus stability and is the major constraint, along with the lateral capsule, to posterolateral rotatory instability (the lateral pivot shift test).

Motion from 30 to 130 degrees is the range most important for activities of daily living.

The radiocapitellar articulation is a pivot or trochoid joint and allows for both flexion and extension of the ulnohumeral joint and forearm rotation of approximately 165 degrees. It permits 80 degrees of forearm pronation and 85 degrees of supination. The anterolateral quadrant of the radial head does not articulate with the radial notch, even in the extremes of pronation and supination, and is a portal for screw or Kirschner-wire fixation. An important relation between the radius and capitellum is the constant axis of rotation. A line drawn along the long axis of the radius transects the center of the capitellum regardless of the degree of elbow flexion (Fig. 10-3). The longitudinal relation of the radius and ulna is maintained by the forearm interosseous membrane, the triangular fibrocartilage complex distally, and the radiocapitellar articulation proximally. Excision of a fractured radial head when the interosseous ligament is torn will lead to proximal migration of the radius. When a collateral ligament is torn, radial head excision without replacement will lead to elbow instability.

The radial head serves as a restraint to valgus stresses across the elbow joint by acting as a fulcrum for the medial collateral ligament. It also transfers stresses from the hand and wrist to the distal humerus. Forces applied in a proximal direction axially along the shaft of the radius result in tightening of the central tendinous portion of the interosseous membrane. These forces are then transmitted from the radius through the interosseous membrane to the ulna and eventually to the trochlea. When the radial head has been removed, proximally directed stresses result in ulnar shift of the radius as opposed to tightening of the interosseous membrane, thereby altering stress transmission to the ulna and the mechanics of the distal radioulnar joint.

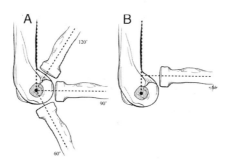

FIG. 10-3   *A.* Normal relation of the radial shaft and radial head to the center of the capitellum. *B.* Dislocation of the anterior radial head.

DISTAL HUMERAL FRACTURES

Fractures of the distal humerus account for one-third of humeral fractures. Preservation of painless elbow motion in a functional range is the goal that directs management. The unique anatomy of the distal humerus together with its articulations with the radius and ulna has resulted in a complex classification system of about 27 fracture types and subtypes.

Classification

The radiologic classification recommended by the Orthopaedic Trauma Association (OTA) best describes the fracture types. Table 10-1 divides the three main fracture groups—A (extraarticular), B (partial articular), and C (complete articular)—into subtypes.

Diagnosis and Initial Management

History and Physical Examination

There is pain and possibly instability or crepitus at the elbow. The mechanism of injury is usually a fall from a height onto the outstretched hand or a direct blow to the elbow. Isolated type A1 apophyseal fractures are expected to cause localized pain and swelling without elbow instability. As the complexity of the fracture increases (types B and C), deformity, instability, and crepitus appear. A careful inspection of the skin is essential, as these fractures are often open.

Radiographic Examination

Anteroposterior, lateral, and oblique radiographs with longitudinal traction applied to the extremity show the full extent of the injury. Computed tomography (CT) and other special views are occasionally useful in the assessment of intraarticular fractures (e.g., shear fractures of the trochlea or capitellum).

Initial Management

Initial management consists of improving fracture alignment and providing immobilization in a long arm splint in partial flexion at the elbow to avoid neurovascular complications. Ice packs can help to control swelling of the

---

TABLE 10-1 Definition of Main Fracture Types (OTA/AO Classification)

A. Extraarticular fracture
   1. Apophyseal avulsion of an epicondyle
   2. Metaphyseal, simple circumferential fracture line
   3. Metaphyseal multifragmentary

A

B. Partial articular fracture (part of articular surface remains attached to the diaphysis)
   1. Lateral condyle sagittal
   2. Medial condyle sagittal
   3. Frontal plane fracture of articular surface

B

C. Complete articular fracture (separated from the diaphysis)
   1. Articular simple and metaphyseal simple
   2. Articular simple and metaphyseal multifragmentary
   3. Articular multifragmentary

C

elbow and forearm. Attempts to reduce unstable intraarticular fragments are not necessary.

Associated Injuries

Compartment syndrome of the forearm is the single most important early complication. The signs of compartment syndrome include disproportionate pain at rest, pain with passive stretch of the muscles in the compartment, tense compartments, and paresthesias. Elevated compartment pressures in the forearm confirm the diagnosis of this surgical emergency. The brachial artery as well as the radial, median, and ulnar nerves are structures at risk of injury with these fractures. Radiographs of the entire extremity are helpful in locating other fractures.

Definitive Management

Extraarticular Fracture—Type A (Fig. 10-4)

Lateral epicondylar fracture (A1.1). These are rare injuries seen predominantly in children. The isolated fracture results from a varus stress to the elbow. In most cases, fracture displacement is minimal and elbow stability is preserved. Treatment in these patients consists of immobilizing the elbow at 90 degrees of flexion with the elbow in supination and wrist in mild dorsiflexion. Large displaced fragments are reduced and fixed with screw or Kirschner-wire internal fixation.

Medial epicondylar fracture (A1.2, A1.3). These fractures are usually seen in children with open physes. A valgus stress to the elbow is the most common mechanism. A direct blow is known to cause this fracture in adults. Displace-

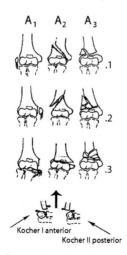

FIG. 10-4   The OTA/AO classification of type A distal humeral fractures. [*From Orthopaedic Trauma Association Committee for Coding and Classification. Fracture and Dislocation Compendium.* J Orthop Trauma *10(suppl): 12–15, 1996.*]

ment of the epicondyle up to 1 cm in children in the absence of valgus stress instability is best treated conservatively with the elbow immobilized to 90 degrees, and the forearm in neutral rotation, and the wrist in neutral position (A1.2). Fragments displaced more than 10 mm or fragments incarcerated in the elbow joint are best treated by open reduction and pin or screw fixation (A1.3). Ulnar nerve dysfunction and elbow instability are more likely to develop in the displaced fracture in adults; therefore open reduction and internal fixation (ORIF) is recommended.

Extraarticular Fractures (Type A2)

These transcondylar or supracondylar fractures are two-part fractures that do not involve the articular surface. They may be classified as high, low, abduction, and adduction. There are also extension or flexion components, as shown in Table 10-2. When there is metaphyseal comminution, the fracture is classified as an OTA group A3 with three subdivisions.

Definitive management. Closed reduction and immobilization in a long arm cast may be possible in some of these fractures, particularly in the elderly person. For the extension injuries, the closed reduction maneuver consists of a longitudinal traction followed by forward pressure on the olecranon process and then acute elbow flexion. Reduction is confirmed with radiographs. The arm is immobilized initially in a splint with elbow flexion at 90 degrees and the forearm in neutral rotation. A radial pulse must be palpable throughout the stages of reduction and immobilization. A minimum of 4 weeks of immobilization is necessary even in impacted fractures. Immobilization is continued in a long arm cast after the first 7 days in a splint.

Failure to hold the fracture adequately reduced requires percutaneous pin fixation or ORIF.

Pin fixation, percutaneous or open, can be used to stabilize an unstable fracture (Fig. 10-5). Open fixation with Kirschner wires and a figure-of-eight tension band can provide adequate stabilization of smaller osteopenic fragments. Transcondylar fractures in the osteopenic bone of an elderly patient are best suited for this treatment.

TABLE 10-2   Extraarticular Supracondylar Fractures (Type A2)

High extension	Oblique fracture line extends from anterodistal to posteroproximal, with posterior displacement of the distal fragment.
High flexion	The oblique fracture line is from anteroproximal to posterodistal, with anterior displacement of the distal fragment.
Low extension	The fracture line is slightly oblique or transverse, with posterior displacement of the distal fragment (OTA subgroup A2.3).
Low flexion	The fracture line is transverse or oblique, with the distal fragment displaced anteriorly.
Abduction	The oblique fracture line extends from distal medially to proximal laterally. The distal fragment displaces laterally (OTA subgroup A2.1).
Adduction	The oblique fracture line extends from proximal medially to distal laterally (OTA subgroup A2.2). The distal fragment displaces medially.

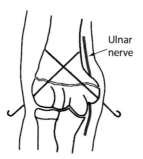

Ulnar nerve

FIG. 10-5   Percutaneous cross-wire fixation.

The Kirschner or Steinmann pins are placed from distal to proximal as crossed pins starting in the medial and lateral epicondyles. Multiple pins are occasionally necessary. Before the pins are placed, the fracture is reduced using closed or open techniques. An image intensifier is used to assist with the reduction and proper placement of the pins, but conventional radiographs, with their better detail, should also be obtained to confim the adequacy of the reduction. The cut ends of the pins are usually left outside the skin for removal after the fracture has healed. A long posterior splint is used for 1 week with the elbow held at 90 degrees of flexion. A long arm cast is then applied for an additional 3 weeks. Prolonged immobilization of the elbow in an adult can lead to permanent elbow stiffness. Pins are removed 6 weeks postoperatively. Elbow motion is started as soon as there is adequate evidence of fracture healing.

Complications

Complications associated with pin placement include nerve damage, wound infection, and loss of reduction. The ulnar nerve may be injured by the placement of the ulnar pin. A 2-cm skin incision over the medial epicondyle can be used to better localize the safest entry point for the medial pin placement and can be extended if tension-band fixation is desired.

Open Reduction and Internal Fixation (Types A2 and A3)

ORIF is the treatment of choice for nearly all adult distal humeral fractures. The goal of treatment is stable fixation allowing early restoration of functional painless elbow motion, which would be endangered by the use of prolonged immobilization or delayed union.

These goals are met by rigid internal fixation of the fracture. The preferred exposure of the distal humerus is by the posterior approach. This can be accomplished by splitting the triceps and elevating it off the humerus, working both medially and laterally as necessary.

Occasionally olecranon osteotomy may be beneficial, although it is usually used for intraarticular fractures. The proximal end of the olecranon process with the triceps tendon insertion is retracted proximally to expose the posterior surface of the distal humerus.

Care is taken to identify and protect the ulnar nerve. Two plates are used to fix the fragments and are placed at 90 degrees to each other so as to maximize fracture fixation. A 3.5-mm reconstruction plate on the lateral column and an LCDP, locking plate, or one-third tubular plate on the medial column provide adequate fixation. In low transcondylar fractures, it may be necessary to use the entire medial epicondyle by contouring the plate and transposing the ulnar nerve anteriorly. Locking plates are useful in patients with osteoporotic bone.

SINGLE-COLUMN FRACTURES (OTA GROUP B1 OR B2)

These uncommon unicondylar fractures extend into the joint. The lateral column is more frequently affected. An oblique fracture of either the medial or lateral column passes through the intercolumnar area of the distal end of the humerus and through the trochlea. The ulna can displace with the fragment if a large portion of the trochlea is involved. The mechanism of the fracture pattern is an asymmetrical axial loading force across the elbow on either the capitellum by the radial head to create a lateral column fracture or the trochlea by the ulna to create a medial column fracture.

Classification

Milch described two types (Fig. 10-6). In type I fractures, the lateral column of the trochlea is intact. In type II fractures, the lateral portion of the trochlea is broken off with the fractured column, which may result in an elbow dislocation. The higher the fracture is on the humerus, the greater the involvement of the trochlea. The OTA/AO classification refers to these fractures as type B partial articular fractures (Fig. 10-7). Type B1, with three subgroups, involves the lateral column, and type B2, with three subtypes, involves the medial column.

Diagnosis and Initial Management

Definitive Management

A nondisplaced single-column fracture can be treated with a splint or long arm cast for 3 or 4 weeks before starting therapy. Displaced or unstable fractures should be treated with ORIF to allow early motion.

Lateral single-column fractures are exposed with Kocher's approach, whereas a medial incision can be used for the medial-column fracture. A pos-

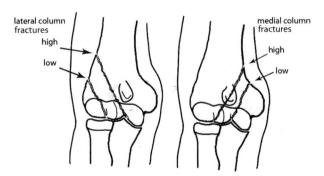

FIG. 10-6   High and low fractures of the lateral and medial columns (OTA B1 and B2).

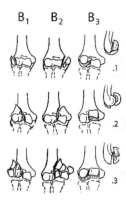

FIG. 10-7   The OTA/AO classification of type B distal humeral fractures. [*From Orthopaedic Trauma Association Committee for Coding and Classification. Fracture and Dislocation Compendium.* J Orthop Trauma *10(suppl): 12–15, 1996.*]

terior incision can also be used with partial elevation of the triceps on the involved side for plate or lag-screw fixation. This permits improved visualization of the joint to assess the articular surface reduction (Fig. 10-8).

FRACTURES OF THE CAPITELLUM (OTA TYPE B3)

The capitellum, an intraarticular structure, articulates with the radial head. The fracture may be associated with other injuries, such as a radial head fracture or a posterior elbow dislocation. The mechanism of injury is usually an axial force, which causes the radial head to compress the articular surface of the capitellum. The result is a shearing off of the articular cartilage and subchondral bone in the coronal plane.

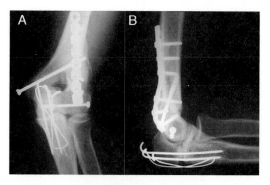

FIG. 10-8   High lateral unicolumn fracture treated with a single plate and screws. *A.* Anteroposterior. *B.* Lateral.

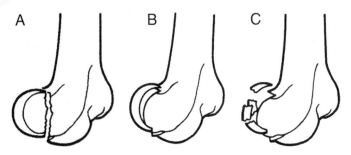

FIG. 10-9   The classification of isolated fractures of the capitellum: *A.* Hahn-Steinthal fracture. *B.* Kocher-Lorenz fracture. *C.* Compression fracture of the capitellum.

Classification

The fractures of the capitellum are divided into three types (Fig. 10-9). Type I, referred to as the **Hahn–Steinthal** fracture, is a single fracture fragment of the **entire thickness** of the capitellum (OTA Type B3.1). Type II is a fracture involving only the **articular surface** and **subchondral bone**. Type III is a compression fracture with **comminution** of the articular surface. The OTA group 3B.2 is a fracture of the trochlea and the lateral part of the capitellum. The OTA 3B.3 is a fracture of the entire capitellum and a separate trochlear fragment. The OTA 3B.2 and 3B.3 fractures are rare.

Radiographic Examination

Anteroposterior and particularly the lateral radiograph confirm the diagnosis (Fig. 10-10). A low single-column fracture may not be easily differentiated from a type I capitellar fracture. CT scan may be helpful in sorting out the exact fracture fragments requiring fixation in the unusual 3B.2 and 3B.3 injuries.

Definitive Management

Type I fractures are most often displaced superiorly, and manipulative reduction of the fracture is usually incomplete. Open exploration of the fracture through a lateral Kocher or Pankovich (anconeus) approach is recommended.

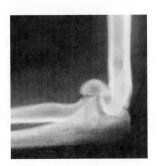

FIG. 10-10   Lateral radiograph of the elbow. This is a type I capitellar fracture.

The single fragment is reduced and temporarily held with smooth Kirschner wires. Percutaneous cannulated screws (2.7 or 4 mm) or headless compression screws are applied over posterior-to-anterior guidewires. The screw end should not extend beyond the subchondral bone as compression is applied to the fracture line. A maxillofacial Y plate has been successfully used to treat type I fractures. Rigid fixation and early mobilization reduce the chance of avascular necrosis and lead to the best recovery of elbow motion. If the capitellar fracture cannot be adequately immobilized or if the fracture fragments during fixation, excision of the capitellum may be necessary.

Type II and III fractures are more difficult to fix because of lack of subchondral bone for screw or wire purchase and due to fragmentation. Here the fragments usually need removal and range of motion is started within the first postoperative week. The results of treatment are less predictable, since joint instability may occur.

When this injury is associated with a radial head fracture, the capitellar fragment is fixed and the radial head fracture is fixed or excised if comminuted. A medial collateral ligament tear may preclude the excision of the radial head: a radial head prosthesis with a soft tissue repair on the medial side is usually needed.

The trochlear fractures (OTA/AO B3.2 and B3.3) are extremely rare as isolated injuries (Fig. 10-11). They are usually part of a more severe bone injury such as a double-column distal humeral fracture, ulnar fracture, or elbow dislocation. Whenever possible, the trochlear fragment is reduced and fixed, as described for the capitellar fractures, with cannulated screws, headless compression screws, or a tension-band Kirschner-wire construct. Invariably a small trochlear fragment is removed if satisfactory reduction and rigid fixation are not possible.

INTRAARTICULAR BICOLUMN FRACTURE (OTA/AO C3)

The incidence of intraarticular bicolumn fractures ranges from 5 to 37% in adults. The mechanism of injury is not clearly established. The most common accepted theory is a blow to the olecranon process with the elbow acutely flexed. The olecranon acts as wedge between the medial and lateral columns of the distal humerus. In one study, type C fractures occurred in 37% of all distal humeral metaphyseal fractures, mainly in females.

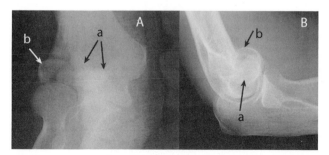

FIG. 10-11   Trochlear (a) and capitellar (b) fracture in a 68-year-old woman (OTA group B3.3). *A.* Anterior view shows lateral subluxation of elbow joint. *B.* Lateral view shows superior displacement of both trochlea and capitellum.

Classification

The OTA/AO classification affords a comprehensive breakdown of these fracture patterns (Fig. 10-12). OTA/AO C1 is a T-condylar fracture without fragmentation. In the OTA/AO C2, there is metaphyseal comminution. The OTA/AO C3 has intraarticular fragments, which may be associated with metaphyseal fragmentation. Some researchers find the AO/OTA radiographic classification to be overly complex in some regions and incomplete in other fracture patterns as determined at the time of surgery. In one large study, the C1, C2, and C3 fractures occurred with equal frequency.

Diagnosis and Initial Management

Initial Treatment

Initial treatment consists of applying a long posterior splint to the extremity. Alignment of the arm is improved without trying to reduce the fracture anatomically. To prevent vascular compromise, the elbow is maintained at 45 degrees of flexion. The extremity is elevated on pillows and ice is applied.

Definitive Management

The primary goal of treatment of intraarticular bicolumnar fractures of the distal humerus (Fig. 10-13) is restoration of painless functional-range elbow motion. Surgical management best accomplishes these goals, although nonoperative or limited surgical treatment options exist.

Nonoperative or Limited Surgical Treatment

Nonoperative or limited surgical treatment includes closed reduction and immobilization, the "bag of bones method," and an external fixator.

Closed reduction and immobilization is not a popular approach. Prolonged immobilization of the elbow at 45 degrees is needed, and invariably this treatment leads to a stiff elbow with malunion or nonunion.

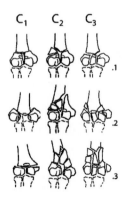

FIG. 10-12   OTA/AO classification of type C fractures. *[From Orthopaedic Trauma Association Committee for Coding and Classification. Fracture and Dislocation Compendium. J Orthop Trauma 10(suppl):12–15, 1996.]*

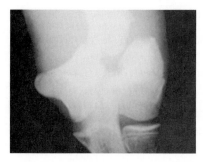

FIG. 10-13   Anteroposterior radiograph of elbow. T-type intraarticular fracture (type C1.1).

The bag-of-bones method for the infirm patient who is not a candidate for a formal surgical intervention consists of reduction of the fracture by compressive manipulation of the distal fragments, followed by "collar-and-cuff strapping" and early joint motion at 2 weeks. This treatment is not for the active patient.

External Fixator

An external fixator can be an excellent alternative to skeletal traction (Fig. 10-14), since mobilization of the patient is possible. Severely comminuted open fractures such as may be seen with gunshot injuries are ideal for this initial management. The fixator is applied laterally on the extremity. It spans the elbow by using humeral and ulnar pins. A hinge in the fixator can afford stable elbow motion. The use of the external fixator can be combined with a limited open reduction of the fracture and fracture fixation with cannulated screws

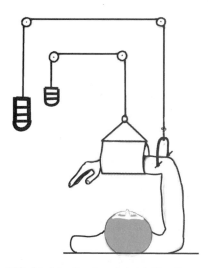

FIG. 10-14   Overhead skeletal traction.

and pins. Care must be taken to avoid the radial nerve, which can be injured when the pins are placed on the distal humerus. This is best accomplished by making a small incision and placing the pins with direct visualization of the humerus.

Open Reduction and Internal Fixation

The best results of treatment of bicolumnar fractures occur with ORIF. A complete set of plates and screws must be available, including a locking plate. Cannulated screws, Kirschner wires, and a minioscillating saw for the olecranon osteotomy are needed. The surgery is best performed during the day, when the regular operating room staff is available; however, open wounds and vascular trauma require more urgent treatment.

Surgical Approach

General anesthesia is required. The patient remains in the supine position, or the lateral decubitus position with the patient supported by a beanbag can be used as an alternative. A sterile tourniquet may be necessary. The extremity is draped free and placed over the chest wall or, if the patient is in the lateral position, over a bolster with the elbow flexed at 90 degrees. Full exposure to the articular surface of the elbow and posterior humerus is necessary. The transolecranon approach is recommended for the type C fracture. The ulnar nerve is mobilized from its anatomic location. An osteotomy is carried out at the midpoint of the olecranon, which is predrilled for screw fixation. The triceps and proximal olecranon are retracted proximally.

The first step in stabilizing the fracture is to reduce and fix the intraarticular components temporarily by using Kirschner wires. The width of the trochlea must be preserved. Compression screws are then inserted from the medial or lateral sides of the condyles, with care to leave room for plates.

Reconstruction plates (3.5 mm), one-third tubular, or specially designed locking plates are used to secure the condylar fragments with the trochlea and capitellum to the lateral and medial columns. For high T or Y bicolumn fractures, the medial plate is placed along the ridge of the medial column down to the medial epicondyle. Anterior transposition of the ulnar nerve is not needed. However, for low fractures, the plate is bent around the medial epicondyle and secured distally with at least two screws. Here the ulnar nerve is transferred anteriorly. The lateral plate is placed at a 90-degree angle to the medial plate to provide the greatest intrinsic stability to the fracture.

The olecranon osteotomy is secured with a large intramedullary compression screw (6.5 mm), which incorporates a tension-band wire. Two Kirschner wires plus a tension-band wire is a popular alternative technique.

Rehabilitation

The postoperative care of the extremity in a cooperative patient will depend on the rigidity of fracture fixation, the condition of the soft tissue, and the presence of other fractures in the extremity. Typically a splint is used for the first week for patient comfort. Splinting the elbow in greater extension may reduce the common complication of loss of elbow extension. When the splint is removed, a hinged elbow brace is used to allow motion in a range that is determined to be stable at the time of surgery. Active and gentle passive motion is started after 1 week. If heterotopic ossification is a concern due to head injury or delayed treatment, indocin or irradiation should be used immediately after surgery.

Adjunctive treatment, such as continuous passive motion or the use of dynamic and static adjustable splints, is supervised as part of the rehabilitation. These devices are most effective during the first 3 months, when the tissue is amenable to stretching. Results are less predictable later. Both stable fracture fixation and a stable joint articulation are prerequisites for dynamic splint therapy.

Arthroplasty

For a severely comminuted distal humeral fracture, total elbow arthroplasty is a possible primary treatment alternative in the elderly. Osteopenia of the fragments or advanced arthritis are conditions that favor a replacement arthroplasty.

Complications

The most common complications of distal humeral fractures are delayed union or nonunion, malunion, ectopic ossification, ulnar nerve injury, elbow stiffness, and wound infection.

Nonunion is associated with failure of the internal fixation. It can result in pain, instability, loss of elbow motion, and arthritis. Revision ORIF with bone grafting is necessary in these cases. A total elbow arthroplasty might be considered if bone stock is inadequate, as in the elderly or patients with advanced arthritis.

Malunion of these fractures can lead to angular deformity at the elbow and elbow arthritis. Undercorrected lateral column fractures can cause cubitus valgus and late ulnar nerve neuritis. Supracondylar osteotomy may be necessary to correct the malunion. Posttraumatic arthritis can occur if there is inadequate reduction of the articular surface or there is residual subluxation of the joint.

Elbow stiffness is the most common complication of any severe elbow injury. Almost all patients will lose some motion regardless of treatment modality. Loss of terminal extension is almost routine in these injuries. Treatment is best directed at prevention, with early motion beginning at 1 to 2 weeks after ORIF, provided that fixation is adequate. In these and other cases of posttraumatic arthrofibrosis, a comprehensive soft tissue release including capsulectomy can be performed after osseous healing. This is also the preferred treatment for heterotopic ossification if it prevents functional range of motion.

Wound infection is treated aggressively with early irrigation and debridement. Stable fixation should be retained, if possible, until fracture healing has occurred.

PROXIMAL FRACTURES OF THE RADIUS AND ULNA AND ELBOW DISLOCATIONS

Diagnosis and Initial Management (Radial Head Fractures)

History and Physical Examination

There is pain, usually localized to the elbow, but it may be deceptively referred into the forearm and wrist. Typically the patient has point tenderness directly over the radial head. The mechanism of injury is usually a fall forward with the elbow extended and the forearm pronated. The necessity for operative or closed management is determined clinically. The two important indications for operative intervention are a significant block to forearm motion and ligamentous instability. The hematoma is aspirated and the elbow injected with local anesthetic. The forearm is actively rotated with the elbow in 60 degrees of flexion. About 50% of elbow rotation and extension-flexion should be restored after aspiration and injection.

Instability is due to disruption of the lateral and/or medial ulnar collateral ligaments or an associated fracture of the coronoid process. Stability is assessed with the forearm supinated and the elbow flexed at 15 degrees, thus relaxing the anterior capsule and removing the olecranon from the olecranon fossae. If the elbow "books" open with a gentle valgus stress, the medial collateral ligament is torn. Posterolateral instability is also determined in supination and extension by axial loading of the forearm against the distal humerus with a valgus stress.

Radiographic Examination

Anteroposterior and lateral radiographs confirm the diagnosis. The radiocapitellar view may provide additional information.

Initial Management

A posterior splint with the elbow flexed at 80 degrees in neutral rotation and a sling provide initial support.

Associated Injuries

Associated neurovascular injuries are uncommon. Radiographs of the humerus, shoulder, and wrist are obtained where indicated.

The distal radioulnar joint is examined for tenderness, instability, and prominence of the distal ulna. If these are present, there may be an associated Essex–Lopresti lesion.

The radiograph is examined for signs of a more extensive injury: a coronoid fracture, an associated fracture of the capitellum, or an avulsion fracture of the medial epicondyle (indicative of an avulsion of the medial collateral ligament).

Diagnosis and Initial Management (Olecranon Fractures)

History and Physical Examination

There is pain localized to the elbow and a history of trauma. Type II fractures are caused by indirect trauma, whereas type III and IV fractures are caused by direct trauma. Type V and VI fractures are high-energy injuries caused by a combination of direct and indirect forces. The physical findings are ecchymosis, swelling, and, if the fracture is displaced, a palpable gap at the fracture site. A break in the skin assuredly communicates with the fracture.

Radiographic Examination

Lateral and anteroposterior views of the elbow are obtained. The lateral view shows the location and direction of the fracture line, the degree of comminution, and whether there is an associated radiocapitellar dislocation. The anteroposterior view shows the presence of an associated radial head fracture and any lateral displacement at the radiocapitellar joint or proximal ulnar angulation (suggestive of an incipient Monteggia injury).

Initial Management

A compression wrap is applied and the arm is placed in a sling for comfort. A splint is optional. If there is an associated radial head subluxation, a closed reduction will not be successful; because of the extent of instability, the fracture must be stabilized.

History and Physical Examination (Coronoid Fractures)

A fall on an outstretched arm driving the coronoid process against the distal humerus is the likely mechanism of injury. A history of associated injuries, such as an elbow dislocation and/or radial head fracture, is important. Palpation over the anterior elbow at the coronoid process causes pain, and there is local swelling. Extension of the elbow increases pain and may result in joint subluxation or dislocation. It may be necessary to extend the elbow and perform stress tests, as previously described, to detect occult elbow instability.

Radiographic Examination

Routine AP and lateral radiographs are necessary to evaluate the extent of the injury. The lateral view is particularly important in determining the size of the fracture fragment. A study by magnetic resonance imaging (MRI) may be helpful in evaluating the integrity of the medial and lateral collateral ligaments.

Initial Management

It is important to determine if the elbow joint is stable by carefully stressing the elbow joint for posterior, posterolateral, and medial instability. Immobilization at 90 degrees of flexion and neutral rotation is recommended for initial care. Surgical intervention is needed for elbow instability associated with type II and III fractures, radial head fractures, or ligament disruption.

Associated Injuries

The most common associated injuries are elbow dislocation, radial head fracture, and medial and lateral collateral ligament injuries.

Diagnosis and Initial Management (Elbow Dislocations)

History and Physical Examination

The patient presents with pain and swelling of the elbow. All elbow dislocations are characterized by loss of the normal relation of the epicondyles to the tip of the olecranon. This physical finding may be obscured by swelling. However, if present, it distinguishes elbow dislocation from other injuries, such as extraarticular supracondylar and transcondylar fractures of the humerus. Posterior dislocations are further characterized by apparent shortening of the forearm and the elbow is fixed in 45 degrees of flexion. In medial and lateral dislocations, the elbow appears wider than normal, and there may be some active and passive motion of the elbow. In anterior dislocations, the elbow is fixed in extension, the forearm is usually supinated, and the capitellum and trochlea are palpable posteriorly. In divergent dislocations, the forearm appears shortened and the elbow is fixed in varying degrees of flexion.

Radiographic Examination

The diagnosis of elbow dislocation is confirmed by true anteroposterior and lateral radiographs.

Initial Management

The elbow is splinted on a pillow or held in a posterior splint until radiographs are obtained and a closed reduction can be performed.

Associated Injuries

Associated injuries of the surrounding neurovascular structures occur. The most clinically significant injury involves the brachial artery. Associated injuries of the median, ulnar, and radial nerves occur with relative frequency; therefore a careful neurologic examination is essential.

Associated bone injuries are also common. The most clinically significant are fractures of the coronoid process and the radial head or neck. The combination of an elbow dislocation with a coronoid process fracture and radial head fracture will render the elbow unstable (known as "the terrible triad of the elbow") and require open reduction and reattachment of the coronoid process fracture and ORIF or replacement of the radial head fracture to achieve stability.

An undisplaced fracture of the radial head or neck may displace during closed reduction. In addition to radial head and neck fractures, there are frequently fractures of the medial or lateral epicondyles. These fractures become clinically significant when they prevent a concentric reduction; if they remain displaced, nonunion is likely. Radiographs of the distal humerus are examined for evidence of intraarticular osteochondral fractures; these can prevent concentric reduction and increase the likelihood of posttraumatic arthritis.

RADIAL HEAD FRACTURES

Classification

Fractures of the radial head are classified according to displacement, extent of involvement, and associated dislocations (Fig. 10-15). Type I fractures are displaced <2 mm. Type II fractures are displaced fractures involving only part of the joint surface. The comminuted type III fractures involve the entire head or neck (Fig. 10-16). Type IV fractures are radial head fractures associated with elbow instability or radioulnar dissociation (i.e., the Monteggia equivalent or Essex–Lopresti lesion).

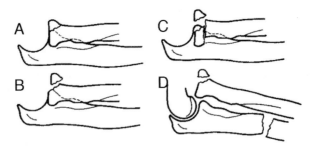

FIG. 10-15   The classification of radial head fractures: *A.* Type I. *B.* Type II. *C.* Type III. *D.* Type IV, showing an associated ulnar fracture (Monteggia fracture-dislocation).

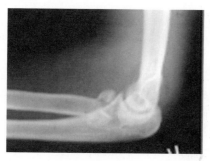

FIG. 10-16   Lateral radiograph of elbow: type III comminuted radial head fracture.

Definitive Management

The type of fracture determines management. Type I fractures (undisplaced) and type II and III fractures without a mechanical block (60 degrees each of active pronation and supination and 70 degrees of total assisted extension/flexion after local anesthetic elbow block) are treated nonoperatively. The patient is placed in a sling for 3 weeks and gentle active range of motion is encouraged. At 3 weeks, the sling is discontinued and more aggressive physical therapy is initiated.

Fractures associated with elbow instability, a loose body, or a mechanical block to elbow motion require operative intervention. The decision to reduce and internally fix the fracture or to excise the radial head, with or without prosthetic replacement, is made after examination of stability under anesthesia and once the fracture is exposed. Circumstances against fixation of the radial head are an elderly patient, injury of the capitellum (if undisplaced or repairable), and preexisting osteoarthritis. Circumstances for fixation include a young patient, involvement of only part of the radial head (i.e., type II), and associated instability (i.e., type IV). In patients with associated instability, there are two alternatives: reduction and fixation of the radial head or excision and replacement of the head with a metallic prosthetic spacer, followed by ligament repair.

Exposure through the **anconeus approach** is used only when the elbow joint is stable and no additional repairs (coronoid or capsule and collateral ligaments) are anticipated. The interval between the anconeus and flexor carpi ulnaris is developed. The insertion of the anconeus is reflected from the ulna and joint capsule by blunt dissection. If the capsule and synovium are not torn, they are incised longitudinally. One should not hesitate to incise the annular ligament to obtain wider exposure. In addition, the proximal or distal portion of the capsular incision can be opened in the shape of a T. As the forearm is pronated and supinated, the entire radial head is visualized. Some associated fractures of the ulna and capitellum can be reduced and stabilized through the same surgical approach.

Fragments are reduced and fixed with very small cortical screws (Fig. 10-17), headless compression screws, or Kirschner wires. Ideally, the implants are buried below the articular cartilage. It is important to remember that the anterolateral quadrant of the radial head does not articulate with the ulna and is

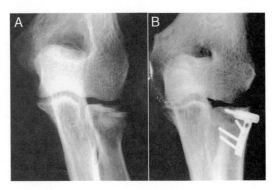

FIG. 10-17 Fracture of the radial head (*A*), treated by open reduction and internal fixation with a miniplate and screws (*B*).

therefore the optimal portal for fixation (Fig. 10-18). If depression of the articular surface is present, elevation and bone grafting are performed.

If the radial head is resected, the neck is preserved. The edges of the metaphysis are smoothed, and bony spikes are removed. If a metallic prosthesis is inserted, the size should match that of the excised radial head. A metal prosthesis, made of vitallium or titanium, is preferred over the once popular Silastic implant (Fig. 10-19). A more recent two-piece modular design has several choices of radial head and stem sizes. The stem is made to spin within the radial canal with forearm rotation. Silicone synovitis and poor force-bearing properties have ended the use of silicone prostheses.

Radial Head Fracture Associated with Elbow Instability

Prior to the incision and fixation or replacement of the radial head, the elbow and forearm are put through a range of motion and stability is tested. If the elbow subluxates posteriorly with the forearm in neutral rotation in the arc between 20 and 130 degrees, a lateral capsular disruption, lateral collateral ligament rupture, or coronoid process fracture will need repair along with fixation or replacement of the radial head. This requires an extended lateral incision and, if needed, a medial incision to repair the medial collateral ligament. Alter-

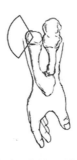

FIG. 10-18 "Safe zone" of radial head for plate or screw placement.

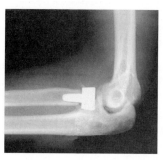

FIG. 10-19   Fracture of the radial head treated with metallic prosthetic replacement. Lateral radiograph of the elbow.

natively, a universal posterior incision with dissection laterally (and medially) can be used.

The repair starts with the coronoid fracture, then the anterior capsule, the radial head, and finally the lateral ligaments along with the posterior lateral capsule and extensor origin. Medial collateral ligament repair and the use of a hinged external fixator follow sequentially if instability persists.

In addition to elbow stability, the stability of the distal radioulnar joint is assessed. If radioulnar dissociation is present, the distal ulna will sublux dorsally with pronation of the forearm. This requires fixation, as discussed further on.

Postoperatively, the arm is placed in a sling or, if an associated ligamentous injury was repaired, a splint with the elbow at 90 degrees and the forearm in pronation or neutral rotation. The sling or splint is removed three times a day for supervised active assisted range-of-motion exercises. Flexion and extension are done with the forearm in pronation if lateral capsular/ligamentous repair was necessary. Rotation is done with the elbow at 90 degrees. At 3 to 4 weeks, the sling or splint is discontinued. Patients with associated radioulnar dissociation present a unique set of problems. In these injuries, the interosseous membrane and distal radioulnar joint capsule are disrupted and pronation and supination exercises may result in displacement. Therefore, after ORIF of the radial head, the distal radioulnar joint is pinned with the forearm in neutral rotation. Four weeks postinjury, the pin is removed. The splint is continued but is removed three times a day for range-of-motion exercises. At 6 weeks, the splint is discontinued. In cases in which a prosthesis has been used, consideration can be given to removal of the prosthesis 1 year postinjury in young patients. At this time, the radius should not migrate proximally.

Complications

The complications following radial head fracture include loss of motion, posttraumatic arthritis, instability, and shortening of the radius with resultant wrist pain.

Loss of motion is the most common complication seen with either nonoperative or operative management. Surgical removal of displaced or angulated small fragments or radial head excision for an incongruous radiocapitellar or proximal radioulnar joint often can improve joint motion.

Posttraumatic arthritis is managed with nonsteroidal anti-inflammatory drugs (NSAIDs) and local steroid injection; occasionally, excision of the radial head is required.

Radial shortening can follow excision of the radial head. The patient complains of pain at the distal radioulnar joint, made worse by grip and attempting to rotate the forearm. In many cases, there is obvious proximal migration of the radius in relation to the ulna. An MRI study may be required to demonstrate disruption of the ligamentous portion of the interosseous membrane. In symptomatic patients, when conservative treatment has failed, ulnar shortening is usually ineffective, as are most other methods of surgical reconstruction leveling the distal radioulnar joint.

In instances in which damage to the interosseous membrane is suspected, radial head resection must be avoided. When the radial head fracture is too comminuted to achieve internal fixation, a delayed radial head excision, the use of a radial head prosthesis, and stabilization, repair, or reconstruction of the central band of the interosseous membrane must be considered.

OLECRANON FRACTURES

Olecranon fractures involve the ulna proximal to the coronoid process. The majority of olecranon fractures are intraarticular. There may be an associated fracture of the radial head or displacement of the ulna with a dislocation of the radiocapitellar articulation.

Classification

Olecranon fractures are classified into six types based on the presence of displacement, intraarticular involvement, comminution, radial head fracture, and radiocapitellar dislocation (Fig. 10-20). Type I fractures are displaced less than 2 mm, without an intraarticular stepoff. Type II fractures are extraarticular and involve the proximal portion of the olecranon. These fractures involve

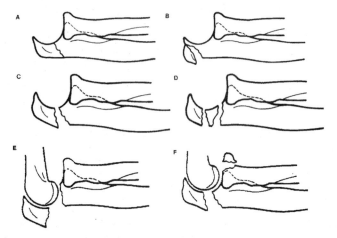

FIG. 10-20   The classification of olecranon fractures: *A.* Type I. *B.* Type II. *C.* Type III. *D.* Type IV. *E.* Type V. *F.* Type VI.

an avulsion of the triceps tendon from the proximal ulna. Type III fractures are simple intraarticular fractures with a transverse or oblique pattern. Type IV fractures are comminuted. The fracture lines may extend distal to the olecranon, and there may be depression of an intraarticular segment. Type V and VI fractures are either an olecranon fracture with an associated dislocation of the radiocapitellar articulation or an associated radial head fracture. The olecranon fracture in a type V or VI fracture is invariably displaced and intraarticular (i.e., a type III or IV fracture).

Definitive Management

The goal of management is an elbow with a functional, painless range of rotation and flexion/extension. It is important to preserve flexion even at the cost of losing some extension. The articular surface should be anatomically reduced to minimize the incidence of posttraumatic arthritis.

Undisplaced fractures (type I) are managed by splinting the elbow at 90 degrees for 3 weeks. The splint is removed once a day for active assisted range of motion. Radiographs are obtained at weekly intervals to confirm that the fracture fragments have not displaced. At 3 weeks, the splint is discontinued, and a sling is used for the next 3 weeks.

Type II, III, IV, V, and VI fractures are managed surgically. Type II to V fractures are approached by way of a straight posterior incision over the subcutaneous border of the olecranon. Type II and transverse type III fractures can be stabilized by using the tension-band technique with 2.0-mm Kirschner wires and an 18-gauge wire. A 6.5-mm cancellous screw and washer can be substituted for the Kirschner wires.

Oblique type III fractures and all type IV and V fractures are stabilized with a plate and screws. A 3.5-mm reconstruction or dynamic compression plate should be used on the dorsal (subcutaneous) surface and frequently needs to be contoured around the proximal end of the olecranon process for orthogonal screw placement to achieve stable proximal fragment fixation. Contoured anatomic plates are also manufactured. Fixation with a plate as opposed to a tension-band wire is indicated for two reasons: first, to prevent shortening of axially unstable fractures (i.e., oblique type III fractures and type IV fractures), and second, to provide rigid stabilization of the olecranon and prevent displacement of the radial head in patients with type V fractures. Type VI fractures have an associated fracture of the radial head. The radial head fracture may have to be reduced and stabilized or replaced with a prosthesis (Fig. 10-21).

Early postoperative motion is encouraged after 4 or 5 days of splint support to control pain and swelling.

Complications

Complications include loss of fixation, nonunion, infection, posttraumatic arthritis, and radioulnar synostosis.

Loss of fixation is often the result of underestimation of the personality of the fracture and inadequate initial fixation. This should be managed by revising the fixation in accordance with principles laid out above. Excision of the proximal fragment and attachment of the triceps tendon to the remaining olecranon is suitable for type II fractures and some types III and IV. Before the fragment is excised, it must be confirmed that the elbow is stable without the fragment (i.e., that the radial head and remaining olecranon will not sublux

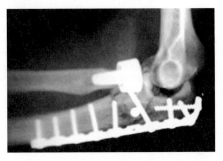

FIG. 10-21   Comminuted olecranon process fracture treated by plate fixation. Type III radial head fracture replaced with a prosthesis. Note proximal contouring of the plate and orthogonal screw fixation.

anteriorly once the fragment is removed). If a minimum of 30 degrees of the trochlear notch remains, the elbow will probably be stable, but this must be confirmed intraoperatively by removing all fixation, flexing the elbow to 90 degrees, and gently stressing the elbow.

Nonunion may be asymptomatic due to fibrous tissue between the fragments. Symptomatic nonunions are managed with reduction, plate fixation, and autogenous cancellous bone grafting.

Infection occurs occasionally because of the subcutaneous location of the fracture. Aggressive management is important because of elbow joint proximity. Fixation providing stability is maintained along with debridement and irrigation of the wound and joint; unstable fixation and necrotic tissue are removed. Parenteral antibiotics are required and an infectious disease consultation is prudent.

Posttraumatic arthritis is managed conservatively with NSAIDs or steroid injection.

Radioulnar synostosis occurs most frequently after type IV, V, or VI fractures. Management alternatives include doing nothing, resection of the osseous bridge, or osteotomy to place the hand in a more functional position.

CORONOID FRACTURES

The coronoid process is important as a restraint against posterior displacement of the ulna and as the attachment of the medial collateral ligament. The anterior capsule inserts at its base 5 mm distal to the intraarticular tip. Isolated coronoid fractures are uncommon. They usually occur in association with elbow dislocations and radial head fractures.

Classification

The Regan-Morrey classification of coronoid fractures describes three types (Fig. 10-22). In type I, the tip of the process fractures. This is believed to be a sign of posterior elbow displacement (a shearing fracture of the coronoid against the distal humerus) and not an avulsion fracture. Type II involves about 50% of the coronoid and can be comminuted or a single fragment. The type III fracture involves most of the coronoid process. A type IV fracture is either a type II or III fracture with extension along the medial cortex to involve

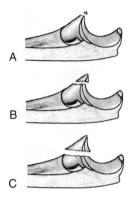

FIG. 10-22 Regan-Morrey classification of isolated coronoid process fractures: *A.* Type I. *B.* Type II. *C.* Type III.

the attachment of the medial collateral ligament.

Definitive Management

Type I

The fracture is usually treated conservatively because sufficient coronoid process is intact to maintain ulnohumeral joint stability. The extremity is immobilized in a long posterior splint with the elbow flexed at 90 degrees and the forearm in neutral rotation. Active elbow range of motion is started after 7 days and full extension is avoided for the first 3 weeks. A removable prefabricated splint or sling between exercise sessions may be useful. Later, progressive resistive exercises are started and continued until the patient reaches maximum medical improvement. Since an isolated fracture is unlikely, ligament damage due to elbow subluxation or dislocation must be determined. Treatment of an associated injury is usually more important than the type I coronoid fracture.

Type II

When about 50% of the coronoid is fractured, the elbow joint is potentially unstable. This can be evaluated by checking for posterior displacement of the forearm as the elbow is extended beyond 60 degrees. A grossly unstable joint is an indication for surgical reduction and fixation of the coronoid fracture. Surgery is also indicated for the "terrible triad" injury. Here the type II coronoid fracture is associated with a radial head fracture and an elbow dislocation. Reducing and fixing the coronoid and radial head fractures and the torn lateral collateral ligament complex are necessary to restore elbow joint stability. Prosthetic replacement of the radial head may be needed for unrepairable type III radial head fractures (Fig. 10-23).

Type III

Elbow instability is expected with this fracture. ORIF with a suture, pins, and/or screws is the treatment of choice. An articulated external fixator can be used if it is not possible to repair the coronoid process or if, in spite of the

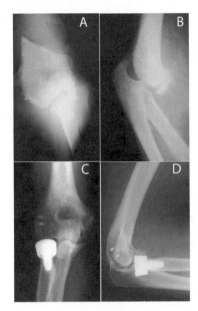

FIG. 10-23   "Terrible triad" of the elbow injury: unstable posterior dislocation with fractures of the coronoid process and radial head and disruption of the
lateral collateral ligament complex. *A* and *B*. Preoperative anteroposterior and
lateral radiographs. *C* and *D*. Radiographs after repair of the coronoid process,
radial head prosthetic replacement, and repair of the lateral collateral ligament-
capsular complex with suture anchors. (*Courtesy of Dr. John A. Elstrom.*)

repair of associated radial head and ligamentous injuries, the elbow joint remains unstable.

Surgical Management

The surgical approach to the coronoid process depends on the associated
injuries. If there is lateral collateral ligament complex disruption and/or the
radial head fracture requires prosthetic replacement, an extended lateral surgical approach can be used. If there is disruption of the medial collateral ligament complex, a medial approach may also be needed. The important consideration is to use the soft tissue defects created by the trauma and avoid
creating additional surgical damage. (See also "Radial Head Fracture Associated with Elbow Instability," above.)

A medial approach exposes and protects the ulnar nerve. The flexor-pronator muscle mass is released from the medial condyle if not disrupted. The
brachialis muscle is reflected off the anterior capsule, which is incised to expose the coronoid fracture. Screw fixation provides the best stabilization. This
can be accomplished with a cannulated headless compression screw placed
over a guide pin inserted from a posterior ulnar incision or directed posteriorly
from the site of reduction. Heavy nonabsorbable sutures around the coronoid
fragment and through drill holes in the ulna is an alternative method when
the fragment is not congenial to screw fixation.

Postoperative management depends on the stability achieved with joint and fracture fixation. Early motion is desirable, but joint stability is essential. The rehabilitation protocol outlined above for radial head fractures with associated ligamentous instability and/or coronoid fracture applies here. An external fixator is usually removed after 6 weeks.

Complications

Complications consist of stiffness, instability, pain, and ectopic ossification.

Stiffness of the elbow is the most common complication. The loss of motion is minimal for type I fractures. Loss of 80 degrees of total elbow motion is associated with type III fractures. Early dynamic splinting can minimize contractures. Capsular releases and a hinged external fixator may be necessary to increase elbow motion after fracture and ligamentous healing.

Instability following adequate surgical treatment must be addressed promptly by obtaining congruous elbow joint alignment and applying a hinged external fixator to allow joint motion. This can provide joint stability while capsular and ligamentous injuries heal and minimize the loss of motion seen with the neglect of cast immobilization.

Pain is commonly associated with instability, posttraumatic arthrosis, and elbow stiffness. Treatment is directed at the underlying cause.

Ectopic ossification is seen in patients with head injury or in whom surgery is delayed more than several days after a fracture-dislocation. Indocin can be used prophylactically to minimize the potential for ectopic ossification. Excision of the ectopic ossification is indicated if elbow stiffness prevents elbow flexion beyond 90 degrees. Low-dose irridation is advisable within the first 48 h after excision.

ELBOW DISLOCATIONS

This section reviews elbow dislocations, excluding Monteggia fractures and isolated dislocations of the radial head.

Classification

Elbow dislocations are classified according to the position of the radius and ulna in relation to the distal humerus. The types of elbow dislocations are posterior, medial, lateral, anterior, and divergent.

Posterior dislocations are by far the most common type of elbow dislocation. In addition to being posteriorly displaced, the radius and ulna may be displaced slightly laterally (Fig. 10-24) or medially. The presence of medial or lateral displacement does not affect the management or the prognosis.

The presence of a fracture of the radial head or coronoid process will frequently render the reduction unstable and thus require open fixation of these fractures (Fig. 10-25).

Medial and lateral dislocations are rare injuries. These have a poorer prognosis than the more common posterior dislocation. Frequently, a medial or lateral dislocation is, in reality, a subluxation (i.e., in a medial dislocation, the trochlear notch articulates with the medial epicondyle and the radial head articulates with the trochlea; in a lateral dislocation, the trochlear notch articulates with the capitellum.

Anterior dislocations of the elbow are extremely rare injuries. The mechanism of injury is either traction on the forearm with the elbow extended or a

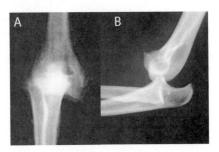

FIG. 10-24 Posterior dislocation of elbow. *A.* Anteroposterior radiograph shows some lateral displacement. *B.* Lateral radiograph shows the posteriorly displaced radius and ulna.

blow to the posterior aspect of the flexed elbow.

Divergent dislocations are also rare injuries. They are distinct from other types of elbow dislocations because there is dissociation of the radius and ulna. The annular ligament and interosseous membrane must be torn for a divergent dislocation to occur. There are two varieties, anteroposterior and mediolateral. In anteroposterior divergent dislocations, the radial head is dislocated anteriorly into the coronoid fossa and the ulna is dislocated posteriorly, with the coronoid process in the olecranon fossa. In mediolateral divergent dislocations, the radial head articulates with the trochlea and the trochlear notch articulates with the capitellum.

Definitive Management

In most cases, management is closed reduction under local anesthesia followed by splinting. Regional or general anesthesia with fluoroscopic monitoring is used if there is an associated undisplaced fracture of the radial head or neck. Open reduction is indicated if there are any of the following: an interposed os-

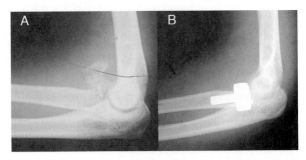

FIG. 10-25 *A.* Lateral radiograph of unstable fracture dislocation of elbow, reduced but grossly unstable due to type III radial head fracture, type III coronoid process fracture, and disrupted medial collateral ligaments. *B.* Open reduction of coronoid process fracture, replacement of radial head with Evolve modular radial head implant, and repair of collateral ligaments.

teochondral fragment preventing concentric reduction, irreducible dislocation, displacement of a fracture of the radial head/neck, or dislocations presenting for treatment more than 1 week following injury.

Closed reduction is performed as atraumatically as possible. This requires adequate analgesia and muscle relaxation. The specific reduction maneuver depends on the type of dislocation.

Posterior dislocation is reduced by traction in line with the deformity after correcting any medial or lateral displacement of the forearm to align the olecranon with the distal humerus. This method allows the coronoid process to slip distally past the humerus, and the elbow is flexed to 90 degrees. There should be immediate relief of pain and increased motion. If this maneuver fails, the patient is placed prone on a stretcher, with the arm and forearm hanging over the edge; a 5- to 10-lb weight is suspended from the wrist. After 5 min, the arm is lifted while flexing and reducing the elbow.

Failure to adequately reduce the fracture in the emergency room requires a repeat attempt in the operating room under general or regional anesthesia, with complete muscle relaxation. Soft tissue or incarcerated loose fragments (i.e., an incarcerated medial epicondyle) may block reduction, necessitating an arthrotomy.

Dislocations more than 10 days old are best treated by open reduction. The Kocher incision will provide access to the radial capitellar joint, and a medial approach will provide access to the medial epicondyle and the ulnar humeral joint.

Fracture of the radial head can be associated with an elbow dislocation and disruption of the medial collateral ligament. A displaced radial head can block motion in any plane. Because the radial-capitellar articulation is a secondary stabilizer to valgus stress, it is preferable to repair the radial head so as to avoid valgus instability. If repair is not possible, radial head replacement with medial collateral ligament repair is indicated.

Large displaced fractures of the coronoid process are associated with recurrent dislocation and need surgical repair.

Medial and lateral dislocations are reduced by traction and medial or lateral pressure.

Anterior dislocations are reduced by applying longitudinal traction to the forearm. A posteriorly directed pressure is applied to the anterior aspect of the forearm, while counterpressure is applied to the posterior aspect of the humerus.

Anteroposterior divergent dislocations are reduced by reducing first the ulna and then the radius. The ulna is reduced as if it were a posterior dislocation. The radial head is reduced by direct pressure and supination of the forearm. Mediolateral dislocations are reduced with traction and by pressing the radius and ulna together.

Complications

The complications of elbow dislocation include chronic instability, posttraumatic arthritis, loss of motion, and heterotopic ossification.

Chronic ligamentous or capsular instability after elbow dislocation can cause chronic subluxation, redislocation, valgus instability, or rotatory instability. Chronic subluxation and redislocation are best prevented by careful primary diagnosis and complete surgical repair. Late diagnosis is managed with repair or reattachment of the anterior capsule and coronoid process, repair or prosthetic replacement of a fractured radial head, and repair or tendon reconstruction of the medial and/or lateral (ulnohumeral) lig-

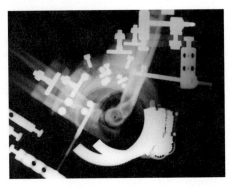

FIG. 10-26   Hinged external fixator used to stabilize a chronic elbow dislocation.

aments in conjunction with a hinged brace or hinged external fixator (Fig. 10-26). Valgus instability is managed by repair or reconstruction of the anterior portion of the medial collateral ligament; posterolateral instability is managed by repair or reconstruction of the lateral collateral ligaments and lateral capsule.

Heterotopic ossification usually involves the collateral ligaments, capsule, or brachialis. Initially, it is managed by discontinuing all passive motion exercises and administering indomethacin. Heterotopic bone can be excised after it has matured, as indicated by a cold bone scan and normal serum alkaline phosphatase levels. Preoperatively, CT or MRI helps to delineate the relation of the heterotopic ossification to surrounding neurovascular structures.

SELECTED READINGS

Muller ME, Nazarian S, Koch P, Schatzer J. Comprehensive classification of fractures of long bone. Berlin: Springer-Verlag, 1990.

Orthopaedic Trauma Association Committee for Coding and Classification. Fracture and Dislocation Compendium. *J Orthop Trauma* 10(suppl 1):v–ix, 1–154, 1996.

Pankovich AM. Anconeus approach to the elbow joint and the proximal part of the radius and ulna. *J Bone Joint Surg* 59A:124–126, 1977.

Distal Humeral Fractures

Cobb TK, Morrey BF. Total elbow arthroplasty as primary treatment for distal humeral fractures in elderly patients. *J Bone Joint Surg* 79A:826–832, 1997.

Grantham SA, Norris TR, Bush DC. Isolated fracture of the humeral capitellum. *Clin Orthop* 161:262–269, 1981.

Milch H. Fractures and fracture dislocations of the humeral condyles. *J Trauma* 15:592–607, 1964.

Pajarinen J, Bjorkenheim JM. Operative treatment of type C intercondylar fractures of the distal humerus: results after a mean follow-up of 2 years in a series of 18 patients. *J Shoulder Elbow Surg* 11:48–52, 2002.

Perry CR, Gibson CT, Kowalski MF. Transcondylar fractures of the distal humerus. *J Orthop Trauma* 3:98–106, 1989.

Robinson CM, Hill RM, Jacobs N, et al. Adult distal humeral metaphyseal fractures: epidemiology and results of treatment. *J Orthop Trauma* 17:38–47, 2003.

Radial Head Fractures

Coleman DA, Blair WF, Shurr D. Resection of the radial head for fracture of the radial head. Long-term follow-up of seventeen cases. *J Bone Joint Surg* 69A:385–392, 1987.

Esser RD, Davis S, Taavao T. Fractures of the radial head treated by internal fixation: late results in 26 cases. *J Orthop Trauma* 9:318–323, 1995.

Harrington IJ, Sekyi-Otu A, Barrington TW, et al. The functional outcome with metallic radial head implants in the treatment of unstable elbow fractures: a long-term review. *J Trauma* 50:46–52, 2001.

Olecranon Fracture

Colton CL. Fractures of the olecranon in adults: classification and management. *Injury* 5:121–129, 1973.

Karlsson MK, Hasserius R, Karlsson C, et al. Fractures of the olecranon: a 15- to 25-year follow-up of 73 patients. *Clin Orthop* 403:205–212, 2002.

Nork SE, Jones CB, Henley MB. Surgical treatment of olecranon fractures. *Am J Orthop* 30:577–586, 2001.

Dislocations

Lill H, Korner J, Rose T, et al. Fracture-dislocations of the elbow joint—strategy for treatment and results. *Arch Orthop Trauma Surg* 121:31–37, 2001.

Pugh DMW, Wild LM, Schemitsch EH, et al. Standard surgical protocol to treat elbow dislocations with radial head and coronoid fractures. *J Bone Joint Surg* 86A:1122–1130, 2004.

Complications

Gelberman RH, Garfin SR, Hergenroeder PT, et al. Compartment syndromes of the forearm: diagnosis and treatment. *Clin Orthop* 161:252–261, 1981.

Ilahi OA, Bennett JB, Gabel GT, et al. Classification of heterotopic ossification about the elbow. *Orthopaedics* 25:1075–1077; discussion 1077–1078, 2001.

Morrey BF. Complex instability of the elbow. *Instr Course Lect* 47:157–164, 1998.

O'Driscoll SW, Bell DF, Morrey BF. Posterolateral rotatory instability of the elbow. *J Bone Joint Surg* 73A:440–446, 1991.

Coronoid Process Fractures

Regan W, Morrey B. Fractures of the coronoid process of the ulna. *J Bone Joint Surg* 71A:1348–1354, 1989.

11 | Fractures of the Forearm

John A. Elstrom

The fractures of the forearm discussed in this chapter include fractures of both the radius and ulna, isolated fractures of the radius and ulna, the Monteggia fracture (fracture of the ulna with dislocation of the radial head), the Galeazzi fracture (fractures of the distal radius with displacement of the distal radio-ulnar joint), and the Essex–Lopresti injury (radioulnar dissociation with injury at the radial capitellar joint).

ANATOMY

Important anatomic features of the forearm include the radius, ulna, proximal and distal radioulnar articulations, interosseous membrane, muscles, nerves, and arteries. The proximal and distal radioulnar articulations are described in Chaps. 10 and 12.

The **radius** is an extension of the hand. It has an apex lateral bow, which, if allowed to heal unrestored (i.e., straightened) after a fracture, will result in loss of forearm rotation. The shaft of the radius is triangular in cross section, with its ulnar corner serving as the attachment of the interosseous membrane. The blood supply of the diaphyseal cortex of the radius is through periosteal and intramedullary vessels. The intramedullary vessels originate from a single nutrient artery that enters the radius through a foramen on the anterior surface of the radius in its proximal third.

The **ulna** is an extension of the arm; it has a slight posterior curve at its apex. The proximal half of the ulna has an apical dorsolateral curve, and the distal half has an apical volar curve. The radial border of the ulna serves as the attachment of the interosseous membrane. The posterior, or subcutaneous, surface is the origin of the deep fascia of the forearm. The blood supply of the ulna is through periosteal and intramedullary vessels, which originate from a single nutrient artery entering the ulna through a foramen on its anterior surface just proximal to its midpoint.

The **interosseous membrane** is a fascial sheet whose fibers are directed fanwise from the radius to the ulna. A condensation of fibers in its midsubstance is termed the **interosseous ligament**. Gaps in the interosseous membrane transmit the anterior and posterior interosseous vessels. The interosseous membrane separates the flexor and extensor compartments and serves as the origin of both flexor and extensor muscles. It also dampens the transmission of proximally directed forces along the radius to the capitellum. An intact interosseous membrane is strong enough to resist proximal migration of the radius, making possible resection of the radial head.

The **muscles** of the forearm are divided into flexor and extensor compartments (Fig. 11-1). The flexors are further divided into superficial flexors originating from the humerus and deep flexors originating from the radius, ulna, and interosseous membrane. The superficial group includes the pronator teres and the flexors carpi radialis, palmaris longus, carpi ulnaris, and digitorum superficialis. The deep flexor group includes the flexors digitorum profundus, pollicis longus, and pronator quadratus. All the flexors are innervated by the median nerve or its anterior interosseous branch except the flexor carpi ulnaris

144

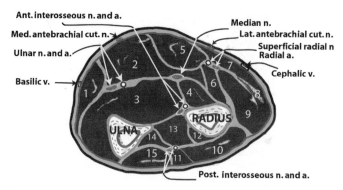

FIG. 11-1   Cross section through the middle of the forearm showing the interosseous membrane and the superficial and deep flexor and extensor compartments. Superficial flexor compartment: (1) flexor carpi ulnaris, (2) flexor digitorum superficialis, (5) flexor carpi radialis, (6) pronator teres. Deep flexor compartment: (3) flexor digitorum profundus, (4) flexor pollicis longus. Superficial extensor compartment: (7) musculus brachioradialis, (8) extensor carpi radialis longus, (9) extensor carpi radialis brevis, (10) extensor digitorum, (11) extensor digiti minimi (v), (15) extensor carpi ulnaris. Deep extensor compartment: (12) supinator, (13) abductor pollicis longus, (14) extensor pollicis longus.

and the ulnar side of the flexor digitorum profundus. These are innervated by the ulnar nerve.

The **anterior interosseous nerve** arises from the posterior aspect of the median nerve in the proximal forearm and supplies the flexors pollicis longus and digitorum profundus, part of the flexor superficialis, and the pronator quadratus. It has terminal sensory fibers to the joints that make up the wrist. Injury to the anterior interosseous nerve is usually indicated by weakness or loss of interphalangeal joint flexion of the thumb and index finger.

The **extensor** compartment is divided into superficial and deep groups. The muscles of the superficial group originate from the humerus and common extensor tendon. The superficial group includes the brachioradialis, extensors carpi radialis longus and brevis, extensor digitorum, extensor digiti minimi, and extensor carpi ulnaris. The deep extensor group includes the supinator, abductor pollicis longus, extensors pollicis longus and brevis, and extensor indicis. With the exception of the supinator, the muscles of the deep extensor group originate from the radius, ulna, and interosseous membrane. The muscles of the extensor compartment are innervated by the radial nerve or its terminal muscular branch, the posterior interosseous nerve.

Three muscles span the radius and ulna: the pronator teres, pronator quadratus, and supinator. Following a forearm fracture, they narrow the interosseous space, resulting in loss of forearm rotation.

The **brachial artery** divides into the **radial** and **ulnar arteries** 1 cm distal to the elbow joint. The radial artery runs along the radial side of the forearm to the wrist, where it lies between the flexor carpi radialis tendon and the radius. It is most easily palpated in this location. The radial artery terminates in the deep palmar arch. The ulnar artery runs along the ulnar side of the forearm until it reaches the wrist. Along the way, it gives off several branches, the most important of which is the common interosseous artery. This, in turn, gives off the anterior and posterior interosseous arteries. The anterior interosseous artery runs on the anterior surface of the interosseous membrane with the anterior interosseous branch of the median nerve. It gives off muscular branches and the nutrient arteries supplying the radius and ulna. The posterior interosseous artery traverses the interosseous membrane proximally to reach the extensor compartment, where it runs between the superficial and deep groups of muscles, giving off numerous muscular branches.

Classification

Injuries of the forearm are broadly classified into two groups: simple and complex. **Simple injuries** are fractures without associated ligamentous disruption. Included in this group are isolated fractures of the radius and ulna (the "nightstick" fracture) (Fig. 11-2) and fractures of both the radius and the ulna (the "both-bone" fracture) (Fig. 11-3). Simple injuries are the result of direct trauma (e.g., a blow to the forearm). They are described as being closed or open, uncomminuted or comminuted, and undisplaced or displaced; if displaced, then shortened or angulated. Isolated fractures of the proximal ulna are more likely to be complex injuries.

Complex injuries are characterized by ligamentous disruption. These injuries disrupt either the proximal, distal, or both radioulnar articulations or a significant portion of the interosseous membrane. The soft tissue component of these complex injuries, in many cases, is more significant than the fracture.

The **Monteggia's fracture** in adults is substantially different from the same injury in children. These injuries are frequently the result of high-energy trauma, and posterior dislocation of the radial head (Bado type II) (Fig. 11-4) is more common than anterior dislocation of the radial head (Bado type I). In addition, comminuted fractures of the radial head, fractures of the coronoid process, and a small osteopenic proximal fragment can make the goal of a stable anatomic reduction of all the components of the fracture difficult to achieve. Ipsilateral diaphyseal fracture of the humerus (floating-elbow injury) requiring stable plate fixation may be seen with the high-energy Bado type I injuries.

The **Galeazzi's fracture and fracture of the distal ulna with ligamentous disruption** are fractures of the distal third of the radius or ulna and a dislocation of the distal radioulnar articulation (Fig. 11-5). Both of these fractures are

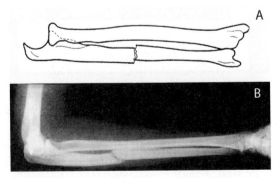

FIG 11-2 *A*, and *B*. Nightstick fractures of the ulna.

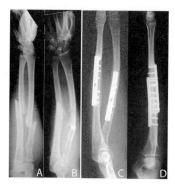

FIG 11-3   *A to D.* Fracture of both bones of the forearm treated with open reduction and internal fixation.

short oblique fractures occurring at the distal metaphyseal diaphyseal junction. The mechanism of injury of the Galeazzi's fracture is forced pronation (usually during a fall on the outstretched hand) or a direct blow. The mirror injury, fracture of the ulna with dislocation of the distal radioulnar articulation, has also been described. Both injuries include disruption of the distal radioulnar joint and a tear of the interosseous membrane from its most distal extent to the fracture of the radius or ulna.

Essex–Lopresti injury (radioulnar dissociation) is a fracture or dislocation of the radial head with disruption of the distal radioulnar articulation and

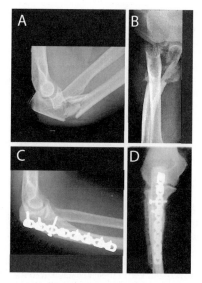

FIG. 11-4   *A to D.* Monteggia's fracture of the proximal ulna associated with posterior dislocation of the radial head, Bado type II. Treated by open reduction and internal fixation. (*Courtesy of Dr. Robert F. Hall, Jr.*)

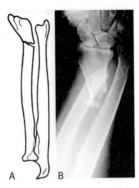

A   B

FIG. 11-5   Galeazzi's fracture: a fracture of the distal radius associated with disruption of the distal radioulnar joint.

tearing of the entire interosseous membrane. Attention may be focused on the injury at the lateral elbow or a Galeazzi-type fracture–dislocation in the distal forearm, but the major component of the injury, radioulnar dissociation, is frequently overlooked. Early diagnosis and appropriate treatment (maintaining a radial capitellar articulation to prevent proximal migration of the radius) is important to obtaining a satisfactory result.

Associated Injuries

Injuries associated with fractures of the forearm include fractures and dislocations of the elbow and wrist, neurovascular injuries, and compartment syndrome. Radiographs of the wrist and elbow determine whether there are associated fractures or dislocations.

Laceration, compression, or stretching of arteries and nerves frequently occurs at the time of the injury. The greater the initial displacement of the fracture, the greater the chance of an associated neurovascular injury. Although the presence of pulses distal to the fracture and capillary refill of the nail beds suggest adequate vascularity, disproportionate unremitting pain, positive stretch signs with passive finger motion, unexplained numbness, and a penetrating injury with excessive swelling are indications for the measurement of compartment pressure or an arteriogram.

The nerve most frequently injured in association with a forearm injury is the posterior interosseous nerve. This is particularly true of Monteggia's fractures. Nerve injury is not uncommon in association with forearm fractures and differs greatly with the type of fracture and the forces creating it. Neurologic injury is identified by a careful neurologic examination of the radial, ulnar, and median nerves before treatment is started.

Compartment syndrome most frequently involves the flexor compartment, but the extensor compartment can also be involved. The patient usually complains of severe pain with dysesthesia. The forearm is tense, and any attempt at passive stretch of the muscles in the compartment is intolerable, with disproportionate exacerbation of the pain. Surgical compartment decompression can be carried out with this clinical picture alone. Repair or stabilization of the skeletal trauma is accomplished at the same time. Measurement of the compartment pressures is done when the patient is unconscious or the clinical picture is uncertain. Compartment pressures above 30 mmHg or high enough to fall within 30 mmHg of the mean diastolic pressure are indications for immediate surgical decompression. This should include the release of the bicipital aponeurosis proximally and the carpal tunnel distally. Since the consequences of a neglected compartment syndrome are so onerous, it is sound advice to proceed with surgical decompression if the question arises.

Diagnosis and Initial Management

History and Physical Examination

There is a history of trauma with pain and swelling in the forearm. There may be deformity. The skin is examined for wounds that may communicate with the fracture. The elbow and distal radioulnar articulation are examined to determine whether they have been injured. Neurologic deficit is infrequent except with penetrating injuries and high-energy open fractures.

Radiographic Examination

Radiographs in the anteroposterior and lateral projections of the forearm, wrist, and elbow are adequate to evaluate most injuries of the forearm. Occasionally, comparison views of the opposite wrist or computed tomography (CT) imaging are helpful in evaluating the relative positions of the distal radius and ulna.

Magnetic resonance imaging (MRI) to obtain axial T2-weighted images with fat suppression as well as ultrasound can be used to determine the integrity of the interosseous membrane when an Essex–Lopresti injury is a consideration.

Initial Management

Initial management involves aligning and splinting the forearm. Displaced or angulated fractures are aligned by administering parenteral analgesia and applying traction across the forearm by suspending the hand from finger traps and hanging 5 to 10 lb of counterforce weight from the arm. Anatomic alignment of fractures that will be managed operatively is not necessary. Some shortening or angulation is acceptable because it will be corrected at surgery. A splint extending from the proximal humerus across the elbow to the metacarpophalangeal joints is applied. The elbow is flexed to 90 degrees with the forearm in neutral rotation. If the radial head cannot be reduced with closed methods following a Monteggia's fracture, open reduction and stabilization are performed within 24 h of injury to minimize the incidence of neurovascular compromise.

Definitive Management

Simple Injuries of the Forearm

Isolated fractures of the ulna (nightstick fractures) that are displaced less than 50%, angulated less than 15 degrees, and in which the interosseous space is maintained are managed nonoperatively. A splint is applied that extends from the elbow to the metacarpophalangeal joints along the ulnar side of the forearm. At 4 weeks, the splint is removed and the forearm lightly wrapped in a compression bandage. A short arm cast is not necessary. Radiographs are obtained at 1, 2, 3, and 6 weeks to confirm that alignment has not changed and the fracture is healing. Isolated undisplaced fractures of the radius can be managed in a long arm cast but must be carefully followed because they tend to displace. Any displacement or angulation that occurs should be treated by immediate open reduction and internal fixation because it will invariably progress. Isolated fractures of the radius and ulna that are displaced or angulated or in which the interosseous space is compromised are treated with open reduction and internal fixation (Fig. 11-3). Fractures of the proximal half of the radius can be approached dorsally, as described by Thompson (1918), or preferably volarly, as described by Henry (1950); fractures of the distal half of the radius are approached volarly. Fractures of the ulna are approached along the subcutaneous border. The fracture is reduced and stabilized with a dynamic compression plate (DCP). If more than half the cortex is comminuted, the fracture is grafted with autogenous cancellous bone.

Intramedullary nailing can be used for segmental fractures and fractures of the proximal radius, in which the posterior interosseous nerve is vulnerable to injury during the exposure. The nails are inserted ulnar to Lister's tubercle for fractures of the radius and through the olecranon for fractures of the ulna. The nails are bent to restore the normal bow of the radius and ulna, thus reestablishing the interosseous space. Intramedullary nailing does not provide fracture fixation equal to plate fixation; thus rehabilitation is delayed. Its main advantage lies in its ability to provide fracture alignment in situations where the conditions for solid plate fixation do not exist (i.e., extreme comminution).

Postoperatively, active range of motion of the forearm, wrist, and elbow is encouraged. If the fracture has been plated, it is assessed as being healed when trabeculae cross the fracture radiographically. This may take up to 6 months. Displacement or angulation indicates loss of fixation. The appearance of callus suggests that fixation is tenuous, but it will also be seen with comminution and bone grafting. Healing of fractures that have been stabilized with an intramedullary nail may be easier to assess because the fixation is not rigid and the patient's symptoms correlate with the amount of healing.

Complex Injuries

An important part of management of complex injuries is adequate treatment of all the components.

A Monteggia's fracture is managed operatively (Fig. 11-4). The ulnar fracture must be anatomically reduced and plated with a 3.5-mm DCP (tension-band fixation and semitubular plates are inadequate). Since the proximal fragment is usually short and osteopenic, application of this plate to the subcutaneous surface of the ulna with contouring around the proximal end of the olecranon is critical.

The fracture of the coronoid process and comminuted fracture of the radial head frequently associated with Bado type II fractures requires anatomic reduction and stable fixation of the coronoid process and preservation of the radial head with reduction and fixation if possible. Excision of the radial head without prosthetic replacement will be problematic: for those fractures that are severely displaced and comminuted, radial head excision and replacement is required.

Intraoperative radiographs are obtained to confirm that the reduction is anatomic and that the coronoid process and radial head are reduced. Postoperatively, a long arm splint is applied with the elbow in 90 degrees of flexion and the forearm in neutral rotation. Early mobilization of the elbow and forearm within the limits imposed by the soft tissue injury is important so as to reduce the risk of synostosis.

The less common Bado type I fracture is frequently a high-energy injury with neurovascular damage, compartment syndrome, and ipsilateral fracture of the humerus. Reduction and fixation of the ulnar fracture with a 3.5-mm DCP will usually result in reduction of the radial head dislocation. Any associated fracture of the humerus should be treated with open reduction and internal fixation. Galeazzi's fractures and fractures of the distal ulna with radioulnar joint disruption are managed with rigid plating. The surgical exposure is from a volar approach for the radius and through a skin incision parallel with its subcutaneous border for the ulna. When the ulnar styloid is avulsed with the triangular fibrocartilage, it is reduced and stabilized with Kirschner wires and a figure-of-eight tension band. The distal radioulnar joint is usually reduced when the radial fracture is plated and radial length is restored. If the distal radioulnar joint is unstable, it can be reduced by supinating the forearm. If it is still unstable in this position, Kirschner-wire fixation between the ulna and radius is carried out just proximal to the sigmoid notch. Inability to reduce the distal radioulnar joint is associated with interposition of the triangular fibrocartilage. A short arm splint is applied unless the distal radioulnar joint requires additional protection with immobilization in supination.

Radioulnar dissociation (Essex–Lopresti injury) is an injury to the distal radioulnar joint and ipsilateral radiohumeral joint associated with disruption of the interosseous membrane. Excision of the radial head for a comminuted fracture when there is an associated injury at the distal radioulnar joint is contraindicated because proximal migration of the radius is likely to occur. It is recommended that the acute injury be treated with repair of the radiohumeral joint, open reduction and internal fixation of any distal forearm fractures, and immobilization of the distal radioulnar joint in a long arm cast with the forearm in supination. Open reduction with Kirschner-wire fixation of the ulna to the radius and repair of the distal radioulnar ligaments should be undertaken if the distal radioulnar joint is unstable.

Open Fractures of the Radius and Ulna

Open fractures of the forearm are classified into three types. Type I is associated with a clean wound and the laceration is shorter than 1 cm. Type II is associated with a laceration longer than 1 cm but without extensive soft tissue damage. The usual cause of type I and type II wounding is penetration from the inside out by one of the fractured bone ends. Type III open fractures are associated with extensive soft tissue damage or a segmental fracture and have been subdivided into type IIIA injuries from gunshots with adequate soft tissue coverage and type IIIB contaminated environment injuries such as farm or lake injuries with extensive soft tissue damage and significant periosteal stripping associated with significant contamination that is not necessarily visible. There may be foreign material hidden in the depths of the wound, or the environment itself may be associated with large numbers of bacterial organisms, as will be present in a polluted lake or farmyard. Type IIIC open fractures are associated with vascular injury necessitating reanastomosis.

The primary consideration in treating these wounds is to prevent soft tissue and bone infection. For this to be accomplished, immediate adequate exploration and debridement of the wound must be performed. Tetanus pro-phylaxis is crucial. The wound should be cleaned and dressed in the emer-gency room and intravenous antibiotic treatment started. The patient is taken to the operating room, where a general anesthetic or an adequate regional anesthetic that allows the use of the tourniquet is given. After limb prepara-tion, the wounds are extended so that an adequate exploration of the soft tissue and bone injury can be performed. Devitalized skin, fascia, muscle, and bone are removed, and an extensive fasciotomy is performed both proximal and dis-tal to the wound so that devitalized soft tissue and foreign material will not go unnoticed. Neurovascular structures in the vicinity of the wound are ex-posed so that their integrity can be determined. The wound is thoroughly irri-gated with an antibiotic solution.

Type I, II, and IIIA open fractures can generally be stabilized with primary internal fixation by using a plate and screws, as described for closed frac-tures; however, the wounds should be left open for delayed wound closure in 3 to 5 days. Primary wound closure of an adequately explored and cleaned type I or type II inside-out fracture in a clean environment in an otherwise healthy patient is acceptable. Intravenous antibiotics are continued for 4 to 5 days unless a wound infection occurs.

Type IIIB and IIIC open fractures are generally not suitable for internal fixation. A half-pin external fixator or pins and plaster can be used to maintain reduction of these fractures. After the soft tissues have healed without infec-tion, delayed cancellous bone grafting or delayed open reduction and internal fixation with plate and screws and cancellous bone grafting can be performed.

COMPLICATIONS

The complications of injuries of the forearm include malunion, nonunion, syn-ostosis (associated with heterotopic ossification), infection, refracture, and subluxation or posttraumatic arthrosis of the distal or proximal radioulnar joints.

Nonunion of these fractures occurs most frequently when an inadequate internal fixation has been performed. It is also associated with more severe injuries (e.g., open fracture, comminution), failure to do primary cancellous bone grafting when indicated, and infection. To avoid failure of internal fixa-tion, 3.5-mm dynamic compression plates should be used, with an adequate number of cortices (generally six cortices: three screws) fixed proximal and distal to the fracture. Semitubular plates do not provide adequate fixation. Symptomatic nonunions are reduced, stabilized with an adequate dynamic compression plate, and grafted with autogenous cancellous bone. Segmental defects of the radius and/or ulna with an adequate soft tissue environment of healthy muscle and minimal scarring can also be managed this way with bridge plating.

Malunion should be prevented by performing open reduction and internal fixation for most diaphyseal forearm fractures. The major cause for malunion following a fracture of the shaft of the radius or ulna is failure to obtain ade-quate radiographic follow-up and perform open reduction and internal fixation as soon as an undisplaced fracture begins to displace (Fig. 11-6). Corrective osteotomy is most efficacious when performed as soon as possible after the in-jury. Satisfactory osseous contact for stable internal fixation can be difficult to obtain. Complications increase, and gains in range of forearm rotation de-crease in patients undergoing operative treatment more than 1 year after the

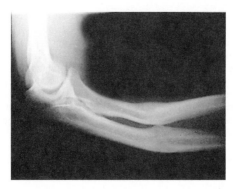

FIG. 11-6   This malunion of a fracture of both bones of the forearm was initially undisplaced. It resulted in a severe cosmetic deformity, with the forearm fixed in neutral rotation.

initial fracture. The usual indications for corrective osteotomy are loss of forearm rotation, cosmetic deformity, and instability of the distal radioulnar joint.

Wound infection is managed by returning the patient to the operating room, where the wound can be adequately opened and cleaned. Cultures are obtained. If a plate and screws are still providing adequate fixation, they are left in place. The wound is left open and supported with a splint. Delayed wound closure is performed after 5 days if the infection is under control. In some instances, the wound will be left open and allowed to heal secondarily, with skin grafting as required. The fracture should unite if infection is controlled; however, cancellous bone grafting may be required.

In instances where bone is avascular and fixation is inadequate, priority must be given to preserving or restoring the soft tissue environment (the envelope) by removal of loose implants and debridement of all devitalized tissue. In this situation, the wound is left open and the fracture stabilized with an external fixator that will prevent shortening and allow for local wound care. The assistance of an infectious disease specialist is often helpful.

Nerve injuries are uncommon except for penetrating wounds (i.e., gunshot fractures). The prognosis for these injuries is frequently poor without surgical exploration and repair. This is usually done as a secondary procedure because the extent of nerve damage at the time of primary exploration is difficult to determine.

Compartment syndrome after forearm fracture is not uncommon. It is very important, in performing open reduction and internal fixation, to deflate the tourniquet and provide adequate hemostasis prior to wound closure. The forearm fascia must not be closed.

If the functional impairment is significant, synostosis can be treated by resection after the synostosis has had a chance to mature. Indications of maturity are a well-ossified mass with corticalized margins, a cold bone scan, a normal serum alkaline phosphatase, and the passage of approximately 12 months since the time of the injury.

Heterotopic ossification with synostosis is more frequently encountered following injuries resulting from high-energy trauma or in patients with concomitant head injury. The synostosis is more likely to recur after excision when located in the proximal or distal paraarticular part of the forearm.

Painful subluxation and posttraumatic osteoarthritis of the radioulnar articulations are managed with anti-inflammatory medication or local steroid injection. If these measures fail, distal radioulnar arthrosis can be managed by (1) hemiresection arthroplasty; (2) arthrodesis of the distal radioulnar joint with resection of a 1-cm section of distal ulnar metaphysis to produce a nonunion, thus preserving forearm rotation (Sauve–Kapandji procedure); or (3) a Darrach resection of the distal ulna.

Routine removal of a diaphyseal plate after fracture fixation is not usually necessary or desirable because bone mineral density and grip strength are not affected. Plate removal can be complicated by neurovascular injury and refracture.

SELECTED READINGS

Elstrom JA, Pankovich AM, Egwele R. Extraarticular low velocity gunshot fractures of the radius and ulna. *J Bone Joint Surg* 60A:335–341, 1978.

Grace TG, Eversman WW Jr. Forearm fractures: treatment by rigid fixation with early motion. *J Bone Joint Surg* 62A:433–438, 1980.

Henry AK. *Extensile Exposure Applied to Limb Surgery.* Edinburgh: E and S Livingstone, 1950:53–64.

Kapandji procedure in the treatment of chronic posttraumatic derangement of the distal radioulnar joint. *J Bone Joint Surg* 80A:1758–1769, 1998.

Lamey DM, Fernandez DL. Results of the modified Sauve-Kapandji procedure in the treatment of chronic posttraumatic derangement of the distal radioulnar joint. *J Bone Joint Surg* 80A:1758–1769, 1998.

Pollack FH, Pankovich AM, Prieto JJ, Lorenz M. The isolated fracture of the ulnar shaft. Treatment without immobilization. *J Bone Joint Surg* 65A:339–342, 1983.

Reckling FW. Unstable fracture–dislocations of the forearm (Monteggia and Galeazzi lesions). *J Bone Joint Surg* 64A:857–863, 1982.

Rettig ME, Raskin KB. Galeazzi fracture-dislocation: a new treatment-oriented classification. *J Hand Surg* 26-A:228–235, 2001.

Ring D, Allende C, Jafarnia K, et al. Ununited diaphyseal forearm fractures with segmental defects: plate fixation and autogenous cancellous bone-grafting. *J Bone Joint Surg* 86A:2440–2445, 2004.

Ring D, Jupiter JB, Simpson NS. Monteggia fracture in adults. *J Bone Joint Surg* 80A:1733–1744, 1998.

Ring D, Tavakolian J, Kloen P, et al. Loss of alignment after surgical treatment of posterior Monteggia fractures: salvage with dorsal contoured plating. *J Hand Surg* 29A:694–702, 2004.

Starch DW, Dabezies EJ. Magnetic resonance imaging of interosseous membrane of the forearm. *J Bone Joint Surg* 83A:235–238, 2001.

Trousdale RT, Amadio PC, Cooney WP, Morrey BF. Radio-ulnar dissociation. A review of twenty cases. *J Bone Joint Surg* 74A:1486–1497, 1992.

Trousdale RT, Linscheid RL. Operative treatment of malunited fractures of the forearm. *J Bone Joint Surg* 77A:894–902, 1995.

12 | Fractures of the Distal Radius and Injuries of the Distal Radioulnar Joint

Santiago A. Lozano C.   Jesse Bernard Jupiter

This chapter comprises fractures of the distal radius and dislocations of the distal radioulnar joint (DRUJ).

FUNCTIONAL ANATOMY

Anatomic considerations of the distal radius with regard to the skeleton, ligaments, and other soft tissue structures are important to understanding mechanisms of trauma, diagnosis, biomechanics, classifications of injury, and treatment alternatives.

The distal radius is an essential articular component of the wrist joint. This articulation depends on the integrity of both the ligamentous and osseous structures responsible for wrist mobility and the capacity to support an axial load.

Anatomically, the thickness of the cortical bone of the radius decreases at the metaphyseal flare, while the amount of cancellous bone increases. This structural transition of bone tissue forms a weak zone, predisposing this region to fracture, especially in osteoporotic patients.

The dorsal surface of the distal radius is thin and convex, serving as a fulcrum for the extensor tendons. Lister's tubercle represents an additional prominence functioning as a fulcrum for the extensor pollicis longus. The dorsal radiocarpal ligaments originate from the dorsal rim of the radius and course obliquely and ulnarly toward the scaphoid and triquetrum, attaching distally on their dorsal aspect. There is also a significant dorsal intercarpal ligament (Fig. 12-1).

The palmar surface of the radius is flat and extends volarly in a gentle curve. The pronator quadratus covers most of the distal metaphyseal flare, extending to insert on the volar surface of the distal ulna. The intracapsular palmar radiocarpal ligament has three parts: the radioscapholunate ligament (ligament of Testut, which controls scaphoid rotation) arises from a tubercle in the middle of this radiopalmar aspect, while the radiotriquetal and radioscaphocapitate ligaments arise from the volar radial styloid. The radial collateral ligament originates from the volar ridge of the styloid (Fig. 12-2).

The articular end of the radius slopes in an ulnopalmar direction; as a result, the proximal carpal row has a natural tendency to slide in an ulnar direction. The distal radial articular surface has three articular facets covered by hyaline cartilage: the scaphoid fossa, the lunate fossa, and the sigmoid notch. A central ridge, traversing from the dorsal to the palmar surface, divides the scaphoid and lunate facets. Each facet is concave in both anteroposterior and radioulnar planes (Fig. 12-3). The third distinct articular surface of the distal radius is the sigmoid notch. It is semicylindric in shape and is oriented parallel to the convexity of the ulnar head. It articulates with the ulnar head, whose articular surface (two-thirds of the circumference, or 270 degrees) is covered by hyaline cartilage (Fig. 12-4). This trochoid articulation is responsible for

155

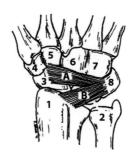

FIG. 12-1   Posterior view of the wrist. (1) Radius. (2) Ulna. (3) Scaphoid. (4) Trapezium. (5) Trapezoid. (6) Capitate. (7) Hamate. (8) Triquetrum. *A.* Dorsal intercarpal ligament. *B.* Dorsal radiocarpal ligament. (*Reproduced by permission of* J Am Acad Ortho Surg.)

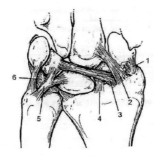

FIG. 12-2   Anterior view of the wrist. (1) Radial collateral ligament. (2) Radioscaphocapitate ligament. (3) Radiolunotriquetral ligament. (4) Radioscapholunate ligament. (5) Ulnolunate ligaments. (6) Meniscus homologus. (*Reproduced by permission of* J Am Acad Ortho Surg.)

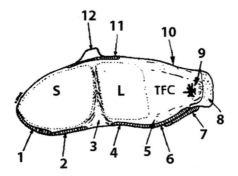

FIG. 12-3   Distal articular aspect of the radius. (S) Scaphoid fossa. (L) Lunate fossa. (TFCC) Triangular fibrocartilage complex. (1) Radioscaphocapite ligament. (2) Radiolunotriquetral Ligament. (3) Interfossal ridge. (4) Radioscapholunate ligament. (5) Palmar radioulnar ligament. (6) Ulnolunate ligament. (7) Ulnocapitate ligament. (8) Ulnar styloid. (9) Prestyloid recess. (10) Dorsal radioulnar ligament. (11) Dorsal radiocarpal ligament. (12) Lister's tubercle. (*Reproduced by permission of the American Society for Surgery of the Hand.*)

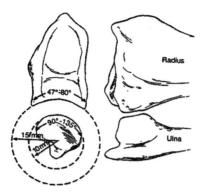

FIG. 12-4 Radioulnar joint. Articulation between the sigmoid notch of the radius and the ulnar head. The arc covered with articular cartilage is greater for the ulnar head than for the sigmoid notch, while the radius of curvature is greater for the sigmoid notch than for the ulnar head. (*Reproduced by permission of the American Society for Surgery of the Hand.*)

pronosupination of the distal forearm and wrist. Rotation of the radius about the ulna is accompanied by a translational displacement of the ulna. During supination, the ulnar head displaces anteriorly in the sigmoid notch; during pronation, it moves dorsally.

The final relevant structure is the triangular fibrocartilage. This important stabilizer originates from the ulnar side of the lunate fossa and extends to the base of the ulnar styloid process. Its palmar and dorsal edges are thickened, blending into the dorsal and volar radioulnar ligaments, which represent major stabilizers of the DRUJ (Fig. 12-3). Other stabilizers of the DRUJ include the joint capsule, the triangular fibrocartilage, the interosseous membrane, the ulnocarpal ligaments, and the sheath of the extensor carpi ullnaris.

Dynamic and static stability of the radiocarpal joint is the result of both the extrinsic and interosseous ligaments of the wrist. The interosseous scapholunate and interosseous lunotriquetral ligaments stabilize the proximal row of carpal bones as a unit.

The flexor and extensor tendons pass across the distal aspect of the radius to make insertions on the metacarpal bases or the phalanges (only the flexor carpi ulnaris inserts on the carpus at the pisiform). The brachioradialis muscle, through its insertion on the distal radius, can act as a deforming force on fracture fragments.

The extensor system is organized into six retinacular compartments through which the extensor tendons run. Although rarely injured in the acute setting, total or partial ruptures of the extensor pollicis longus occur occasionally in association with distal radial fractures.

The volar distal radius is located just proximal to the carpal tunnel. Fractures of the distal radius can increase the pressure inside this structure and directly affect the median nerve (by inflammation, accumulation of blood, compression by displaced fragments, or laceration), producing symptoms and signs of acute median nerve dysfunction. It is axiomatic that neurovascular examination is necessary during the initial assessment of a patient.

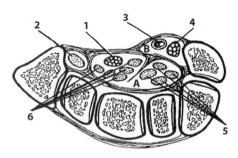

FIG. 12-5   Carpal (*A*) and Guyon's (*B*) tunnels. (1) Median nerve. (2) Flexor pollicis longus. (3) Ulnar artery. (4) Ulnar nerve. (5) Deep flexor tendons. (6) Superficial flexor tendons.

On the ulnar side, the flexor carpi ulnaris, ulnar artery, and ulnar nerve lie volar and ulnar to the distal radius. The ulnar nerve and artery pass through Guyon's canal into the hand (Fig. 12-5).

The anatomic relationship of the components described above and their functional interaction ensure wrist mobility and stability. It is therefore important to restore these anatomic characteristics in treating a fracture of the distal radius.

BIOMECHANICS OF THE WRIST

Kinematics

For clinical purposes, wrist motion is evaluated in two cardinal axes that compose the cone of combined movements in all four directions known as circumduction: palmar flexion, wrist extension, and radioulnar deviation. There are variations in the angular displacement measured in degrees, but normal wrist mobility will fall in the ranges described in Table 12-1.

Several investigators have attempted to define the "minimal functional range of motion" required by a patient to perform activities of daily living for self-care and independent functioning. These studies revealed that most functional activities could be accomplished with 40 degrees of extension, 40 degrees of palmar flexion, and 40 degrees of combined radioulnar deviation.

Palmar Flexion-Extension

The greater axis of motion of the wrist is that of flexion and extension. During normal wrist motion, there is a difference in movement between the proximal and distal rows of carpal bones as well as between the bones of the proximal

TABLE 12-1 Wrist Motion Range

Movement	Normal range	Functional range
Flexion	80 ± 5 degrees	40 degrees
Extension	70 ± 5 degrees	40 degrees
Radial deviation	20 ± 5 degrees	40° of combined
Ulnar deviation	40 ± 5 degrees	radioulnar deviation

row itself. In extension, the wrist deviates radially; in flexion, ulnar deviation occurs.

Radioulnar Deviation

As seen in the flexion-extension arc, the distal row and hand displace as a unit during radioulnar deviation. During radial deviation, the proximal row (triquetrum, lunate, and scaphoid) flexes and deviates radially. In contrast, during ulnar deviation, the proximal carpal row extends, deviates ulnarward, and pronates. The extension-flexion motion is greater than that of radioulnar deviation.

Residual deformity following a distal radial fracture, such as increased dorsal or volar angulation, shortening, and/or losses of angular inclination can significantly affect the kinematics of the wrist. In normal conditions, approximately 80% of the force is transmitted across the radiocarpal joint and 20% across the ulnocarpal joint space; some movements, such as forearm pronation, increase the transmission of ulnocarpal joint force. This phenomenon seen in pronation has been explained by the relative distal prominence of the ulna that occurs in the forearm while it pronates. During ulnar deviation, ulnocarpal forces increase up to 30%, while the radiocarpal forces increase up to 87% during radial deviation.

When a radial fracture heals with increased dorsal angulation as well as loss of normal ulnar inclination of the distal articular surface, forces placed on the distal ulna proportionally increase, resulting in ulnar wrist pain and impingement as well as degeneration or ruptures of the triangular fibrocartilage complex (TFCC). These changes may occur with as little as 10 to 20 degrees of alteration in distal radial alignment. Shortening of the radius as it relates to the distal ulna also affects load patterns, leading to ulnar impingement and TFCC disruption.

EPIDEMIOLOGY

Distal radial fractures have a bimodal distribution in the population regarding prevalence. Osteopenic women in their fifties or sixties who experience low-energy trauma after a fall represent the dominant group. The most common pattern in this group is an extraarticular "bending" type injury. Conversely, younger males in their teens and twenties, with denser bone, characterize the second group. These fractures result from higher impact and typically have more comminution and displacement.

IMAGING DIAGNOSIS

Accurate diagnosis and careful preoperative planning are crucial in the treatment of distal radial fractures. Standard initial radiographs must include the anteroposterior (AP), lateral (Lat), and oblique (Obl) views to reveal the fracture pattern as well as the extent and direction of the initial displacement.

Oblique projections are very useful to identify displacement of fractures that involve the articular surface. The AP projection will help to define whether a fracture involves the intraarticular surface and to verify the presence of associated intracapsular or interosseous injuries to the carpal ligament. Associated intracarpal lesions may be suspected if there is a scapholunate space greater than 2 to 3 mm (the "Terry Thomas sign"); a loss of symmetry in the articular surface of the proximal carpal row (Gilula's lines); or shortening or translation of the carpus (Fig. 12-6).

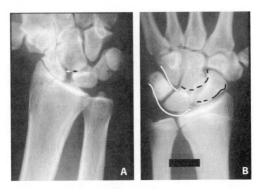

FIG. 12-6   Radiographic findings of soft tissue lesion. *A.* "Terry Thomas" sign (interosseous rupture of the scapholunate ligament). *B.* Disruption of Gilula's arches (rupture of interosseous ligament).

Cardinal measurements in the AP projection include radial height (normal average 12 mm), ulnar tilt of the radius (average 23 degrees), radial width (usually within 1 mm of that of the contralateral side), and the alignment of the distal radioulnar joint (Fig. 12-7). On the lateral view, volar tilt is the relevant measurement. It is always important to be certain that the lateral projection is a "true" lateral view. The best criterion to confirm that the radiograph is a true lateral view is to observe the palmar cortex of the pisiform, lunate, and capitate, in this order, from the volar to the dorsal aspect of the radius. **(For radiographic measurement parameters, see Table 12-2 and Fig. 12-7).** Films taken after a fracture has been reduced help to quantify residual deformity and comminution to determine if further treatment is necessary.

In cases of severe comminution with complex intraarticular patterns of fracture, imaging by computed tomography (CT) allows for more accurate assessment of displacement as well as the number and orientation of fragments. New technologies such as three-dimensional CT reconstruction offer a better understanding of the fracture and allow more accurate planning of treatment for complex injuries.

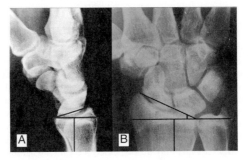

FIG. 12-7   Radiographic measurement technique. *A.* Lateral view, palmar tilt (average 11 degrees). *B.* Anteroposterior view, radial inclination (average 23 degrees).

TABLE 12-2 Radiographic Measurements

Measure	Description	Normal values
Radial inclination (PA view)	Angle between a line drawn from the tip of the radial styloid to the most distal ulnar aspect of the lunate facet and a line perpendicular to the longitudinal axis of the radius	22 ± 3 degrees
Radial length (PA view)	Longitudinal difference between a line perpendicular to the long axis of the radius drawn at the radial styloid and another line tangential to the distal articular surface of the ulna.	11 ± 3 mm
Ulnar variance (PA view)	Perpendicular line to the radius long axis at the sigmoid notch. Then quantify how much ulnar head is distal to that line.	Axial shortening Grade 0: <3 mm Grade 1: 3–5 mm Grade 2: >5 mm
Radial tilt (lateral view)	Line through the volar and dorsal margins of the distal radius compared to a perpendicular line to the long axis of the radial shaft	11 ± 3 degrees
Radial shift (PA view)	Distance between the longitudinal axis of the radius and a line drawn tangential to the radial styloid	Bilateral comparison

MECHANISM OF INJURY

Distal radial fractures can be subdivided by their mechanism of injury in five groups: (1) bending extraarticular fractures, (2) shearing intraarticular fractures, (3) compression intraarticular fractures, (4) avulsion fractures of the radial or ulnar styloid with radiocarpal subluxation, and (5) complex high-energy fractures.

Bending fractures (Colles' and Smith's fractures) are the result of forces over the thin metaphyseal cortex (the bone fails in tension on one cortex as the opposite cortex is compressed). Commonly the scapholunate complex transmits the force of the impact to the dorsal rim of the radial articular surface, creating comminution in the dorsal cortex as the volar cortex fails in tension.

Shearing fractures (volar Barton, dorsal Barton's, and chauffeur) result from axial transference of forces into the distal radius through the proximal carpal bones. It has been postulated that these shearing forces occur when the wrist is locked in either palmar flexion (gripping handlebars of a bike or motorcycle) or when it is fixed in extension (driving a car). These forces lead to dorsal Barton or volar (reverse) Barton's fractures respectively. The cardinal feature is a coronal plane articular fracture with subluxation of the carpus from the remaining (intact) articular surface. The chauffeur fracture is a shear fracture involving the radial styloid.

Compression fracture mechanisms have been described since the midnineteenth century, when Voillemier in 1842 reported the injury of a patient who fell from a three-story height. In 1929, Stevens described a postero-medial impaction fracture of the radius that occurred with the arm in full pronation. Later, Scheck (who coined the term *die punch* to describe the lunate fossa fracture) suggested that both compression and bending forces occur with the lunate facet fracture. Melone extended the analysis of this mechanism and developed the concept of the "medial complex" to describe the compromise of the lunate fossa (with dorsal and volar medial facets), ligamentous attachments, the proximal carpal row, and the ulnar styloid. The lunate is very often the focus of direct compression, and it has been suggested that the injury to the hand with the wrist extended drives the lunate into the dorsal aspect of the distal radius, causing the fracture on the dorsal side. At high velocities wider separation of the lunate fossa can be expected; translation and rotational displacements of 180 degrees of the palmar medial facet fragment can be seen.

Avulsion fractures of ligamentous attachments include radial and ulnar styloid fractures. A torsional force has been implicated in this mechanism of trauma. Carpal displacement is common with this injury, making treatment difficult.

High-energy fractures are a combination of the bending, shearing, compression, and avulsion forces outlined above, with greater comminution.

CLASSIFICATION SYSTEMS

Several formal systems have been proposed to classify distal radial fractures according to the mechanism of trauma and/or morphologic characteristics, recommended treatment, and prognosis. The more comprehensive classifications include that proposed by Castaing (1964) and another by Frykman (1967); the latter unfortunately fails to provide relevant details about the extent and direction of articular fracture displacement. Melone proposed a system including the impaction type of injury of the end of the radius, considering four components: the radial shaft, radial styloid, dorsomedial portion of the lunate facet, and palmar medial portion of the lunate facet.

The most versatile and detailed classification system is perhaps that established by Muller et al. (1990). The basis of this method is the division of all fractures of a bone segment into three types, with further subdivision in three groups, each one with subgroups. This system has an ascending order of severity defined by the morphologic findings, difficulties of treatment, and prognosis related to the fracture.

Type A

Distal radial fractures not involving the articular surface (Colles' and Smith's fractures) fall into this type (Fig. 12-8*A* and *B*).

Type B

This group comprises are distal radial fractures involving part of the articular surface (Fig. 12-9). These shearing fractures are subdivided into three groups: B1: fractures involving injuries in the sagittal plane (radial styloid, cuneiform and lunate facet fractures); B2: fractures in the coronal plane affecting the dorsal aspect (Barton's fracture), and B3: fractures of the volar aspect, or reverse Barton's fracture. The number of fracture fragments (Fig. 12-10*A* to *C*) determines an additional subdivision of these subgroups.

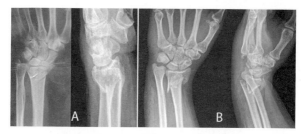

FIG. 12-8   AO fractures group A (extraarticular fractures). *A.* Colles' fracture, anteroposterior and lateral radiographs. *B.* Smith's fracture, anteroposterior and lateral radiographs. (*Courtesy of David Ring, M.D.*)

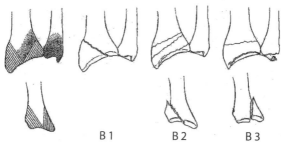

FIG. 12-9   Muller classification (AO) of intraarticular shearing fractures group. Group B1: Fractures involving the sagittal plane. Group B2: Fractures of the dorsal margin, or Barton's fracture. Group B3: Fractures of the volar margin, or reverse Barton's fracture.

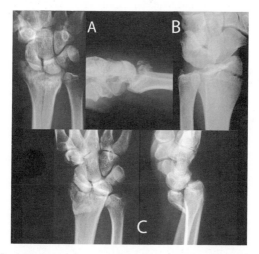

FIG. 12-10   Muller classification (AO) intraarticular shearing fractures group (AO group B). *A.* Dorsal Barton's fracture. Group B2: anteroposterior and lateral radiographs. (*Courtesy of Dr. Mark S. Cohen.*) *B.* Chauffeur fracture. Group B1: radial styloid fracture. Anteroposterior radiograph. *C.* Volar Barton's fracture. Group B3: anteroposterior and lateral radiographs.

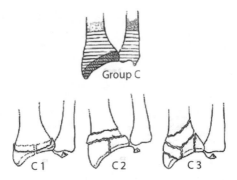

FIG. 12-11   Muller classification (AO) intraarticular compressive fractures group. C1: Two fragment intraarticular fracture without multifragmented metaphysis. C2: Intraarticular fracture with multifragmented metaphysis. C3: Comminution of articular surface.

Type C

These are distal radial fractures involving a complete articular surface injury (Fig. 12-11). The mechanism in general is compressive. They are classified as follows: C1, two-fragment intraarticular fracture without metaphyseal fragmentation; C2, two-fragment intraarticular fracture with multifragmented metaphysis; C3, fractures with comminution of the articular surface. Comminution is defined as involvement of more than 50% of the metaphysis as seen on any radiograph, comminution of at least two cortices of the metaphysis, or greater than 2.0-mm shortening of the radius. These C1, C2, and C3 groups are further divided according to the number of fragments (Fig. 12-12*A* and *B*).

TREATMENT

Initial Treatment

Treatment decisions will be based on an understanding of the fracture pattern, any associated soft tissue injury, and the functional status of the patient. The

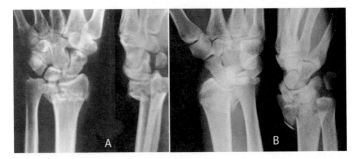

FIG. 12-12   Muller classification (AO) intraarticular compressive fractures group. *A*. C1 Anteroposterior and lateral radiographs. *B*. C3 Anteroposterior and lateral radiographs.

open fractures will require debridement and irrigation in the operating room plus the use of parenteral antibiotics. Highly displaced fractures will benefit from early reduction, even if it is not definitive, because it allows the achievement of reasonable alignment that may reduce the incidence and severity of neurovascular damage.

Neurovascular conditions such as acute carpal tunnel and compartment syndrome require early decompression.

The next step is to have a good understanding of the fracture itself. The mechanism of trauma, the fracture pattern, the displacement of the fragments and their position, and the degree of stability are key points of consideration in determining whether surgical treatment is needed as opposed to closed reduction and cast immobilization.

Anatomic correction of displaced articular surfaces is crucial, as there is strong evidence from clinical and biomechanical studies that arthrosis may develop with articular displacement of 2 mm or greater. Pathologic consequences such as posttraumatic wrist arthritis, midcarpal instability, pain, stiffness, reduction in grip strength (more than 50%), and carpal subluxation with wrist instability may result because of a malunited intra- and/or extraarticular fracture.

Useful parameters to determine whether the anatomy of a fracture indicates instability and will need surgical stabilization are cited in Table 12-3. Surgical intervention becomes an important consideration when an acceptable reduction cannot be either achieved or maintained with cast immobilization.

Definitive Treatment

Different options exist for each type of fracture. An analysis of important points and recommendations for treatment of each type of fracture is offered below.

Nondisplaced Intra- and Extraarticular Stable Fractures

These patients are best treated with short casts unless the fracture is associated with severe soft tissue swelling. Initial evaluation is usually followed by temporary immobilization in a sugar-tongs splint. Clinical and x-ray follow-up should be done within 1week. If the position is maintained, a short arm cast is applied; it is used for a period of 4 to 6 weeks.and then removed (Fig. 12-13).

Displaced Extraarticular Fractures

This type of fracture can be displaced dorsally (Colles' fracture) (Fig. 12-8A) or volarly (Smith fracture) (Fig. 12-8B). Displaced volar or Smith's fractures are intrinsically unstable. Flexor muscles across the wrist exert shearing forces over the fracture site. Once the displacement is evident on the initial films, reduction and fixation are indicated. The option for treatment with unstable volar fractures includes a closed reduction and percutaneus Kirschner-wire fixation with a cast or an external fixator or open reduction and plate-and-screw fixation. Radiographs are taken weekly to verify no displacement for the

TABLE 12-3 Factors Associated with Instability

1. Excessive comminution[a]
2. Initial loss of 15 mm or more of radial length
3. Initial dorsal tilt of 20 or more degrees

[a]Comminution in the volar and dorsal cortex is seen in postreduction films.

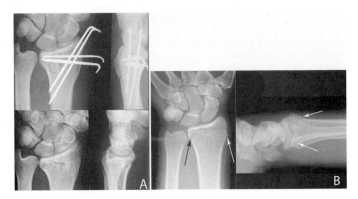

FIG. 12-13 Nondisplaced fractures. *A.* Intraarticular nondisplaced fracture, anteroposterior and lateral radiographs. *B.* Extraarticular nondisplaced fracture. Anterposterior and lateral radiographs.

first 3 weeks. If alignment is maintained after 3 weeks, the cast and K wire are maintained for an additional 3 weeks. At this point, the cast is removed and physical therapy is undertaken to gain range of motion during the next 6 to 8 weeks.

Dorsally displaced Colles' fractures should be reduced if greater than 5 mm of radial length is lost or more than 10 degrees of dorsal tilt is present. Reduction is done under parenteral analgesia, hematoma block, and regional or general anesthesia. Fracture reduction starts with finger-trap traction, suspending the limb by the thumb and index finger with countertraction of 10 to 20 lb for a period of 5 to 10 min to disimpact the fracture.

Manipulation starts with maximum extension of the wrist and then flexion while the surgeon's thumbs mold the distal radius by pressing it over the dorsal and radial surfaces. The distal fragment is pushed volarly until volar cortical apposition is achieved. The wrist is splinted in modest flexion (10 to 20 degrees) and ulnar deviation with a sugar-tongs splint. If a cast is to be applied, it is prudent to split it to allow for swelling and thus avoid complications. After complete reduction and immobilization, postreduction films are taken to confirm the quality and stability of the reduction. The patient should receive instructions regarding cast care, antiswelling measures such as elevation and digital range of motion, and signs of neurovascular compression and excessive soft tissue reaction to the injury.

Displaced distal radial fractures are unstable and often redisplacement in the cast can occur. Factors associated with instability are (1) initial loss of radial length greater than 15 mm, (2) excessive comminution, (3) initial dorsal tilt greater than 20 degrees, or (4) comminution of both volar and dorsal cortices (seen in the postreduction films). If these characteristics are present, percutaneus fixation after closed reduction or open reduction plus internal fixation are indicated (Fig. 12-14).

Postreduction follow-up is done weekly for 3 weeks after manipulative reduction of the fracture due to the possibility of redisplacement. If alignment is adequate at this point, the patient is placed in a short arm cast. After 6 weeks, the cast is removed and the rehabilitation protocol is similar to that described for the volar (Smith's) fracture.

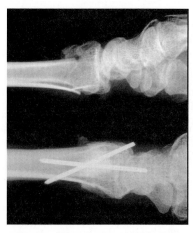

FIG. 12-14   Displaced extraarticular fracture (AO group A) (Colles's fracture) treated with closed reduction and percutaneus pin fixation.

Redisplacement of the fracture requires remanipulation and possibly percutaneus fixation. Attempts at remanipulation after initial reduction should be done in the OR under anesthesia and should be performed within 3 weeks postfracture; closed reduction beyond this time may be not successful. Second reductions are done with the same technique described for fresh fractures; assistance through fluoroscopy is useful while manipulating the fracture. When alignment is achieved, stabilization is done via percutaneus Kirschner-wire fixation. Two 0.062-in. wires are utilized. The first one is inserted through the radial styloid and driven across the fracture focus and out the proximal metaphysis. The second one is placed ulnarly over the dorsal radial cortex and driven perpendicular to the former through a different region than the fracture area, ending in the volar radial metaphysis. Usually, two Kirschner wires are enough, but additional pin fixation may be required. Even though percutaneus fixation had been done, casting or an external fixator is necessary to maintain stability. The pins are cut beneath the skin and removed later in the office.

Intrafocal Kirschner-wire fixation creates a dorsal buttress that counteracts recurrence of the dorsal tilt. Two Kirschner wires are inserted through small dorsal incisions about 2 cm apart at the proximal dorsal margin of the fracture and out the proximal fragment volar cortex at an angle of 45 degrees to buttress the distal fragment (Kapandji technique). An additional pin through the radial styloid can augment the fixation achieved.

Open or Severely Comminuted Extraarticular Fractures

These fractures require initial management, like all open fractures, according to their severity, with debridement and irrigation, antibiotics, and a tetanus toxoid booster. Grades I and II can be reduced closed and fixed percutaneously; grade III injuries require management with an external fixator or open reduction plus internal fixation. Comminution causes instability, and maintenance of reduction by casting only is almost impossible in highly comminuted fractures. Additional measures are necessary; their selection depends on bone quality. In young patients with adequate bone stock, percutaneous pinning might be sufficient. Otherwise, if bone quality is not good, open reduction and plate fixation or external fixation is the best option. Finally, if large defects are seen during open reduction or on fluoroscopy/radiographs, treatment options such as bone grafting and/or bone substitutes should be considered.

Displaced Intraarticular Fractures

The styloid, volar, and dorsal margin shearing fractures make up group B in the AO classification. Treatment options vary according to the subtype. The B1 group (styloid) is subclassified in three types as comminution and instability increase: B1.1 (one fragment), B1.2 (if comminution is present), and B1.3 (if a vertical shear fracture of the lunate facet is seen) (Fig. 12-9). The aims of treatment in this group are the restoration of radial articular congruity, length, alignment, and maintenance of the integrity of supporting volar wrist capsular ligaments. Nondisplaced fractures can be treated with casting above the elbow, with the forearm positioned in supination and the wrist in slight ulnar deviation. Close follow-up with radiographs during the initial 3 weeks is required. Percutaneous fixation after reduction of displaced fractures should be done with Kirschner wires or cannulated screws. The surgeon is obliged to use small skin-only incisions, spread with a hemostat to bone, and insert a drill sleeve in this procedure due to the proximity of sensory branches of the radial nerve. If reduction cannot be achieved with closed maneuvers or if carpal injuries are associated, open reduction and internal fixation is recommended through the dorsoradial aspect approach, taking special care of structures such as the superficial radial nerve, radial artery, and extensor pollicis longus. If comminution is present, dorsal wrist capsulotomy is necessary to define an anatomic reduction.

Dorsal rim fractures (B2) are commonly accompanied by styloid fractures. Failure to recognize intraarticular impaction can be avoided by obtaining a CT scan for surgical planning. Stability after closed reduction and casting is unpredictable. Therefore, if possible, percutaneus fixation protected with an external fixator is the treatment of choice. Alternatively, through a dorsal approach between the second and third extensor compartments, the articular involvement can be directly visualized. Fixation is done with a T or L plate according to the fragment size to restore anatomy and prevent recurrence of deformity.

Volar fractures (reverse Barton's or B3) are intrinsically unstable. If plain radiographs suggest the possibility of more than one fracture line, CT imaging is useful for surgical planning of the management of small impacted fragments. Volar subluxation of the carpus is always associated with shortening and palmar displacement of the fragment. Open reduction and internal fixation is the most reliable method to achieve realignment of articular surface and the radiocarpal joint. The operative approach is through a volar radial incision, developing the interval between the flexor carpi radialis and the radial artery, followed by reflection of pronator quadratus. When symptoms of acute median nerve compression are present, the carpal tunnel is released through an additional palmar incision. In fractures without intraarticular conmination, hyperextension of the wrist over a rolled towel with the forearm in maximal supination is a very useful reduction maneuver. Definitive treatment is done with a volar T plate. The proximal screw is applied first; the second screw goes distally to increase the buttress effect. Multiple fragments can be secured using screws within or outside the plate (Fig. 12-15A and B), with closure over a suction drain for B type fractures.

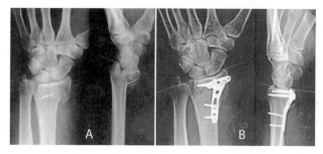

FIG. 12-15   Displaced intraarticular B3 fracture (volar Barton's) treated with a palmar locking plate. *A.* Preoperative radiographs. *B.* Postoperative radiographs.

A bulky dressing and additional splint immobilization is maintained for 14 days. Generally, the patient can resume manual work and some sports about 2 months after surgery.

Compression fractures are known as Group C in the AO classification (Fig. 12-11). The objectives of treatment are relocation of displaced fragments, maintenance of relationship between radial length and distal ulna, and, last, restoration of the normal angulation of the distal metaphyseal segment of the radius. In many fractures, the patterns of compression are predictable. Fractures without comminution are best treated with manipulative reduction via longitudinal traction alone or manipulation and subsequent pinning. These fractures should be treated in the OR under proper anesthesia. The patient should have the iliac crest prepared in case autologus bone grafting is required. Closed reduction manipulation is done through longitudinal traction, wrist flexion, and ulnar deviation. As in the B1 type, reduction and fixation is done with 0.062-in. smooth Kirschner wires if the radial styloid is involved. The wire is obliquely drilled from the radial styloid, which is palmar to slightly ulnar to the metaphyseal flare of the distal radius. When the fracture includes a "die punch" fragment of the lunate facet, reduction is achieved by traction and fixation is done with a transverse subchondral pin from the radial styloid to the sigmoid notch. It provides a buttress effect under the reduced lunate fragment; however, penetrating the sigmoid notch with the pin must be avoided. If satisfactory reduction is not achieved, the fragment can be manipulated through a small incision (1 to 2 cm) with a small elevator.

Intraoperative fluoroscopy is required to guide the elevator and confirm reduction. Bone for grafting should always be available to fill any defects that may be present after the disimpaction of fragments. Small amounts of bone are usually required; thus, bone graft taken with trephine biopsy needles may be sufficient.

When the fracture pattern includes sagittal splits of the two major fragments, reduction and compression assisted with large reduction bone clamps can be done while interfragmentary fixation is completed with Kirschner wires. When closed reduction or minimal open reduction is possible, postoperative management includes long arm casting for 3 weeks, followed by short arm plaster for an additional 3 weeks. Wires are left in place during the complete 6-week period. If the operative reduction required manipulation of impacted fragments or soft tissue swelling is substantial, protection with an external fixator

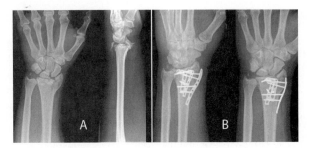

FIG. 12-16   Severely displaced intraarticular C2 fracture treated with plate system (T and L plates, 2.4 mm) *A.* Preoperative radiographs. *B.* Postoperative radiographs.

is preferred rather than the plaster; it should be in place from 4 to 6 weeks (Fig. 12-16).

When the fracture involves the volar lunate facet, this fragment will tend to rotate when traction is applied to the upper limb; as a result, this type of fracture requires reduction through an anterior approach. Continuous intraoperative traction with an external fixator is useful to restore axial length and realign the radial styloid, which is then fixed with Kirschner wires. The volar fragment can be exposed with an ulnar-based incision. The pronator quadratus might be approached through an interval between the ulnar neurovascular bundle and the flexor tendons. This muscle is partially incised and retracted while volar reduction is done without dissecting additional soft tissue. If the fragment is small, fixation takes place via a small Kirschner wire that is retrieved over the dorsum of the radius. If the fragment is large enough, fixation is accomplished with a small (2.7-mm) L or T plate (Fig. 12-17). Finally, if proximal metaphyseal comminution is present, bone grafting and external fixation are crucial to maintain radial length.

It is becoming apparent that with newer, more precise anatomic methods of distal radial fixation, comminuted dorsally displaced and angulated type C fractures can be reduced and stabilized by a volar approach through the bed of the flexor carpi radialis (FCR) tendon with ulnar reflection of the pronator quatratus (Fig. 12-18*A* to *D*).

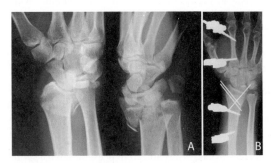

FIG. 12-17   Severely displaced intraarticular C3 fracture treated with percutaneous fixation and an external fixator.

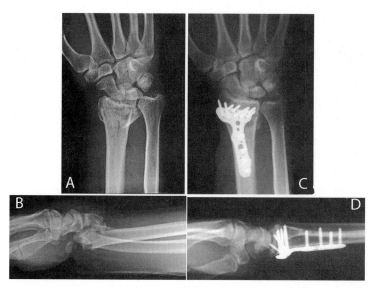

FIG. 12-18   Severely comminuted, dorsally displaced, and angulated type C fracture treated through a volar approach with an anatomic locking plate that permits precise radial styloid fixation. (*Courtesy of Robert F. Hall, Jr., M.D.*)

Complications

Inadequate reduction, loss reduction or fixation, instability of the DRUJ, loss of wrist and forearm motion, neurovascular problems such as acute median nerve compression, compartment syndrome, and complex regional pain syndrome are recognized complications following distal radial fractures.

Acute complications such as median nerve compression or compartment syndrome require immediate surgical decompression. Pain, intense swelling, pain with passive motion, and sensory disturbances in the hand are warning signs of compartment syndrome, in which case compartmental pressures should be measured and/or fasciotomies undertaken. Neglected compartment syndrome has catastrophic consequences for both patient and surgeon.

Complex regional pain syndrome (reflex sympathetic dystrophy) is another well-known but often underrecognized complication of injury; it is characterized by disproportionate pain, trophic processes (stiffness, tissue atrophy, diffuse osteopenia, swelling), autonomic dysfunction (vasoconstriction or dilatation), and impairment of function. Early detection by clinical examination and bone scintigraphy is important. Aggressive physical therapy, tricyclic antidepressants, and stellate ganglion blocks are some options of treatment.

Severe initial articular surface trauma, inadequate articular fracture reduction, and healing with excessive dorsal tilt are demonstrated causes of posttraumatic arthritis with pain, loss of motion, and weakness of grip. Malunion may benefit from a corrective osteotomy.

In general, outcomes following fractures of the distal radius are satisfactory, but careful management is necessary to reduce the number and severity of complications, permit maximum recovery of function for the activities of daily living, and restore patients to their occupations and avocations.

Distal Radioulnar Joint Dislocations

Anatomy

The DRUJ is separated from the carpus by the TFCC. Described by Palmer and Werner (1981), this includes the articular disk (or triangular fibrocartilage proper), the dorsal and palmar radioulnar ligaments, the meniscus homolog, and the extensor carpi ulnaris sheath (or the floor of what is known as the ulnar collateral ligament).

TFCC collagen fibers are oriented along lines of stress; dorsal and palmar radioulnar ligaments are formed by longitudinal fibers.

The articular disc is a fibrocartilage structure that originates from the hyaline cartilage of the distal radiolunate fossa. This hyaline cartilage surrounds the edge of the distal radius and is continuous with the cartilage of the sigmoid notch. The complete hyaline cartilage layer has a different signal during MRI than does fibrocartilage. This difference in signal intensity should not be misinterpreted as a rupture of the articular disc.

In terms of vascularity, dorsal and palmar branches of the anterior interosseous artery and the dorsal and palmar radiocarpal branches of the ulnar artery supply extrinsic vascularity to the DRUJ.

Interosseous vessels from the head of the ulna also vascularize the TFCC through the foveal area. The dorsal and palmar radioulnar ligaments and the peripheral 20% portion of the articular disk have a good blood supply, while the inner 80% of the surface is avascular. These anatomic details are crucial to understand the behavior and prognosis of TFCC ruptures (traumatic or degenerative) described and classified by Palmer, but they are beyond the scope of this chapter.

Last, the stability of the DRUJ is due to a number of different structures. The dorsal and volar radioulnar ligaments and the TFCC are primary considerations; however, the extensor carpi ulnaris subsheath, the interosseous membrane, the pronator quadratus, the ulnocarpal ligaments, and the osseous architecture of the joint have been recognized as additional stabilizers. The importance of each in terms of stability is still being worked out.

Initial diagnosis

Isolated distal radioulnar dislocations are extremely rare; often they are associated with distal forearm fractures such as the Galeazzi fracture. These dislocations associated with fractures are covered in Chap. 11; thus the focus here on isolated dislocations.

The initial presentation of these patients is characterized by ulnar-sided wrist pain associated with crepitation and snapping when the forearm is moved in the pronosupination axis; another typical scenario is ulnar-sided wrist pain with the forearm locked (inability to rotate the forearm).

Dislocations are defined according to the direction in which the ulnar head displaces in relation to the radius. It is very important to appreciate that the ulna is the static bone whereas the radius is the mobile structure. The mechanisms of injury are, in general, extreme pronation for a dorsal subluxation and extreme supination for a palmar dislocation. Typical signs in the physical exam for dorsal dislocation include reduced supination, prominence of the ulnar head, and decreased mobility of the DRUJ. Common findings for volar dislocation are narrowing of the wrist, apparent absence of the ulnar head, and difficulties in pronation. The diagnosis is largely based on physical findings, as the radiographic images are often unsatisfactory due to problems with positioning.

Imaging studies

Radiographs remain the initial diagnostic study. The standard PA view allows evaluation of the fovea and ulnar styloid in "ulnar variance position"; this projection is taken with the shoulder abducted 90 degrees, the elbow flexed at 90 degrees, and the wrist placed in neutral pronosupination. Comparative true lateral views are useful in evaluating alignment of the ulnar head and sigmoid notch. Oblique views are routinely taken in a semipronated and semi-supinated positions. The semisupinated position is very useful to visualize the pisotriquetral joint and the hook of the hamate. Metal markers pointing out the specific area of pain are helpful in identifying sources of wrist pain. X-rays must be comparative. Often, when the diagnosis remains in doubt, CT imaging is necessary.

CT is the imaging modality of choice for evaluating DRUJ subluxation or dislocation. Magnetic resonance imaging (MRI) and MRI arthrography demonstrate better soft tissue detail.

Initial management

Once the diagnosis of subluxation or dislocation of the DRUJ is made, closed reduction should be attempted. This is done under sedation or with regional anesthesia. The maneuver for dorsal dislocation is reduction with the forearm in supination, with the opposite force for a volar dislocation. Articular stability is evaluated after reduction and, if stable, a long arm cast is used for 6 weeks with the forearm immobilized in supination for cases of dorsal dislocation and pronation for volar cases. If closed reduction cannot be accomplished or if postreduction instability remains, open management is indicated.

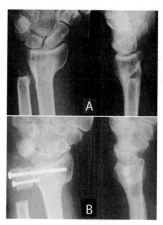

FIG. 12-19 *A.* Darrach procedure. *B.* Sauve-Kapandji procedure

Volar dislocations are approached volarly and the ulna is levered to it original position from under the volar surface of the radius. Dorsal dislocations are approached dorsally. Soft tissue interposition is often the cause of failed closed reduction. This may include osteochondral fragments or tendinous tissues in the sigmoid notch. If the ulnar styloid needs to be repaired, small compression screws or Kirschner wires can be used as internal fixation. If a volar approach is required, internal fixation of the styloid may require an additional incision.

Once reduction is achieved, the wrist is held in neutral rotation, with immobilization maintained for 6 weeks with long arm casting. Radioulnar pinning with Kirschner wires to maintain neutral rotation is best avoided, as complications are frequent.

Complications

Chronic instability, posttraumatic arthrosis, pain and limitation of forearm rotation are the main complications of this injury. Other phenomena such as extensor tendon entrapment and compression of the dorsal ulnar sensory nerve branch have been seen.

Treatment for the principal complications includes excision of the ulnar head (Darrach procedure) (Fig. 12-19A), arthrodesis of the ulnar head to the radius at the sigmoid notch with a more proximal 2-cm resection of the distal ulna to reproduce a nonunion (Sauve-Kapandji procedure) (Fig. 12-19*B*), and hemiresection of the ulnar head (Bowers procedure).

SELECTED READINGS

Chidgey LK. The distal radioulnar joint: problems and solutions. *J Am Acad Orthop Surg* 3:95–109, 1995.

Fernandez DL, Palmer AK. Fractures of the distal radius. In Green DP (ed). *Green's Operative Hand Surgery.* New York: Churchill Livingstone, 1999:929–985.

Fernandez DL, Ring D, Jupiter J, et al. Surgical management of delayed union and nonunion of distal radius fractures. *J Hand Surg* 26:201–209 2001.

Graham TJ. Surgical correction of malunited fractures of the distal radius. *J Am Acad Orthop Surg* 5:270–281, 1997.

Jupiter JB. Complex articular fractures of the distal radius: classification and management. *J Am Acad Orthop Surg* 5:119–129, 1997.

Jupiter JB, Fernandez DL. Complication following distal radial fractures. *J Bone Joint Surg* 83A:1244–1265, 2001.

Jupiter JB, Fernandez DL, Whipple T, et al. Intra–articular fractures of the distal radius: contemporary perspectives. *Instr Course Lect* 47:191–202, 1998.

Knirk JL, Jupiter JB. Intra-articular fractures of the distal end of the radius in young adults. *J Bone Joint Surg* 68:647–659, 1986.

Melone CP Jr. Distal radius fractures: patterns of articular fragmentation. *Orthop Clin North Am* 24:239–253, 1986.

Palmer AK, Werner FW. The triangular fibrocartilage complex of the wrist anatomy and function. *J Hand Surg* 6:153–162, 1981.

Simic PM, Weiland AJ. Fractures of the distal aspect of the radius: changes in treatment over the past two decades. *Instr Course Lect* 52:185–195, 2003.

Strohm PC, Muller CA, Boll T, Pfister U. Two procedures for Kirschner wire osteosynthesis of distal radial fractures. *J Bone Joint Surg* 86A:2621–2628, 2004.

Trumble TE et al. Intra-articular fractures of the distal aspect of the radius. *Instr Course Lect* 48:465–480, 1999.

13 | Fractures and Dislocations of the Wrist

John J. Fernandez

ANATOMY AND KINEMATICS

The unique functional nature of the wrist lets it transmit loads between the hand and forearm in a stable manner while allowing for a wide range of motion in three planes. Because there are no direct tendon attachments to the mobile carpus, the dual functions of stability and mobility are based on the interrelationship of the carpal bones, their shapes, and their ligamentous attachments.

The wrist is defined by the structural and functional anatomy of the distal radius, the distal ulna, and the carpal bones. It begins at the metaphyseal flare of the distal radius and the adjacent ulna, including the distal radioulnar joint. It terminates with the distal row of carpal bones at the carpometacarpal joints of the hand.

Multiple anatomic joints together form the three functional joints of the wrist: the radiocarpal joint, the midcarpal joint, and the distal radioulnar joint. The eight carpal bones are functionally organized into two carpal rows (Fig. 13-1). The proximal carpal row is made up of the scaphoid, lunate, triquetrum, and pisiform. The distal carpal row is made up of the trapezium, trapezoid, capitate, and hamate. The radiocarpal joint is the articulation of the distal radius and ulna and the proximal carpal row. The midcarpal joint is the articulation of the proximal carpal row and the distal carpal row. The distal radioulnar joint is the articulation of the distal radius and distal ulna.

The articular surface of the distal radius is composed of two fossae. The scaphoid fossa is concave and has a triangular outline. The lunate fossa is also concave but, in contrast, has a rectangular outline. The sagittal ridge, a linear elevated area in the sagittal plane of the distal radius, separates the two fossae. The distal articular surface of the radius is inclined ulnarly approximately 22 degrees and tilted palmarly approximately 11 degrees. During power grip, the wrist positions itself optimally into extension and ulnar deviation. The loads placed across the carpus drive it radially and dorsally. This unique angular alignment allows the radius to act as a mechanical buttress countering those forces.

There is a concavity at the ulnar portion of the distal radius, the sigmoid notch, which articulates with the head of the distal ulna, forming the distal radioulnar joint. This joint is principally stabilized by the **triangular fibro-cartilage complex** (TFCC). The TFCC is a fibrocartilage structure that has a triangular shape and originates from the base of the ulnar styloid attaching to the ulnar rim of the distal radius along the lunate fossa. It has a variable thickness and is interposed between the lunate and triquetrum distally and the head of the ulna proximally.

The ligaments of the wrist can be described as intrinsic or extrinsic and are located dorsal or volar. The **intrinsic ligaments**, also known as the interosseous ligaments, have their origins within the carpus itself, linking the carpal bones directly to one another (Fig. 13-1). The most dynamic and important are the scapholunate and lunotriquetral ligaments. These ligaments link the proximal

175

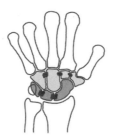

FIG. 13-1   Intrinsic ligaments interconnect the carpal bones, forming a distal carpal row (*light gray*) and a proximal carpal row (*dark gray*).

carpal row together. The **scapholunate interosseous ligament** (SLIL) is U-shaped and composed of three sections: dorsal, proximal, and palmar. The dorsal section, the thickest and strongest, is composed primarily of oriented collagen fibers. The proximal part, the membranous portion, is predominantly fibrocartilage with little structural significance. The **lunotriquetral interosseous ligament** (LTIL), like the SLIL, is also U-shaped and has three similar sections. In contrast to the SLIL, the palmar region of the LTIL is the thickest and strongest.

The **extrinsic ligaments** are defined by dorsal and volar thickenings in the wrist capsule outside the synovial cavity. These link the distal radius and ulna to the carpus. The dorsal extrinsic ligaments form a V-shaped complex with the apex on the triquetrum (Fig. 13-2). The proximal limb, the **dorsal radiocarpal ligament** (DRC), originates from the dorsal rim of the distal radius and extends ulnarly to the dorsum of the triquetrum, with attachments to the underlying lunate and lunotriquetral ligament. The distal limb, the **distal intercarpal ligament** (DIC), originates from the dorsum of the triquetrum and travels radially to the dorsal groove of the scaphoid and trapezium, with attachments to the underlying lunate. This dorsal ligamentous complex helps to stabilize the scaphoid and lunate.

The palmar extrinsic ligaments are arranged in a double-V configuration with the apices pointing distally (Fig. 13-3). The proximal V links the distal

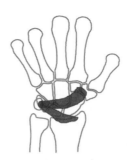

FIG. 13-2   Dorsal extrinsic ligaments arranged as an ulnarly based V. The distal limb is the distal intercarpal ligament. The proximal limb is the dorsal radiocarpal ligament.

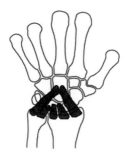

FIG. 13-3 Palmar extrinsic ligaments arranged in a double-V configuration. Ligaments from left to right: ulnotriquetral-triquetrocapitate, ulnolunate, short radiolunate, long radiolunate, and radioscaphocapitate. The "space of Poirier" is the relative weak spot over the midcarpal joint between the capitate and lunate.

radius and ulna to the proximal carpal row. The radial limb is the long radiolunate ligament. The ulnar limb includes the short radiolunate ligament and the ulnolunate ligament. The distal V, also known as the deltoid ligament or arcuate ligament, links the distal carpal row to the proximal carpal row and distal radius and ulna. The radial limb is the radioscaphocapitate ligament, while the ulnar limb includes the triquetrocapitate ligament and the ulnotriquetral ligament. At the capitolunate joint, there is a relative weak area in the capsule, known as the **space of Poirier** that is not well supported by the ligaments. The bony and ligamentous constraints of the wrist define the kinematics. The center of rotation in the sagittal and coronal planes is not fixed and varies depending on the position of the wrist. For the most part, the center of rotation is within the head of the capitate distal to its proximal cortex, near its longitudinal axis.

The carpal bones act as two distinct units: a distal carpal row (trapezium, trapezoid, capitate, hamate) and a proximal carpal row (scaphoid, lunate, triquetrum). The distal carpal bones are bound very securely to one another by their interosseous ligaments. These make the distal carpal row a single functional unit. There is a similar secure ligamentous interconnection between the distal carpal row and the second and third metacarpals. The combination of the relatively immobile distal carpal row and the second and third metacarpals creates the **fixed hand unit** (Fig. 13-4). In effect, the distal carpal row is part of the hand. In contrast, the proximal carpal row moves independently of the hand and forearm. The proximal carpal row becomes an **intercalated segment** between the distal carpal row and hand distally and the radius and ulna proximally (Fig. 13-4).

The scaphoid traverses the midcarpal joint and is aligned 45 degrees to the longitudinal axis of the wrist. By virtue of this anatomy, the distal carpal row exerts influence over the scaphoid. The scaphoid has a dynamic tendency to flex, particularly with radial deviation and flexion. The triquetrum is controlled through its semihelicoid articulation with the hamate. The triquetrum has a dynamic tendency to extend, particularly with ulnar deviation and extension. The lunate, by virtue of its location between the scaphoid and triquetrum, is under the influence of both the scaphoid and triquetrum. In its normal state, the lunate lies in a neutral position, canceling the opposing forces of the scaphoid and triquetrum.

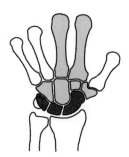

FIG. 13-4   Fixed hand unit composed of index and middle metacarpals bound to distal carpal row (*light gray*). Intercalated segment composed of proximal carpal row is seen between radius and ulna proximally and fixed hand unit distally (*dark gray*).

Approximately 40 to 60% of wrist motion comes from the midcarpal joint, contributing more to flexion, and 40 to 60% comes from the radiocarpal joint, contributing more to extension. Of the total forces transmitted through the wrist, roughly 50% travel through the scaphoid fossa, 30% through the lunate fossa, and the remaining 20% through the TFC. The forces across the TFC relatively increase with ulnar deviation, pronation, and extension.

If the normal relationship between the carpal bones is interrupted through injury, the alignment of the proximal carpal row is disturbed. This can lead to abnormal motion and force distribution. These abnormal kinematics lead to pain and premature arthrosis.

Recognition of the complex anatomy and kinematics of the wrist allows the pathologic states of fractures, dislocations, and instability to be better understood. Through restoration of the normal anatomy, improved treatment outcomes can be anticipated.

DISLOCATIONS OF THE WRIST

Classification

The precise injury pattern is determined by the amount and direction of force applied across the wrist. The mechanism is usually a high-velocity injury, resulting in an axial load with the wrist in extension. Dislocations of the wrist usually lead to some type of carpal instability. The International Wrist Investigators have proposed a classification for wrist ligament injuries. This broad classification of instability takes into account six categories: duration, severity, direction, etiology, pattern, and location.

Duration is acute, subacute, or chronic. Injuries under 6 weeks are acute. Between 6 weeks and 3 months, the injury is considered subacute. Over 3 months, the injury becomes chronic.

Severity is defined by the radiographic appearance and the results of stress testing. Static instability appears abnormal on x-rays without the need for stress testing. Dynamic instability appears normal on regular x-rays but reveals abnormal findings during stress testing. Balanced instability appears normal on x-rays with or without stress testing.

Direction refers to the radiographic appearance of the lunate relative to the capitate and the scaphoid. With *dorsal intercalated segment instability*

(DISI), the lunate assumes a dorsally angulated position relative to the capitate (see Fig. 13-16). With *volar intercalated segment instability* (VISI), the lunate assumes a volarly angulated position relative to the capitate (see Fig. 13-18). Ulnar translation refers to the radiographic appearance in which less then 50% of the body of the lunate is centered over the radius and the distance between the radial styloid and the scaphoid is increased (see Fig. 13-14).

Etiology is variable but can generally be expressed as traumatic, inflammatory, or degenerative.

The *pattern* describes the actual source of the mechanical instability. Instability in the presence of an interruption in the continuity of the proximal carpal row is defined as a pattern of *carpal instability dissociative* (CID). This refers to a dissociation within the proximal carpal row. If there is no interruption in the proximal carpal row, the pattern is defined as *carpal instability nondissociative* (CIND).

Location refers to the actual anatomic structures implicated in the cause of the instability. Most acute dislocations can be described by their location alone including perilunate, radiocarpal, and axial.

Perilunate Dislocations

These are the most common of the wrist dislocations; they include a variety of injuries that involve the area around the lunate. Some of these are purely ligamentous injuries (dorsal and palmar perilunate), while others include fractures (transscaphoid, transradial styloid perilunate, and scaphocapitate syndrome).

The pattern of injury observed in perilunate dislocations has been well described by Mayfield et al. The spectrum varies from a minor scapholunate sprain to a complete dislocation of the lunate. This pattern of injury progresses around the lunate from radial to ulnar in a clockwise direction. There are four stages of *progressive perilunar instability*: stage 1, scapholunate dissociation; stage 2, capitolunate dissociation; stage 3, lunotriquetral dissociation; and stage 4, lunate dislocation (Figs. 13-5 and 13-6).

If the application of force concentrates ulnarly instead of radially, a reverse injury pattern can be observed, reverse perilunate instability. This is similar to what Mayfield described but in an opposite direction, affecting the lunotriquetral joint first.

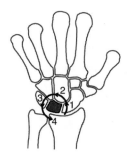

FIG. 13-5 Stages of progressive perilunate instability: (1) scapholunate dissociation; (2) capitolunate dissociation; (3) lunotriquetral dissociation; (4) lunate dislocation.

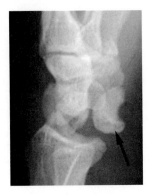

FIG. 13-6 Perilunate dislocation, palmar lunate dislocation. Note lunate dislocated palmarly with scaphoid and capitate dorsal.

If the injury is purely ligamentous, it is referred to as a ***lesser-arc injury*** (Fig. 13-7). If there is a fracture involving one or more of the bones around the lunate, it is known as a ***greater-arc injury*** (Fig. 13-8).

Axial Dislocations and Fracture-Dislocations

These are rare and have been described by Garcia-Elias and colleagues. The mechanism of injury is usually a high-energy crush or blast injury creating an axially oriented injury to the hand and carpus.

The hand and carpus are divided into columns: radial and ulnar. With injuries involving the ulnar column, the fourth and fifth metacarpals usually remain attached to the hamate (Fig. 13-9). A dissociation or fracture occurs between the capitate and the hamate and in some cases the triquetrum or pisotriquetral joint proximally. Radial column injuries involve the thumb and trapezium (Fig. 13-10).

Radiocarpal Dislocation

This is an unusual injury in which the entire carpus as a unit dislocates from the radius. There is no injury to the proximal carpal row or midcarpal joint. These are often associated with radial styloid fractures.

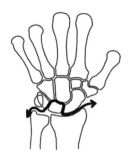

FIG. 13-7 Injuries of the lesser arc involve only the ligaments surrounding the lunate.

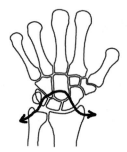

FIG. 13-8 Injuries of the greater arc involve not only the ligaments but also the bones surrounding the lunate.

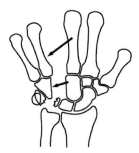

FIG. 13-9 Axial fracture-dislocation to ulnar column. These injuries can also present without an associated fracture and with variable involvement of the triquetrum.

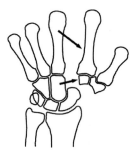

FIG. 13-10 Axial dislocation of the radial column. These injuries can also present with associated fractures of the trapezium and with variable involvement of the trapezoid.

Ulnar translocation is a radiographic finding and type of radiocarpal dislocation in which the entire carpus translates ulnarly. This can be seen following a traumatic radiocarpal dislocation secondary to injury of the palmar extrinsic ligaments, but it is most commonly the result of chronic ligamentous attenuation. This is encountered mostly in inflammatory conditions such as rheumatoid arthritis.

Diagnosis

History

Many wrist dislocations present themselves on a delayed basis. Neither the patient nor the initial treating physician may initially appreciate their severity. At times the symptoms can be relatively subtle and the radiographs misleading or initially nondiagnostic. The history is usually one of a high-energy injury such as a fall from a significant height or a motor vehicle collision. The mechanism is an axial load with the wrist in pronation, ulnar deviation, and extension.

There is always some element of pain, swelling, deformity, and loss of motion. The amount varies according to the severity of the initial trauma and the amount of bone and soft tissue damage. Because of this, there should always be an index of suspicion during the evaluation of any patient with wrist pain after trauma.

Because these injuries are usually related to high-energy mechanisms, other associated injuries must be ruled out. These include injuries to head, chest, abdomen, and other extremities. A careful assessment of the ipsilateral extremity is mandatory, as the wrist injury may distract from other injuries to the adjacent hand, elbow, and shoulder.

Physical Examination

The skin should be inspected for wounds possibly communicating with a fracture or joint. Injuries associated with open wounds tend to be more severe and are often linked with injuries to the nerves and arteries. The vascular integrity of the hand must be judged before and after treatment. Because there is a relatively high incidence of nerve involvement, particularly the median nerve, a careful neurologic exam of the hand, including two-point discrimination, is needed.

The palpatory exam may reveal points of maximum tenderness, which indicate the areas of principal involvement. Unfortunately, in most cases, there is a diffuse, nonspecific tenderness over the dorsum of the wrist.

A history of specific actions or maneuvers that increase symptoms can be helpful. The patient may be able to elicit or increase the symptoms by moving the wrist in a particular manner. Sometimes the wrist must be axially loaded, as when gripping or pushing against something, to duplicate the symptoms.

Active and passive range of motion should first be assessed without any forces across the wrist. Range of motion is again assessed while placing loads across the wrist. The wrist is loaded actively by having the patient make a tight fist and passively by axially pushing the hand against the radius and ulna. Attention should focus on an increase in discomfort or a change in the normally smooth transition of motion. Associated noises may be heard or palpated such as crepitus, clicking, snapping, and popping.

There are special provocative maneuvers or stress tests that can be performed to help diagnose instability. **Watson's maneuver**, or the **scaphoid shift test**, assesses the stability of the scapholunate ligament. Direct pressure is placed with the thumb over the scaphoid tubercle in a dorsal direction. The wrist is then moved from full ulnar deviation into radial deviation. A positive result is elicited if the proximal scaphoid subluxates over the dorsal rim of the distal radius. This can be felt as a sudden dorsal shift of the carpus on the distal radius and is associated with pain.

Volar and dorsal shift tests and the ***midcarpal shift test*** assess the midcarpal joint. With volar and dorsal shift tests, the forearm is stabilized and the wrist is held in neutral position. The hand is then pushed volar or dorsal and the amount of motion and discomfort is assessed against the contralateral side. With the midcarpal shift test, the hand is pushed volar and the wrist is moved from ulnar deviation into radial deviation and repeated. A positive finding is a "catch-up clunk," in which the wrist suddenly jumps and pushes dorsally when going into ulnar deviation.

The lunotriquetral joint can also be tested with provocative testing. ***Reagan's test***, or ***lunotriquetral ballottement***, is performed by stabilizing the lunate dorsally and volarly with one hand by grasping it between the thumb and index finger. The triquetrum is then held in a similar fashion with the other hand and pressure is applied dorsally and volarly to the triquetrum against the lunate. An increased laxity and increase in pain is a positive finding. The ***lunotriquetral shear test*** is executed by placing volar-directed pressure on the dorsal lunate with one thumb and then placing dorsal-directed pressure on the volar pisiform with the other thumb. This places shear stress along the lunotriquetral joint, causing an increase in pain.

Diagnostic Studies

Radiographs should be utilized for the initial evaluation. A routine series includes neutral posteroanterior (PA), ulnar deviation PA, true lateral, and a 45-degree pronation PA view. Similar views of the contralateral wrist should be obtained for comparison. The information from these x-rays is dependent upon their quality. Check to make sure the alignment is accurate in each view. If the initial series is not diagnostic then additional special views can be obtained: a PA view in full radial and ulnar deviation and a clenched-fist AP view.

The intercarpal spaces between the carpal bones are measured and should not exceed 2 to 4 mm, particularly in comparison with the contralateral wrist (Fig. 13-11). There should be a smooth transition without significant step-off between the carpal bones of the distal and proximal rows along a set of curved lines, *Gilula's lines*, drawn along the articular surfaces (Fig. 13-12).

The scaphoid is shaped like a cylinder. Its normal appearance is slightly oblong on the PA view, particularly in ulnar deviation. If the scaphoid is flexed abnormally, the x-ray will project the cylindrical shape down its axis as a circular shadow known as the ***cortical ring sign*** (Fig. 13-11). The lunate normally has a rectangular shape with some small overlap with the capitate. If the lunate flexes or extends abnormally, the overlap with the capitate will increase and the shape of the lunate will appear triangular.

With dislocations and instability of the wrist, the height of the carpus can become shortened as the proximal carpal row rotates out from underneath the capitate. The ***carpal height ratio*** evaluates the carpal height (Fig. 13-13). The height of the carpus is measured from the proximal lunate to the distal capitate. This number is divided by the length of the third metacarpal. The normal ratio is ***0.54 ± 0.03***. If the result is abnormal, there may be a dislocation or fracture of the wrist.

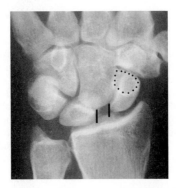

FIG. 13-11   PA "grip view" radiograph showing scapholunate gap in excess of 4 mm, also known as the "David Letterman sign" and cortical ring sign (*dotted lines*).

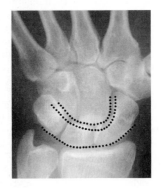

FIG. 13-12   Gilula's lines drawn along the articular surfaces of the proximal and distal carpal rows. Normally there should be no significant breaks in the congruity of the lines.

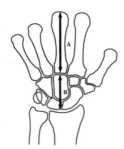

FIG. 13-13   Carpal height ratio divides the height of the carpus (*B*) by the length of the third metacarpal (*A*). The normal ratio is 0.54 ± 0.03. A ratio less than this signifies some level of carpal collapse.

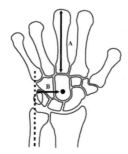

FIG. 13-14 Ulnar translocation ratio divides the distance between the center of the capitate and a line drawn down the ulnar shaft (*B*) and the length of the third metacarpal (*A*). The normal ratio is 0.30 ± 0.03. A number below this signifies some level of ulnar translocation.

Ulnar translocation can be appreciated on the PA view if the carpus appears to be translated ulnarly relative to the radius (Fig. 13-14). The ulnar transloca-tion ratio can be identified radiographically from the ratio of the distance be-tween the center of the capitate and a line along the longitudinal axis of the ulna divided by the length of the third metacarpal. The normal ratio is *0.30 ± 0.03*. If the result is less than this, ulnar translocation should be suspected.

On the lateral view, the alignment of the lunate and the interrelationship of the scaphoid and the lunate are evaluated. The *scapholunate angle* is measured between a line drawn down the axis of the scaphoid and a line drawn down the axis of the lunate (Fig. 13-15). This angle should be between 30 and 60 degrees. The axis of the lunate should be within 15 degrees of the axis of the capitate and the axis of the radius. If the lunate is dorsally tilted with a scapholunate angle greater than 60 degrees and a capitolunate angle greater than 15 degrees, DISI must be suspected (Figs. 13-16 and 13-17). If the lunate is volarly tilted with a scapholunate angle less then 30 degrees and a capitolunate angle greater then 15 degrees, VISI must be suspected (Figs. 13-18 and 13-19).

Fluoroscopy can be utilized to assess dynamic instability when the static ra-diographs appear normal. Stress testing is performed while looking at the wrist in real time.

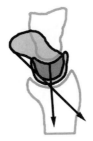

FIG. 13-15 Normal scapholunate angle of 30 to 60 degrees. The scapholu-nate angle is measured between a line parallel to the axis of the scaphoid and a line down the axis of the lunate perpendicular to its distal surface.

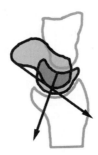

FIG. 13-16   Instability of the dorsal intercalated segment with the scapholunate angle in excess of 60 degrees. Notice that the lunate surface is tilted dorsally.

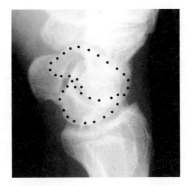

FIG. 13-17   Radiograph demonstrating dorsal angulation of the lunate with relative flexion of the scaphoid (DISI).

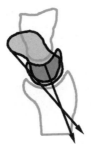

FIG. 13-18   Instability of the volar intercalated segment with a scapholunate angle of less than 30 degrees. Notice that the lunate surface is tilted volarly.

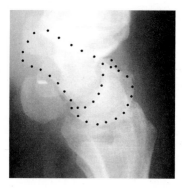

FIG. 13-19 Radiograph demonstrating volar angulation of the lunate with relative extension of the scaphoid (VISI).

Arthrography can be used to detect tears of the scapholunate and lunotriquetral ligaments as well as tears of the TFC.

Unfortunately, the incidence of false-negative and false-positive results confers poor specificity and a poor predictive value to arthrography. This is particularly true in patients above age 50.

Magnetic resonance imaging (MRI) has a relatively poor sensitivity in assessing injuries to the carpal ligament. It may be best utilized to assess and rule out other possible causes of wrist pain, like Kienböck's disease and occult carpal fractures. If utilized, MRI should be performed with a 1.5-tesla magnet and a dedicated wrist coil (Fig. 13-20). To increase sensitivity, gadolinium can be injected, using a technique similar to that used in obtaining a triple-compartment arthrogram.

Bone scanning is best used to rule out significant wrist pathology. Because of its sensitivity, a negative result greatly reduces the possibility of significant wrist pathology. However, positive results are nonspecific and may not provide much useful information.

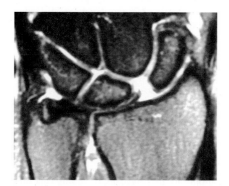

FIG. 13-20 MRI of a wrist with scapholunate dissociation. Note the large gap between the scaphoid and lunate, with a remnant of the scapholunate ligament still attached to the lunate.

Wrist arthroscopy is the "gold standard" for the diagnosis of ligamentous injury and instability. It can be used to confirm and stage the diagnosis. Additionally, arthroscopy can be used to effect treatment with repair or debridement.

Treatment

Initial Management

Dislocations of the carpus should be reduced as soon as possible. An initial assessment and examination should be performed prior to reduction to document any deficits. The reduction technique is the same for *perilunate dislocations*, *transscaphoid fracture-dislocations*, and *radiocarpal dislocations*. *Scapholunate dissociations*, *axial dislocations*, and *ulnar translocations* cannot be treated with closed reduction alone and require more definitive management.

Adequate anesthesia is critical and should be planned. A simple hematoma block or local block is usually not sufficient, particularly without deep sedation. Preferably, the anesthesia team is consulted in the emergency department. The anesthetist can monitor the patient and administer a regional block and any needed sedation. This allows the orthopedist to focus on the reduction itself. A regional block—such as an axillary, supraclavicular, infraclavicular, scalene, or Bier block—is preferred. These blocks provide analgesia and muscle relaxation, both of which are very important for a successful reduction.

The patient is placed in a supine position. Finger traps are applied to at least two digits and suspended with the elbow bent 90 degrees and the hand directed toward the ceiling. Traction is applied with 15 lb of weight suspended from the upper arm, with appropriate padding. Traction is maintained for 10 min prior to any attempts at reduction.

The reduction maneuver has been described by Tavernier. The hand is removed from the traction setup to perform the reduction maneuver. An assistant should help stabilize the proximal forearm. The surgeon grasps the patient's hand as if to shake it and manual traction is applied. The contralateral thumb applies a dorsally directed force to the palmar part of the lunate at the carpal canal. The patient's hand is then brought into hyperextension and gradually back into flexion, pulling the head of the capitate over the dorsal rim of the lunate.

Postreduction radiographs or fluoroscopy is used to assess the reduction and the injury pattern, including possible associated fractures.

Initial attempts at reduction may not be successful. There may be excessive swelling or soft tissue interposition blocking the reduction. If closed reduction is not possible, the wrist should be splinted in a neutral position and open reduction planned as soon as possible.

After the reduction, a long arm thumb spica splint is applied with the wrist in neutral position and the elbow flexed 90 degrees. Strict elevation is critical, and the patient should be hospitalized at least overnight for neurovascular checks and frequent applications of ice packs. Definitive management should be planned and executed within 2 to 3 weeks of the injury. If there are persistent median nerve symptoms after the closed reduction, surgical treatment should be performed as soon as possible.

Definitive Management

Various treatment options are available, including cast immobilization, percutaneous pinning, and open reduction and fixation. Long-term results with cast immobilization are poor; therefore this treatment should be reserved for individuals in whom surgery is contraindicated. For similar reasons, percutaneous pinning is not usually recommended as definitive management; it is usually reserved for cases where an open reduction cannot be performed. This includes severely injured patients who are not stable enough for a lengthier procedure or in whom surgical incisions are contraindicated because of soft tissue injury, such as burns or open wounds.

Percutaneous pin-fixation technique. The goal of percutaneous pin fixation is an accurate reduction and stable fixation. If an acceptable reduction cannot be achieved, open reduction and fixation is necessary.

The pinning technique is the same whether it is executed percutaneously or with an open incision (Fig. 13-21). The technique is dependent on good-quality fluoroscopy. The patient is positioned supine with the hand on an arm table. The assistant stabilizes the forearm proximally.

The lunate is first reduced and fixed to the capitate. A 0.062-in. smooth K wire is preplaced in the capitate. This K wire is driven from distal to proximal starting at the very distal, dorsal edge of the capitate near the carpometacarpal joint. The K wire should be angled minimally relative to the capitate. If the pin is angled too much, it will pass palmar to the lunate. Once the pin is preplaced in the capitate, the lunate is reduced relative to the capitate. The lunate is usually dorsally angulated relative to the capitate. The lunate is reduced by volarly translating, not angulating, the hand relative to the forearm. With the forearm stabilized by the assistant, a volar translation force is applied to the dorsal hand. This pushes the capitate volarly against the volar lip of the lunate, tipping it back into a neutral position. During this maneuver, the hand is radially deviated to place at least 50% of the capitate over the lunate. Once the lunate is reduced, the pin is advanced across the capitolunate joint.

The scaphoid is then reduced and fixed to the capitate and the lunate. A 0.045-in. K wire is preplaced near the snuffbox through the waist of the scaphoid, aiming toward the capitate. A second 0.045-in. K wire is placed in a similar fashion across the proximal pole of the scaphoid directed toward the lunate. A 0.065-in. K wire is placed into the dorsal scaphoid from slightly distal to proximal and radial to ulnar to act as a joystick. The joystick K wire is then pulled proximally and ulnarly to pull the scaphoid into extension and push it

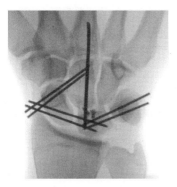

FIG. 13-21 Radiograph of a stage 4 injury exhibiting pinning technique. Note the capitolunate pin fixing the lunate in its reduced position relative to the capitate. If this were a stage 1 or stage 2 injury, only the radial pins and capitolunate pin would be necessary.

against the lunate, which has been fixed to the capitate. Once the reduction of the scapholunate joint is verified fluoroscopically, the pins in the scaphoid are then advanced across the scaphocapitate and scapholunate joints. Two additional 0.045-in. K wires are placed alongside these pins for a total of two pins across each joint.

If the injury involves the lunotriquetral joint, the triquetrum is then reduced and fixed to the lunate. Pressure is applied to the dorsal triquetrum in a volar direction. Two 0.045-in. K wires are placed across the triquetrum into the lunate.

All pins are then cut well beneath the level of the skin. A long arm thumb spica wrist splint is applied with the wrist in a neutral position. After 1 to 2 weeks the splint is changed to a cast. A short arm thumb spica cast can be utilized if the patient is felt to be compliant; otherwise a long arm thumb spica cast is used for the first 8 weeks. After 8 weeks, the pins are removed and immobilization in the thumb spica cast is continued for 4 additional weeks. The total time of immobilization is 12 weeks after reduction and fixation.

Beginning almost immediately after surgery and during the first 12 weeks, the patient is regularly seen in therapy for aggressive range of motion of the digits and edema-reducing modalities.

Twelve weeks postoperatively, the cast is discontinued and replaced by a removable short arm thumb spica splint. The therapist then begins gentle active and active assisted range of motion to the wrist.

Eighteen weeks postoperatively, the splint is discontinued and more aggressive passive range of motion is begun, including dynamic splinting. Gentle strengthening can commence, with more aggressive strengthening delayed until 6 months postoperatively.

Open reduction, ligament repair, and fixation.   In most cases, a single, dorsal wrist approach is utilized for the bone reduction and ligament repair. If the patient exhibits median nerve symptoms, a carpal tunnel release should be executed. In these cases, a dual dorsal and palmar approach to the wrist is utilized. If no median nerve symptoms are present, a single, dorsal wrist approach is employed.

The dorsal approach to the wrist is made through a longitudinal incision in line with the third metacarpal and Lister's tubercle, extending from the carpometacarpal joint proximally to Lister's tubercle. The extensor pollicis longus tendon is identified and the extensor retinaculum of the third dorsal compartment is opened longitudinally. The extensor retinaculum is then released radially and ulnarly, exposing the extensor tendons. The joint is exposed through a fiber-splitting capsulotomy, as described by Berger (Fig. 13-22). This ligament-sparing approach preserves the distal intercarpal and proximal radiocarpal ligament through a radially based flap.

The scapholunate ligament is usually avulsed from the insertion on the scaphoid, although avulsions from the lunate can also be observed. If the injury is acute or subacute, there is typically enough scapholunate ligamentous tissue to allow for a direct repair. If the tissues are insufficient for direct repair, a dorsal capsulodesis may be required to reinforce the site.

A repair technique as described by Viegas is preferred (Fig. 13-23). This technique repairs the scapholunate interosseous ligament (SLIL) and the dorsal intercarpal ligament (DIC), both of which have been implicated in the pathogenesis of instability. Small bone anchors are utilized with 3-0 or 4-0 braided suture. Two anchors are placed in the dorsal rim of the proximal scaphoid at the insertion of the SLIL and just radial to it. An additional su-

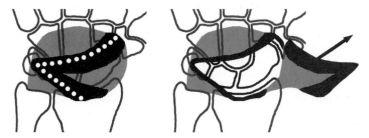

FIG. 13-22   Fiber-splitting capsulotomy approach to gain access to dorsal wrist.

ture anchor is placed in the dorsal rim of the lunate at the insertion of the SLIL. The sutures are then placed through the stump of the SLIL with either the scaphoid or lunate anchor as appropriate. This same suture is then passed through the proximal part of the DIC. The remaining sutures are passed through the DIC in a similar manner. When the sutures are tied, the proximal segment of the DIC will be pulled over the SLIL in a vest-over-pants fashion. This will anchor the SLIL to its insertion and the DIC to the dorsal rim of the scaphoid and lunate. The sutures are not tied until the carpus is reduced and fixed with pins.

The carpal bones are then reduced and fixed utilizing the techniques described under "Percutaneous Pin-Fixation Technique," above. A small elevator may be needed to disimpact the carpal bones or lever them into place. The carpus is then inspected for ligament injuries and associated fractures. There can be related osteochondral injuries to the scaphoid and lunate surfaces, with cartilage loss and loose bodies. These injuries require debridement of all loose fragments. After reduction and fixation of the carpal bones, the previously placed sutures are tied, securing the ligamentous tissue.

Direct repair of the lunotriquetral ligament is not necessary for a good result. This joint is usually well reduced on radiographs without the need for significant reduction maneuvers. The injury to the lunotriquetral ligament and joint is addressed with pin fixation.

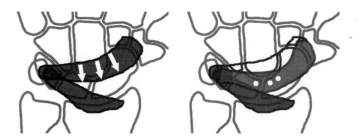

FIG. 13-23   Preferred repair technique using a portion of the distal intercarpal ligament to augment the repair of the scapholunate ligament. Suture anchors placed in the lunate and scaphoid are used to secure the ligament and then the distal intercarpal ligament.

If the median nerve is asymptomatic and the carpus can be suitably reduced, a separate volar approach to repair the volar ligaments is unnecessary. If a carpal tunnel release is required or the carpus cannot be reduced through the dorsal approach, an extended carpal tunnel approach is used to assist in the reduction and decompress the median nerve. The transverse retinacular ligament is released, allowing complete inspection of the median nerve. The flexor tendons and median nerve are carefully retracted to expose the volar capsule. The radioscaphocapitate ligament and palmar lunotriquetral ligament are repaired directly with 4-0 braided sutures. Care must be taken not to place sutures across the tear in the capsule at the space of Poirier just distal to the lunate. This will add nothing to the repair and may promote stiffness.

The carpal bones are reduced and fixed to one another using the technique described in the discussion of percutaneous pinning. After the pins have been placed, the dorsal sutures are tied, anchoring the SLIL and DIC. The remaining dorsal capsule is repaired to itself with 4-0 braided sutures. The dorsal retinaculum is repaired directly with 4-0 braided sutures, leaving the extensor pollicis longus transposed over the retinaculum beneath the subcutaneous layer.

The postoperative rehabilitation program is then instituted as described in the discussion of percutaneous pinning.

Scapholunate dissociation.   Scapholunate dissociation is part of the spectrum of progressive perilunar instability, as described by Mayfield and colleagues. Injury to the scapholunate interosseous ligament and the supporting ligaments, such as the dorsal intercarpal ligament, results in carpal instability. The treatment is the same as described above for perilunate dislocations except for the reduction and pinning of the lunotriquetral joint, which is unnecessary in these cases. If there is any doubt that the injury may have been a perilunate dislocation that reduced itself spontaneously, the lunotriquetral joint should be included in the pinning sequence.

Transscaphoid perilunate fracture-dislocation.   In cases of associated scaphoid fracture, transscaphoid perilunate fracture-dislocation, the scaphoid requires anatomic reduction and fixation and the lunotriquetral joint must be pinned. The scaphoid is usually fractured through its waist, preserving the scapholunate interosseous ligament, but the lunotriquetral ligament and dorsal intercarpal ligaments are also probably ruptured. The fracture can be reduced through a palmar or dorsal approach. If the palmar approach is chosen, this is applied as described by Russe. After reduction and fixation of the scaphoid, the carpus is reassessed. If the scapholunate angle is normal and there is no significant intercarpal gap, the lunate is percutaneously pinned to the capitate with a single 0.062-in. K wire from distal to proximal. The triquetrum is then pinned to the lunate with two 0.045-in. K wires.

We prefer a single, dorsal approach, as described for perilunate dislocations. This allows adequate visualization of the scaphoid for proper reduction and fixation of the fracture. The carpus is then assessed and repaired as needed with pinning as previously described.

Regardless of the approach, the scaphoid is anatomically reduced and bone grafted as necessary. The fracture can be fixed with multiple 0.045-in. K wires, particularly if there is related comminution. If there is minimal comminution, a headless compression screw is the preferred form of fixation.

Transradial styloid perilunate fracture-dislocation.   In cases of associated radial styloid fracture, transradial styloid perilunate dislocation, the radial styloid fragment must first be reduced and fixed. The fracture is approached and reduced through a dorsal ligament-sparing approach, as described previously. The fracture can be fixed with multiple 0.045-in. K wires or cannulated screws. The carpal ligaments are then assessed and repaired as needed.

Radiocarpal dislocation. This is a relatively rare injury. Because of associated injuries to the median and ulnar nerves, it is recommended that the nerves be decompressed through an extended carpal tunnel approach and the volar capsular tears repaired directly. The radiocarpal joint is then fixed with 0.062-in. K wires through the metaphysis of the radius proximally into the scaphoid and lunate distally. The postoperative rehabilitation is similar to that of perilunate dislocations.

Axial dislocations and fracture-dislocations. These are relatively rare and associated with very severe high-energy injuries. Usually there are associated soft tissue injuries to the tendons, nerves, arteries, and skin, requiring repair or debridement. In many cases soft tissue coverage is needed with local or remote flaps. A combined dorsal and volar approach is usually needed to assess and fix the injuries, including decompression of the nerves. The joints and bones are reduced and fixed with pins and screws as needed. The morbidity of these injuries to overall hand function can be significant and carries a guarded prognosis.

Complications

The incidence of complications increases with the severity of the injury and associated injuries to the surrounding soft tissues. The most common complication is residual stiffness and associated weakness of the wrist and hand. This is observed uniformly among patients to varying degrees.

Residual carpal instability, DISI, or VISI, can occur, leading to chronic pain and dysfunction. Posttraumatic arthrosis occurs in up to 56% of patients regardless of early recognition and treatment.

Associated median nerve injury or dysfunction can occur on an acute or delayed basis. Early recognition is important for timely treatment and recovery.

Osteonecrosis of the involved carpal bones can occur but are relatively unusual complications. Nonunions of the fractures can also occur with varying frequency, depending on the energy of the injury.

FRACTURES OF THE WRIST

The unique anatomy of the carpal bones differentiates them from the long bones. The bulk of their surface is enveloped in articular cartilage. As a consequence, there are few areas through which blood vessels can enter. This leaves the blood supply at risk after injury. In addition, the better part of a carpal bone surface articulates with other bones. This magnifies the significance of any fracture displacement, which can result in posttraumatic arthrosis.

Classification

Scaphoid Fractures

Fractures of the scaphoid account for nearly two-thirds of carpal fractures. They tend to occur in younger individuals, most often in males. The mechanism of injury is one of axial load to the radial half of the palm with the wrist in hyperextension. This extended wrist position cradles the proximal pole of

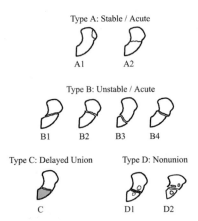

FIG. 13-24 Herbert classification of scaphoid fractures.

the scaphoid while exposing its distal half to a bending moment, which leads to the fracture.

Herbert and Fisher have proposed a system that attempts to incorporate many of the attributes of scaphoid fractures (Fig. 13-24). These characteristics include chronicity, location, orientation, displacement, comminution, and associated injuries. This system attempts to prognosticate the outcome of the fracture based on its features.

Time to treatment affects the prognosis of healing. Fractures treated after a delay in diagnosis have a higher rate of nonunion than those treated early. A delayed union occurs after 4 to 6 months and nonunion after 6 months.

The scaphoid can be geographically defined into thirds: a proximal pole, a middle waist, and a distal head. Roughly 70 to 80% of fractures occur in the middle third or waist of the scaphoid, with 10 to 20% affecting the proximal pole and 5% affecting the distal head. The location of the fracture has prognostic consequences based on the blood supply of the scaphoid. Palmar branches of the radial artery enter the distal tuberosity, accounting for 20 to 30% of the distal blood supply. Dorsal branches of the radial artery enter the dorsal ridge of the scaphoid along its middle third, accounting for 70 to 80% of the remaining blood supply. Because of this arrangement, the location of the fracture and the amount of displacement can disturb the blood supply. Fractures of the proximal pole particularly can lead to a high rate of osteonecrosis and nonunion.

The orientation of the fracture, the initial displacement, and the amount of comminution have been implicated in the stability of the fracture. Russe classified fractures according to the orientation of the fracture line related to the axis of the scaphoid. Transverse fractures made up the bulk, accounting for nearly two-thirds with the fracture plane perpendicular to the axis of the scaphoid. Horizontal oblique fractures made up one-third, with the fracture plane parallel to the plane of the joint and oblique to the axis of the scaphoid. These had the most stable configuration. Vertical oblique fractures made up only 5%, with the fracture plane perpendicular to the plane of the joint and oblique to the axis of the scaphoid. These are the most unstable of the fractures.

The amount of fracture displacement has been implicated in the rate of healing and osteonecrosis. Fracture displacement of as little as 1 mm has been associated with rates of nonunion and osteonecrosis in excess of 50%. In addition, displacement can occur as a volar flexion angulation. More than 20 degrees of flexion at the fracture site or increases in the scapholunate angle indicate greater instability. Sometimes displacement is difficult to judge on radiographs, in which case evaluation by CT becomes necessary.

Lunate Fractures

Traumatic fractures of the lunate that are not associated with Kienbock's disease are relatively unusual. They are classified based on the fracture pattern: fractures of the volar pole (most common), small marginal chip fractures, fractures of the dorsal pole, sagittal body fractures, and transverse body fractures.

Triquetral Fractures

Fractures of the triquetrum are probably underreported, as they may be difficult to diagnose and verify on radiographs. Nonetheless, these fractures comprise the second most common carpal bone fracture. The most common triquetral fracture is a chip or avulsion fracture off the dorsal aspect of the triquetrum. The ulnar styloid can forcefully impinge on the dorsal triquetrum as the wrist goes into hyperextension, shearing the dorsal part of the triquetrum off the main body. In addition, the strong dorsal ligaments originating from the dorsal triquetrum can avulse a portion of the dorsal triquetrum off the body in the later stages of progressive perilunate instability, as described by Mayfield and colleagues. Infrequently, larger fractures through the body of the triquetrum can occur in association with perilunate fracture-dislocations or axial fracture-dislocations.

Trapezium Fractures

Fractures of the trapezium occur as two types: fracture through the body of the trapezium and fractures across the trapezial ridge. Fractures of the body are the result of an axial load and can be associated with thumb metacarpal fracture or subluxation. Fractures of the trapezial ridge are more common and result from an avulsion of the flexor retinaculum incurred during a fall.

Trapezoid Fractures

These are extremely rare secondary to the protected position of the trapezoid within the carpus. Usually these are associated with axial fracture-dislocations resulting from severe blast or crush injuries.

Capitate Fractures

Fractures of the capitate can occur as isolated fractures, fractures associated with other injuries, or as part of scaphocapitate syndrome. As in the case of the scaphoid, the blood supply to the capitate is retrograde, which can complicate healing. In scaphocapitate syndrome, the scaphoid and capitate fracture through their midportion as the wrist gets pushed into hyperextension. As the wrist returns to a neutral position, the distal portion of the capitate rotates the head of the capitate palmarly 90 to 180 degrees. This injury can surprisingly be difficult to appreciate on regular radiographs. Isolated fractures of the capitate are usually minimally displaced and can be effectively treated without surgery. Fractures associated with other carpal injuries, however, are usually displaced, requiring surgical fixation.

Hamate Fractures

Fractures of the hamate occur in two primary forms: through the body and across the hamulus. Fractures of the hamate body occur in a sagittal plane in association with axial fracture-dislocations. Fractures through the hook of the hamate are more common. These occur either through the base of the hook due to an impact injury or near the tip due to an avulsion injury from the flexor retinaculum. These fractures are particularly common among athletes playing golf, tennis, and baseball or laborers like mechanics who are subjected to repetitive impact to the palm.

Pisiform Fractures

These are often associated with other wrist fractures and result from direct impacts. They can occur as small chip fractures, split fractures of the body, or comminuted fractures of the body. There can be associated ulnar nerve symptoms and, because of the pisiform's articulation with the triquetrum, these fractures can result in posttraumatic arthrosis.

Diagnosis

A high index of suspicion is often required to make the diagnosis of a carpal bone fracture. Frequently these fractures are only minimally displaced and, because of the complex three-dimensional anatomy, standard radiographs can appear normal. Persistent wrist pain after a history of injury, particularly higher-energy injuries, requires a careful examination and appropriate diagnostic studies.

Physical Examination

The examination is performed like that for wrist dislocation. Areas of deformity or swelling should be noted. Regions of palpable tenderness are particularly useful in defining the carpal bones involved. Persistent tenderness in the snuffbox distal to the radial styloid raises suspicion for scaphoid fracture. Tenderness near the proximal palm along the hypothenar region indicates a fracture of the hook of the hamate. Similarly, tenderness along the proximal palm in the thenar region indicates a trapezial ridge fracture. Tenderness at the ulnar portion of the wrist flexion crease signifies pisiform injury, whereas tenderness at the radial portion of the wrist flexion crease denotes scaphoid tubercle fracture.

Diagnostic Studies

Several attributes unique to the carpal bones can make their fractures difficult to visualize on plain radiographs. The carpals are relatively compact and overlap in several areas. In addition, the displacement or angulation of the fracture can be relatively subtle. Finally, the carpals are oriented in several planes, making them more difficult to assess on basic frontal and lateral views.

Radiographs, even with their limitations, are helpful for the initial evaluation, utilizing a four-view series: neutral posteroanterior (PA), ulnar deviation PA, true lateral, and a 45-degree-pronation PA view. The lateral and pronated views can reveal dorsal fractures of the triquetrum and lunate. Special 45-degree-supination PA views can reveal injuries to the hamate, triquetrum, or pisiform. A carpal tunnel view can be helpful in disclosing injuries to the hook of the hamate or the trapezial ridge. Multiple oblique views or direct fluoroscopy can sometimes reveal a small fracture fragment off one of the carpal bones. If the initial radiographs are negative, repeat films should be obtained 2 weeks later, as bone resorption may make the fracture site more apparent.

Bone scan is extremely sensitive to fractures but may be nonspecific. The bone scan cannot visualize alignment or quantify displacement.

Magnetic resonance imaging (MRI) is more helpful, as it is also very sensitive to fractures but is much more specific than bone scan. Unfortunately, it is relatively poor at quantifying displacement and alignment.

Computed tomography (CT) or polytomography is the best at visualizing alignment and displacement of the bones and is very specific. CT scan is somewhat less sensitive than bone scan or MRI. CT scans show the fracture best with images at 1-mm intervals and the beam perpendicular to the fracture line. In the case of the scaphoid, the beam would be parallel to the axis of the scaphoid in the sagittal plane. In the case of the hamate, the beam would be in the transverse plane parallel to the carpometacarpal joint.

Treatment

Initial Management

The cornerstone of treatment is an accurate diagnosis. After careful examination and radiographic testing, the diagnosis should be apparent. If the diagnosis is not clear, the wrist should be immobilized in a short arm wrist splint or, in the case of radial-sided pain, a thumb spica splint for 2 weeks.

The wrist is then reexamined and further diagnostic studies are performed as needed to confirm or rule out a fracture. An MRI is preferred for its combination of sensitivity and specificity. If the MRI is positive, a CT scan or polytomogram can be obtained to increase the specificity and visualization of the involved structures.

Definitive Management

Scaphoid fractures. The treatment of nondisplaced scaphoid fractures depends on an accurate diagnosis. The prognosis is significantly affected if the fracture is displaced and is subsequently treated as a nondisplaced fracture. Displacement is defined as any separation or translation greater than 1 mm, an increase in the scapholunate angle greater than 60 degrees, or scaphoid angulation at the fracture greater than 20 degrees. Anything appearing greater then a crack in the bone should be seen as indicating displacement.

The alignment can be difficult to assess because of the fracture orientation and the unique shape and orientation of the scaphoid. This is particularly true in assessing fracture angulation. The radiographs must be of high quality and well aligned. Multiple oblique views in various positions of wrist rotation should be obtained in addition to the standard four-view series. If there is any doubt, a CT scan or polytomography should be employed to verify alignment.

Nondisplaced fractures should be treated with strict immobilization. There has been a good deal of debate over the optimal extent of immobilization, including the position of the wrist, inclusion of the thumb, and inclusion of the elbow. There is clinical and biomechanical evidence to support several options. The cast should be well molded and changed every 2 weeks until the swelling has stabilized.

The mode of treatment also varies with the location of the fracture within the scaphoid. Fractures of the distal third are usually avulsion or impaction fractures involving the tubercle or articular margin of the scaphoid. These should be treated with a short arm thumb spica cast for 4 to 6 weeks, depending on the radiographs and physical examination.

Fractures of the middle and proximal thirds should be treated with a long arm thumb spica cast with the elbow flexed at 90 degrees and the thumb included up to the tip. The position of the wrist should be supinated, extended, and ulnarly deviated. The cast should be well molded and changed every 2 to 3 weeks, depending on the amount of swelling.

After 6 weeks of long arm immobilization, the cast can be changed to a short arm thumb spica cast for an additional 6 weeks. After 12 weeks of immobilization, the radiographs must be carefully assessed. If there appears to be radiographic evidence of healing and there is no tenderness or pain at the fracture site, the casting can be discontinued. If there is any concern or doubt about the appearance of the radiographs, a CT scan or polytomogram should be obtained to verify union. Because of the incidence of nonunion, the radiographs and physical examination must be repeated at 6 and 12 months prior to final discharge.

Minimally invasive internal fixation techniques, which can effectively stabilize the scaphoid securely, have gained interest in the treatment of nondisplaced scaphoid fractures. There can be significant financial and social burdens as a result of the needed immobilization. This is particularly true in laborers and athletes. In addition, fractures of the proximal pole appear to have a higher incidence of nonunion, delayed union, or avascular necrosis with closed treatment. Minimally invasive internal fixation for nondisplaced scaphoid fractures can be offered to selected patients who may benefit.

There is little controversy regarding the treatment of displaced scaphoid fractures. To minimize the rate of nonunion, malunion, and avascular necrosis, displaced fractures must be reduced and surgically fixed.

Several surgical techniques and approaches have been described. If the fracture is minimally displaced with little comminution, a closed reduction can be attempted. If the reduction is successful, the fracture can be fixed with percutaneously placed 0.045-in. K wires or preferably a percutaneously placed headless compression screw (Fig. 13-25).

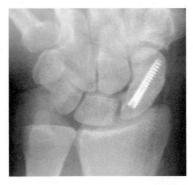

FIG. 13-25 Radiograph demonstrating the use of a headless, variable-pitch compression screw for the treatment of a scaphoid fracture. The screw was placed percutaneously in an antegrade fashion through the dorsal proximal pole of the scaphoid.

If closed reduction is unsuccessful, open reduction is necessary. An open dorsal or volar approach can be utilized to reduce the fracture and bone graft if needed. Volar approaches are preferred for middle- and distal-third fractures. Dorsal approaches are preferred for fractures of the proximal pole. Excessive volar comminution should be treated with a bone graft.

After acceptable reduction, the fracture is stabilized with internal fixation. A headless compression screw is the preferred internal fixation device. The placement of the screw can sometimes be demanding and requires some skill and practice. Multiple K wires can be utilized if comminution and fracture configuration preclude the use of an internal screw. The K wires should be 0.035 or 0.045 in. in size with at least three pins placed in a parallel configuration down the axis of the scaphoid.

Depending on patient compliance, a postoperative long arm thumb spica splint is utilized for the first 2 weeks. After 2 weeks, a short arm thumb spica splint is utilized for 4 to 6 additional weeks or until radiographic and clinical union is achieved.

Other carpal fractures. Nondisplaced fractures of the carpus excluding the scaphoid have a high rate of union with few complications. The wrist should be immobilized in a short arm cast for 4 to 8 weeks or until radiographic and clinical union have occurred.

Displaced fractures must be reduced and fixed in the same way as displaced scaphoid fractures. Many of these fractures are relatively small, requiring the use of K wires or buried minifragment screws. Fractures of the capitate head and neck are ideally suited for fixation with small headless compression screws. Pisiform fractures can initially be treated with casting and the pisiform later excised if complications develop.

Complications

Arthritis

Posttraumatic arthrosis can occur as a result of intraarticular fractures that have healed with displacement or associated osteochondral defects. The remedy depends on the location and extent of involvement. If the midcarpal joint is involved and the radiocarpal joint is spared, a limited arthrodesis of the midcarpal joint can be performed. If the radioscaphoid joint is involved and the midcarpal joint is spared, a proximal-row carpectomy can be performed. If both the midcarpal and radiocarpal joints are involved, a total arthrodesis may be needed.

Nonunion and Avascular Necrosis

Scaphoid fractures have a relatively high rate of nonunion and avascular necrosis. Nondisplaced fractures can have a 15% rate of nonunion and displaced fractures nonunion rates in the range of 50%. The rate of avascular necrosis depends on the location of the fracture and varies from 30 to 100% for middle-third and proximal-pole fractures respectively. Similar complications can be seen with displaced capitate head and neck fractures.

Nonunions can be difficult to address, owing to bone loss and deformity. Vascularized bone grafts, wedge grafts, and corticocancellous bone grafts may be necessary to correct deformity and promote bone healing. If significant collapse or degeneration occurs, the wrist can be reconstructed with a limited arthrodesis or proximal-row carpectomy.

SELECTED READINGS

Berger RA. The gross and histologic anatomy of the scapholunate interosseous ligament. *J Hand Surg [Am]* 21:170, 1996.

Friberg S, Lindstrom B. Radiographic measurements of the radiocarpal joint in normal adults. *Acta Radiol (Stockh)* 17:249, 1976.

Garcia-Elias M, Dobyns JH, Cooney WP, et al. Traumatic axial dislocations of the carpus. *J Hand Surg [Am]* 14:446, 1989.

Gelberman RH, Menon J. The vascularity of the scaphoid bone. *J Hand Surg [Am]* 5:512, 1980.

Gilula LA, Destouet JM, Weeks PM, et al. Roentgenographic diagnosis of the painful wrist. *Clin Orthop* 187:52, 1984.

Herbert TJ, Fisher WE. Management of the fractured scaphoid using a new bone screw. *J Bone Joint Surg [Br]* 66:114, 1984.

Herzberg G, Comtet JJ, Linscheid RL, et al. Perilunate dislocations and fracture-dislocation: a multicenter study. *J Hand Surg* 18A:768, 1993.

Johnson RP. The acutely injured wrist and its residuals. *Clin Orthop* 149:33, 1980.

Kleinman WB. Diagnostic exams for ligamentous injuries. *American Society for Surgery of the Hand, Correspondence Club Newsletter* 51, 1985.

Lichtman DM, Schneider JR, Swafford AR, et al. Ulnar midcarpal instability: clinical and laboratory analysis. *J Hand Surg [Am]* 6:515, 1981.

Mayfield JK, Johnson RP, Kilcoyne RK. Carpal dislocations: pathomechanics and progressive perilunar instability. *Orthop Clin North Am* 15:209, 1984.

Mikic ZDJ. Arthrography of the wrist joint. An experimental study. *J Bone Joint Surg [Am]* 66:371, 1984.

Nicodemus C, Viegas SF. True instantaneous kinematics of the wrist. 10th International Wrist Investigators' Workshop, Mayo Clinic, Rochester, Minnesota, May 22. 1994.

Reagan DS, Linscheid RL, Dobyns JH. Lunotriquetral sprains. *J Hand Surg [Am]* 9:502, 1984.

Ruby LK, Cooney WP, An KN, et al. Relative motion of selected carpal bones: a kinematic analysis of the normal wrist. *J Hand Surg [Am]* 13(1):1, 1988.

Russe O. Fracture of the carpal navicular: diagnosis, non-operative treatment, and operative treatment. *J Bone Joint Surg [Am]* 42A:759, 1960.

Short WH, Werner FW, Fortino MD, et al. Distribution of pressures and forces on the wrist after simulated intercarpal fusion and Keinbock's disease. *J Hand Surg [Am]* 17:443, 1992.

Slade JF III, Moore AE. Dorsal percutaneous fixation of stable, unstable, and displaced scaphoid fractures and nonunions. *Atlas Hand Clin* 8:1, 2003.

Tavernier L. Les deplacements traumatiques du semilunaire. Lyon, France: Thesis, Universite de Lyon, p 138, 1906.

Teisen H, Hjarbaek J. Classification of fresh fractures of the lunate. *J Hand Surg [Br]* 13:458, 1988.

Viegas SF, DaSilva MF. Surgical repair for scapholunate dissociation. *Tech Hand Upper Extrem Surg* 4(3):148, 2000.

Viegas SF, Yamaguchi S, Boyi NL, et al. The dorsal ligaments of the wrist: anatomy, mechanical properties, and function. *J Hand Surg [Am]* 24(3):456, 1999.

Watson HK, Ashmead D IV, Makhlouf MV. Examination of the scaphoid. *J Hand Surg [Am]* 13:657–660, 1988.

Wolfe SW, Crisco JJ, Katz LD. A non-invasive method for studying in vivo carpal kinematics. *J Hand Surg* 22B:147, 1977.

Wolfe SW, Nev C, Crisco JJ. In vivo scaphoid, lunate, and capitate kinematics in flexion and in extension. *J Hand Surg [Am]* 25(5):860, 2000.

Youm Y, McMurtry RY, Flatt AE, et al. Kinematics of the wrist. *J Bone Joint Surg* 60A(4):1913, 1978.

14 | Fractures and Dislocations of the Metacarpals and Phalanges

John A. Elstrom

This chapter covers fractures and fracture dislocations of the metacarpals and phalanges.

ANATOMY

The **metacarpals 2 through 5** have an expanded cuboidal base, with facets for articulation with the carpus and neighboring metacarpals. Dorsal and palmar intermetacarpal ligaments and interosseous ligaments stabilize these articulations. The first **carpometacarpal joint** (CMC) is a biconcave saddle joint stabilized primarily by the anterior oblique ligament and the intermetacarpal ligament.

The **metacarpophalangeal joints** (MCP) are complex hinge joints that allow medial and lateral movement when they are fully extended. The volar aspect of these joints is supported by a volar plate. The collateral ligaments are medial and lateral to the joints and are the primary medial and lateral stabilizers. The metacarpal head is cam-shaped, and the collaterals are under maximal stretch in flexion. The MCP joint is safely splinted in 70 to 90 degrees of flexion. The cam effect of the metacarpal head maintains the length of the collateral ligament and prevents extension contracture (Figs. 14-1*A* and *B*). The MCP joint of the thumb is structurally similar to the other MCP joints, but its intrinsic muscles (adductor pollicis, abductor pollicis brevis, and flexor pollicis brevis) and three extrinsic tendons (flexor pollicis longus, extensor pollicis brevis, and extensor pollicis longus) are dynamic stabilizers. The thumb is splinted in opposition (the position of function) to avoid contracture of these intrinsic muscles (i.e., the first web space).

Proximal and middle phalanges have a slight apex dorsal curve. The **proximal and distal interphalangeal joints** (PIP and DIP) are true hinge joints. Stabilizing ligaments are similar to those of the MCP joint, but unlike the MCP joints, there is no side-to-side motion. The PIP joints are splinted in 0 to 10 degrees of flexion, thereby preventing the development of a check-rein effect about the volar plate with a flexion contracture.

The **extensor hood** is dorsal to the PIP joint; its central slip inserts on the middle phalanx and the lateral bands form the DIP joint extensor. The flexor digitorum sublimis (FDS) inserts on the middle phalanx, and the flexor digitorum profundus (FDP) inserts on the base of the distal phalanx.

FRACTURES OF THE METACARPALS

Classification

Fractures of the metacarpals are classified as involving the base, the diaphysis, the neck, or the head. Additional factors that influence management are

201

A

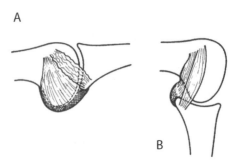

FIG. 14-1   *A* and *B.* The cam shape of the metacarpal head causes the collateral ligaments to be stretched maximally when the MCP joint is flexed.

whether the fracture is open, closed, or the result of a high-energy injury, and whether more than one metacarpal is fractured.

Fractures of the **metacarpal bases** can be associated with dorsal subluxation of the CMC joint (Fig. 14-2). This is particularly true of fractures of the base of the fifth metacarpal, which are displaced dorsally and proximally by the extensor carpi ulnaris (Fig. 14-3).

A torsional force to the finger, axial loading of the metacarpal head, or a direct blow to the dorsum of the hand determines whether a metacarpal shaft fracture is oblique or transverse.

Metacarpal neck fractures, also known as **boxer's fractures**, are due to an axial loading volarly directed force to the metacarpal head. The interosseous muscles maintain the fracture in a flexed position.

Fractures of the **metacarpal head** are due to avulsion of a collateral ligament or to impaction from a longitudinal blow. Fracture of the metacarpal head due to impaction from a tooth during a fistfight is also known as a **fight bite** and is particularly likely to become infected.

Diagnosis and Initial Management

History and Physical Examination

There is pain localized to the area of injury and a history of trauma. Swelling will be present, deformity may be. In particular, correct rotational alignment must be confirmed. Digital scissoring may occur in spiral fractures of the metacarpal diaphysis, and it is essential to flex the injured MCP joint to observe

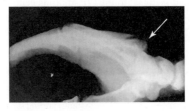

FIG. 14-2   Dorsal dislocation of the fifth MCP joint and a fracture of the base of the fourth metacarpal.

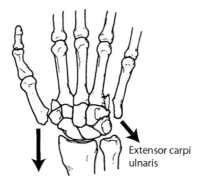

FIG. 14-3   Fracture with subluxation of the base of the fifth metacarpal and Bennett's fracture of the first metacarpal.

rotational alignment. The fingertips of correctly aligned fingers point toward the tubercle of the scaphoid. Alignment of the nail bed can also be compared with the opposite side to check for this deformity. It will not be evident on x-ray.

Radiographic Examination

Anteroposterior (AP), lateral, and oblique views of the hand are obtained. A 30-degree pronation AP view of the fifth CMC joints will show subluxation of this joint. Computed tomography (CT) may help in the evaluation of the CMC joints.

Initial Management

Initial management of a metacarpal fracture that is displaced is reduction and immobilization in a splint. The splint extends from the PIP joints to the elbow. The position of immobilization is as follows: the MCP joints are flexed to 90 degrees, the PIP joints are extended, and the wrist dorsiflexed to 20 degrees. When reduction is required, a metacarpal or hematoma block is administered.

Fracture-dislocations of the **base of the metacarpals (the MC-C joints)** are reduced by longitudinal traction and pressing the metacarpal base volarward. Fractures of the metacarpal diaphysis and neck are usually angulated with the apex dorsal. **Diaphyseal fractures** are reduced with longitudinal traction and application of a corrective force to the apex of the deformity. **Spiral fractures** of the diaphysis are often underestimated. They require immobilization with the MCP joints flexed so that rotational deformity does not occur. **Boxer's fractures** are reduced by flexing the MCP and PIP joints and pushing the proximal phalanx dorsally at the PIP joint to lift the metacarpal head while maintaining volar-directed pressure on the metacarpal proximal to the fracture. Fractures of the **metacarpal head** usually do not require closed reduction and are splinted.

Associated Injuries

A wound over the metacarpal head should raise suspicion of a fight bite. Because of the likelihood of infection, these injuries should be surgically explored, thoroughly irrigated, and closed secondarily. Other injuries associated with metacarpal fractures and dislocations are infrequent.

Definitive Management

Most metacarpal fractures are managed with splinting or casting for 3 to 6 weeks. Immobilization is discontinued when there are clinical (i.e., absence of pain at the fracture site) and early radiographic signs of healing.

There are specific indications for surgery for each type of metacarpal fracture. An unstable fracture or a less than anatomic reduction of a fracture of the **metacarpal base** is an indication for operative reduction and fixation. The fracture is either reduced under direct vision through a dorsal incision or with the aid of fluoroscopy. Kirschner wires are driven across the fracture into the carpus or, in situations involving multiple metacarpals, plate fixation spanning the carpometacarpal joint may be preferable. Postoperatively, the hand is splinted for 3 to 6 weeks. During this time, the splint is removed daily for range-of-motion exercises of the PIP and MCP joints. K wires are removed when fracture or joint stability is assured. Plate fixation has the advantage that it does not interfere with rehabilitation and it can be removed at any time.

Indications for internal fixation of fractures of the **metacarpal diaphysis** areas follows: (1)shortening of more than 3 mm, (2) rotational malalignment resulting in digital scissoring, (3) dorsal angulation of the fourth and fifth metacarpals greater than 40 degrees, (4) dorsal angulation of the second and third metacarpals greater than 10 degrees, (5) multiple metacarpal fractures, and (6) gunshot wounds or crush injuries with comminution or loss of bone (Fig. 14-4). The fracture can be reduced closed using fluoroscopy or exposed through a dorsal incision. Fractures reduced closed are stabilized with percutaneous K wires. Plates and screws, interosseous K wires, and intramedullary K wires are used to stabilize fractures that have been opened. Fractures with a deficient or contaminated soft tissue envelope need stable fixation, especially to prevent shortening; they are managed with plates and screws, an external fixator, K-wire spacers, or polymethylmethacrylate spacers prior to the definitive

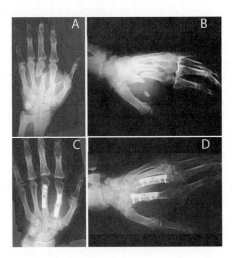

FIG. 14-4   *A* to *D*. Multiple metacarpal fractures resulting from a crush injury to the hand, treated by debridement, immediate internal fixation, and secondary wound closure, thus allowing early motion.

reconstruction. Postoperatively, simple fractures are immobilized for 6 weeks, the splint is removed daily for range-of-motion exercises, and the pins are removed at 6 to 8 weeks. The postoperative management of fractures with loss of bone and severe soft tissue injury is individualized.

Indications for internal fixation of fractures of the **metacarpal neck** are rotational deformity resulting in digital scissoring and excessive dorsal angulation of the apex. Up to 40 degrees of angulation in the fourth and fifth and up to 10 degrees in the second and third metacarpals are acceptable. A greater angulation is acceptable in the fourth and fifth metacarpals than the second and third because the latter CMC joints are more rigid, and significant angulation results in a more obvious dorsal deformity and a prominent metacarpal head in the palm with painful grasp.

The fracture is reduced closed using fluoroscopy and stabilized with percutaneous K wires driven into an adjacent metacarpal or used as intramedullary rods and inserted through the MCP joint. When they are inserted through the MCP joint, they are cut long, and the MCP joint is maintained in flexion until the fracture heals (usually 4 to 6 weeks), at which point the pins are removed.

Undisplaced fractures of the **metacarpal head** are splinted, as described under "Initial Management," above, for 3 weeks. Fractures with large displaced intraarticular fragments are exposed through a dorsal incision, reduced, and stabilized with K wires. Comminuted fractures that cannot be reduced are managed with distraction in an external fixator or dynamic traction.

Collateral ligamentous avulsions are managed with buddy taping. Collateral avulsion with bony displacement of more than 5 mm is managed with open reduction and pinning. **Fight bites** are always explored, debrided, and irrigated through the wound and left open. Parenteral antibiotics are administered for 2 weeks.

Complications

Complications include malunion, nonunion, posttraumatic arthrosis, and joint contractures/tendon adhesions. **Malunion includes digital shortening, unsightly or painful bony prominence, and malrotation (digital scissoring);** these can be managed with osteotomy and internal fixation. **Nonunion** is infrequent and is managed with stable fixation and bone grafting. **Adhesions and contractures** are managed initially with intensive physical therapy and later, if necessary, with surgical release. Arthroplasty of the MCP joints and CMC joint arthrodesis are possible salvage procedures but are rarely needed.

FRACTURES AND DISLOCATIONS OF THE PHALANGES

Fractures of the phalanges are classified as involving the base of the proximal phalanx, the diaphysis of the proximal or middle phalanx, the PIP joint, the DIP joint, or the distal phalanx. Dislocations involve the MCP, PIP, or DIP joints.

Fracture of the **base of the proximal phalanx** is due to avulsion by the collateral ligament (corner fracture) or impaction by the metacarpal head. Pilon fractures are comminuted intraarticular fractures of the base of the proximal or middle phalanx; these are difficult to reconstruct surgically and have a poor prognosis.

Fracture of the **diaphysis of the proximal or middle phalanx** is caused by a direct blow or torsional force. Fractures of the proximal phalanx have apical volar angulation secondary to the pull of the interossei. Deforming forces on the middle phalanx are the FDS tendon and the long extensor tendon. Distal fractures of the middle phalanx tend to have apical volar angulation, proximal fractures, and apical dorsal angulation.

Fractures of the **PIP joint** involve the proximal or middle phalanx. Fractures of the proximal phalanx are condylar, unicondylar, or bicondylar (comminuted); undisplaced; or displaced.

Fractures of the base of the middle phalanx are undisplaced or displaced, involving the volar or dorsal lip; they may be lateral avulsions and comminuted (pilon-type) fractures.

Fractures of the **DIP joint** involve either the condyles of the middle phalanx or the base of the distal phalanx. Fractures of the dorsal lip of the distal phalanx, or **mallet finger**, are caused by avulsion of the extensor tendon. Fractures of the volar lip of the distal phalanx are caused by avulsion of the FDP tendon or volar plate during hyperextension. FDP avulsions occur in contact sports such as rugby or football and most often involve the fourth finger.

Distal phalangeal fractures are caused by a direct blow or by a power tool. These are frequently open and often involve an injury to the nail bed that must be repaired. Radiographically, they are longitudinal, transverse, or comminuted.

Dislocations of the **MCP and DIP joints** are usually dorsal and caused by hyperextension. Dislocations of the PIP joint are most commonly dorsal, but they can also be volar. Volar PIP joint dislocations are associated with an extensor tendon central slip rupture and require special treatment of that injury.

Diagnosis and Initial Management

History and Physical Examination

There is a history of trauma, with pain at the area of injury. There may be swelling and deformity. Malrotation, which can result in digital scissoring, will be evident by flexing the MCP joints while keeping the PIP joint extended or by checking the rotation of the nail bed. Dimpling of the skin associated with a dislocation indicates that reduction may not be possible by closed means. MCP joint dislocations frequently require open reduction.

Radiographic Examination

AP, lateral, and oblique radiographs define the injury. CT imaging can be helpful in characterizing obscure joint injuries, but the proper coils must be available.

Initial Management

The majority of fractures of the phalanx are managed with closed methods. Buddy taping is used for fractures of the proximal and middle phalanges that do not require reduction. In cases where reduction is performed, a metacarpal, digital, or hematoma block is administered and the deformity corrected; this consists of traction and manipulation to correct angulation or malrotation. Immobilization of a reduced proximal phalangeal fracture is done by taping the injured finger to an adjacent digit and applying a cast or splint extending from the proximal forearm to include the involved fingers or terminating the cast at the metacarpal heads and using an Alumafoam extension. The wrist is immobilized in 20 degrees of dorsiflexion, the MCP joint in 80 degrees of flexion, and the PIP and IP joints in extension. Except for splinting to the adjacent digit, uninvolved fingers should not be immobilized. Fractures of the PIP joint and distal phalanx are immobilized in an Alumafoam splint.

The reduction of dislocations of the PIP and DIP joints is usually a matter of correcting deformity and can be accomplished with or without anesthetic block simply by pushing the displaced distal segment palmarward over the stabilized proximal component. Traction can be counterproductive in some instances.

Definitive Management

Small avulsion fractures of the **base of the proximal phalanx** are managed with buddy taping and early protected motion. Displaced fragments comprising more than 30% of the articular surface are exposed through volar or dorsal incisions, depending on location, and fixed with small K wires, or screws. **Impaction** fractures are managed with reduction of the joint surface, elevation of depressed articular segments, and fixation of the joint surface to the diaphysis. The MCP joint is immobilized at 90 degrees to "mold" the fracture to the shape of the metacarpal head. Motion is started at 3 weeks. When a comminuted impaction (pilon) fracture cannot be reduced and stabilized surgically, dynamic traction through the middle or distal phalanx (with or without a limited open reduction and pinning) can provide a qualified reduction and allow early passive motion. The Schenck dynamic splint is useful in this regard (Fig. 14-5).

Undisplaced fractures of the **diaphysis of the proximal and middle phalanges** are managed with buddy taping and supportive casting (or splinting).

Displaced diaphyseal fractures are managed with closed reduction and casting for about 3 weeks. Clinical fracture stabilization occurs rapidly, and prolonged immobilization while waiting for radiographic signs of consolidation is detrimental. Up to 15 degrees of angulation in the plane of motion is well tolerated. Rotational deformity results in digital scissoring, and angulation in the coronal plane results in spaces between the fingers when the hand is cupped. "Bayoneting" of fracture fragments results in a prominent spike of bone that can result in impingement on tendons, limiting motion.

Failure to maintain reduction, open fractures, and injuries with multiple fractures are indications for operative reduction and stabilization. Open reduction is performed through a splitting incision of the dorsal extensor tendon;

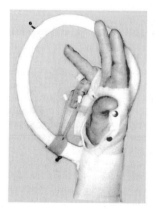

FIG. 14-5   The Schenck dynamic traction device. (*From Sarris I, Goitz R, Sotereanos D. Dynamic traction and minimal internal fixation for thumb and digital pilon fractures. J Hand Surg 29A:39–43, 2004, with permission from the American Society for Surgery of the Hand.*)

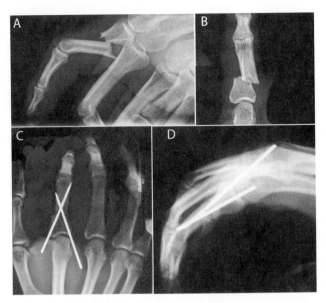

FIG. 14-6   *A to D.* Displaced transverse fracture of the base of the index finger proximal phalanx, treated by percutaneous pinning.

closed reduction is achieved with the aid of fluoroscopy. Fixation is done with K wires, plate and screws, or an external fixator. The typical transverse fracture is fixed with crossed intramedullary K wires (Fig. 14-6) and the oblique fractures with interfragmentary screws or K wires (Fig. 14-7). For comminuted diaphyseal fractures, a miniplate and screws provides fixation that allows immediate motion (Fig. 14-8). Postoperatively, immobilization is maintained for a few days for the wound and fracture to stabilize; if fixation is adequate, active range-of-motion exercises are initiated.

Undisplaced fractures of the **PIP joint** (proximal or middle phalanx) are managed with buddy taping. Displaced unicondylar or bicondylar fractures of the proximal phalanx are reduced open and stabilized. The surgical exposure splits the extensor tendon, thereby preserving the attachment of the central slip tendon on the base of middle phalanx. Stabilization is done with K wires or screws. Barton (1984) described an excellent extraarticular method of reduction and fixation of oblique unicondylar fractures using a midlateral approach, precisely reducing the extraarticular component and fixing it with a transverse K wire or screw. Comminuted fractures are managed with an external fixator or with dynamic traction.

Displaced **volar lip** fractures of the base of the middle phalanx involving more than 30% of the joint surface are often associated with joint instability (Fig. 14-9). They are exposed through a volar Brunner incision, the A-3 pulley is opened, flexor tendons are retracted, and the fragment is reduced and stabilized with K wires. Alternatively, comminuted fragments are excised and the volar plate is sutured into the defect with a pull-out suture. The joint is pinned for 3 weeks or, alternatively, an extension-block K wire can be inserted into the head of the proximal phalanx, maintaining joint reduction by preventing

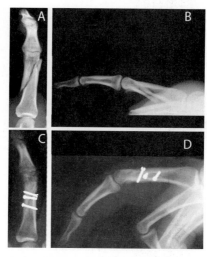

FIG. 14-7   *A* to *D*. Spiral fracture of the proximal phalanx stabilized with transverse 1.5-mm screws.

dorsal displacement of the middle phalanx. Limited protected motion can begin when the situation has stabilized and the pins have been removed. Recently, grafting of the defect with the distal articular surface of the hamate has been described. Agee (1978) described a force coupling device for maintaining joint reduction while allowing motion.

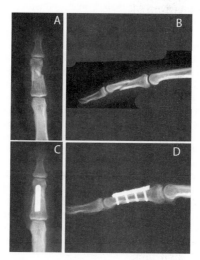

FIG. 14-8   *A* to *D*. Comminuted angulated middle phalangeal fracture treated with a miniplate and screws, thus allowing early motion. (*Courtesy of Robert F. Hall, Jr., M.D.*)

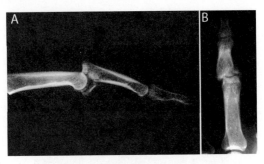

FIG. 14-9   *A* and *B*. Comminuted fracture-dislocation of the PIP joint. (*Courtesy of Robert F. Hall, Jr., M.D.*)

Fractures of the dorsal lip are rare and represent avulsion of the central slip of the extensor tendon. Displacement of more than 2 mm results in an extension lag or boutonniere deformity. If more than 30% of the articular surface is involved, the joint may be unstable. Exposure is through a dorsal approach, and stabilization is done with K wires or a pull-out suture tied over a volar button. Displaced lateral avulsion fractures are the result of collateral ligament avulsion. They are opened, reduced, and stabilized with a pull-out wire, figure-of-eight tension band, or K wires.

The **comminuted** fracture of the middle phalangeal base is also a pilon fracture. Fracture reduction can be difficult to achieve and maintain; the results of open treatment are mediocre. Collapse of the joint surface requires elevation by means of a limited open procedure and, rarely, the support of a bone graft. Severely comminuted fractures can then be managed with an external fixator or dynamic skeletal traction (Fig. 14-5).

Fractures of the **DIP joint** involve the head of the middle phalanx or the base of the distal phalanx. Intraarticular fractures of the condyles of the middle phalanx are similar to condylar fractures of the proximal phalanx. Undisplaced condylar fractures are managed with splinting or buddy taping. Displaced fractures are opened, reduced, and pinned. The DIP joint is immobilized for 3 weeks, but the PIP joint is left unsplinted. A fracture of the **dorsal lip of the distal phalanx**, or **mallet finger**, is an avulsion of the extensor tendon. Most are managed with immobilization of the DIP joint in extension for 6 weeks. Fractures comprising more than 30% of the articular surface may be reduced open and pinned through a dorsal incision, but the complication rate is high: foremost is stiffness. Open reduction is recommended only for those fractures associated with subluxation of the joint. A better alternative is closed extension-block splinting (Fig. 14-10*A* to *C*). In this method the DIP joint is flexed maximally and, using fluoroscopy, a K wire is inserted into the head of the middle phalanx to block retraction of the avulsed bone fragment. The distal fragment is then reduced to both the articular surface and the dorsal avulsed fragment and the joint is pinned longitudinally. In either instance, the joint is pinned for 6 weeks.

Fractures of the volar lip are FDP avulsions and are explored. The tendon is repaired or the fragment of bone is reduced and stabilized with a pull-out wire or small-diameter K wires.

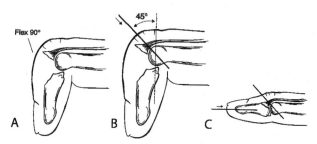

FIG. 14-10 *A to C.* Extension-block pinning for large mallet fractures. (*From Hofmeister E, Mazurek M, Shin A, Bishop A. Extension block pinning for large mallet fractures. J Hand Surg 28A:453–459, 2003, with permission from the American Society for Surgery of the Hand.*)

Undisplaced transverse tuft fractures of the **distal phalanx** are splinted after any subungual hematoma is decompressed. Displaced fractures are often associated with a soft tissue laceration and are pinned if unstable. Disruption of the nail bed must be repaired or nail deformity will ensue with nail regrowth.

Longitudinal fractures may be intraarticular and, when displaced, are pinned percutaneously with the aid of fluoroscopy or under direct vision.

Dislocation of the MCP joint is most commonly dorsal and can be recognized with hyperextension of the digit. This can be reduced by distal and volar-based pressure on the base of the proximal phalanx. Irreducible dislocation is caused by detachment of the volar plate and its interposition between the metacarpal head and the base of the proximal phalanx. The digit is in slight hyperextension, and the volar skin may be puckered. Operative reduction can be through a volar or dorsal incision. The volar plate is divided longitudinally through the dorsal incision, allowing the metacarpal head to reduce. To affect reduction through the volar approach, the A-1 pulley is divided, allowing the tendon to be retracted and permitting the volar plate and proximal phalanx to fall into a reduced position.

Dislocation of the PIP joint is most commonly dorsal but can also occur volarly. Dorsal dislocation is associated with avulsion of the volar plate and is usually stable. This can be treated with immobilization or extension-block splinting for 1 to 2 weeks. Unstable dorsal dislocations with volar fractures can be treated with extension-block splinting for 3 to 4 weeks, extension-block pinning, or open reduction of a large fragment. In extension-block pinning, a K wire is placed through the head of the proximal phalanx, temporarily blocking extension and redisplacement of the middle phalanx.

Volar dislocation of the **PIP** joint can be straight volar or with a rotatory component. Straight volar dislocations usually involve avulsion of the central slip. Reduction is performed with gentle traction, and the **PIP joint** is splinted in extension for 6 weeks to avoid a boutonniere deformity. Rotatory dislocation of the **PIP joint** most frequently involves buttonholing of the condyle of the proximal phalanx between the central slip and the lateral band. This can be irreducible; open reduction is then necessary to extricate the lateral band from the joint and reduce the entrapped condyle.

Dislocations of the **DIP** joint are generally dorsal and are reduced with gentle traction. Irreducible dislocations are rare and are associated with interposition of the volar plate or flexor tendon. Surgery is necessary to extricate the inter-posed structure.

Complications

Complications of phalangeal fractures and dislocations include malunion, chronic subluxation, nonunion, joint stiffness, and posttraumatic arthrosis.

Malunion can be managed with osteotomy and internal fixation to correct deformity; but in special circumstances, such as joint subluxation or Swan-neck deformity, arthroplasty or a soft tissue procedure, respectively, may be indicated. Corrective osteotomy is generally delayed until soft tissue equilibrium has been restored (e.g., edema and swelling are gone and a satisfactory range of motion is present). Neglected joint instability is corrected immediately if the disability warrants.

Nonunion and joint stiffness are addressed with either internal fixation and possibly bone grafting in the first instance or aggressive physical therapy in the second. Occasionally, significant loss of motion will benefit by a soft tissue release.

FRACTURES OF THE THUMB

Two injuries are unique to the first ray: fractures of the base of the metacarpal and gamekeeper's thumb. Other fractures of the first ray are managed as are their counterparts in the second through fifth rays.

Fractures of the base of the first metacarpal are classified as Bennett's fractures, Rolando's fractures, or extraarticular fractures. The **Bennett's fracture** is a fracture-dislocation. The volar lip fragment is held by the anterior oblique ligament and varies in size. The metacarpal shaft is subluxed radially, proximally, and dorsally by the pull of the adductor pollicis brevis and the abductor pollicis longus (Fig. 14-3). The **Rolando's fracture** is a comminuted intraarticular fracture of the base of the first metacarpal. Extraarticular fractures of the base of the first metacarpal are usually transverse fractures within 1 cm of the articular surface.

Gamekeeper's thumb is an avulsion injury of the ulnar collateral of the MCP joint. The collateral ligament is often displaced proximally, allowing the adductor tendon to become interposed between the tendon end and its insertion on the base of the proximal phalanx. This produces the Stener lesion (Fig. 14-11A and B). The collateral ligament can also be avulsed from the proximal phalanx with an osteocartilaginous fragment of the articular surface (a corner fracture) or torn in midsubstance.

Diagnosis and Initial Management

History and Physical Examination

There is a history of injury to the thumb. Pain, swelling, and localized tenderness indicate the area of injury.

Radiographic Examination

Radiographs of the thumb are obtained with a special palm-up metacarpal–carpal joint AP view, if indicated, to delineate a fracture at that joint as being either of the Bennett's or Rolando's type.

Stress radiographs of an injured MCP joint to determine the extent of instability must usually be carried out after a local anesthetic block. This study

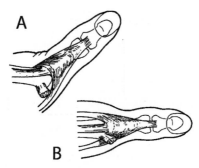

FIG. 14-11   *A* and *B*. Gamekeeper's thumb and the Stener lesion.

might possibly create a Stener lesion and should not be done in the presence of a nondisplaced corner fracture. Stressing of the MCP joint with an ulnar opening of 10 to 15 degrees greater than at the unaffected side is indicative of an ulnar collateral avulsion.

Initial Management

The initial management is typically a well-padded thumb spica splint applied along the radial aspect of the forearm to the tip of the thumb.

Definitive Management

The **Bennett's fracture** is reduced closed under fluoroscopy with longitudinal traction, abduction, and pronation. Finger-trap traction facilitates the procedure. The reduction is stabilized with percutaneous pins. The first metacarpal is pinned with multiple K wires to the carpus, the second metacarpal, or both. It is not necessary to transfix the small volar fragment as long as reduction is maintained. Fragments comprising more than 30% of the articular surface are reduced and pinned to ensure maintenance of reduction of the articular surface. Open reduction may be necessary to achieve a satisfactory result. This is accomplished through an angled incision at the base of the thumb that elevates the thenar musculature from the CMC joint. Postoperatively, the hand is placed in a thumb spica splint from the IP joint to the proximal forearm for 4 weeks. The pins are removed a week later, as rehabilitation progresses.

The **Rolando's fracture** is reduced open through a hockey-stick incision of the volar side of the MCP joint. The fracture is reduced and a mini–T plate or Kirschner wires are used to stabilize the fragments. Severely comminuted Rolando's fractures may not be amenable to open reduction. Reduction with traction, percutaneous pinning of the metacarpal shaft (i.e., distal fragment) through the proximal fragment to the carpus or to the second metacarpal, and application of a mini–external fixator (with pins in the distal first metacarpal and trapezium) can maintain length and an approximate reduction (Fig. 14-12). Postoperatively, the hand is splinted from the IP joint to proximal forearm for 4 weeks.

Extraarticular fractures of the first metacarpal are managed with closed reduction and casting for 4 to 5 weeks. Reduction is obtained by longitudinal traction and pronation of the distal fragment. Casting can be carried out in

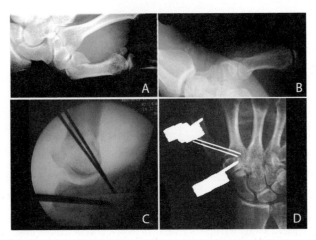

FIG. 14-12 *A to D.* Comminuted intraarticular fracture of the base of the thumb metacarpal (Rolando's fracture), treated with reduction with finger-trap traction, percutaneous K-wire fixation, and static external fixator traction.

finger-trap traction, but when traction is released, the fracture tends to collapse. Diligent radiographic follow-up is important. Fifteen degrees of angulation is acceptable. Occasionally percutaneous pinning or open reduction and internal fixation are needed.

Gamekeeper's thumb is managed with open repair of the ulnar collateral ligament and volar capsule through an ulnar incision. The ligament is repaired or bony avulsions are reduced and stabilized. This is usually accomplished with a transosseus suture (pull-out suture) tied over a button on the side opposite the injury, Kirschner wires, or a figure-of-eight tension-band wire (passed under the ligamentous attachment to the avulsed fragment and through a transverse drill hole just distal to the fracture). Supplemental K-wire fixation of the MCP joint is recommended for purely soft tissue repairs. Postoperatively, the hand is placed in a thumb spica splint for 4 weeks for bony avulsions and 6 weeks for ligamentous repairs.

Complications

The most common complication of Bennett's and Rolando's fractures is MCC joint arthritis. This can be managed conservatively with nonsteroidal anti-inflammatory drugs and local steroid injections. If these measures fail, the joint is arthrodesed. The most common complication of gamekeeper's thumb is chronic instability of the MCP joint due to delay in presentation or failure of the repair. It is managed with ligamentous reconstruction with a tendon graft or **MCP joint** arthrodesis.

SELECTED READINGS

Agee JM. Unstable dislocation of the proximal interphalangeal joint of the fingers: a preliminary report of a new treatment technique. *J Hand Surg* 3:386–389, 1978.
Barton MJ. Fractures of the hand. *J Bone Joint Surg* 66B:159–167, 1984.

Becton JL, Christian JD Jr, Goodwin HN, Jackson JG. Simplified technique for treating the complex dislocation of the index metacarpal-phalangeal joint. *J Bone Joint Surg* 57A:698–700, 1975.

Dinowitz M, Trumble T, Hanel D, et al. Failure of cast immobilization for thumb ulnar collateral ligament avulsion fractures. *J Hand Surg* 22A:1057–1063, 1997.

Eaton RG, Malerich MM. Volar plate arthroplasty for the proximal interphalangeal joint. A ten year review. *J Hand Surg* 5:260–268, 1980.

Gonzalez MH, McKay W, Hall RF Jr. Low velocity gunshot wounds of the metacarpal: treatment by early stable fixation and bone grafting. *J Hand Surg* 18A:267, 1993.

Hofmeister EP, Mazurek MT, Shin AY, Bishop AT. Extension block pinning for large mallet fractures. *J Hand Surg* 28:453–459. 2003.

Mueller JJ. Carpometacarpal dislocations: report of five cases and review of the literature. *J Hand Surg* 11A:184–188, 1986.

Parsons SW, Fitzgerald JAW, Shearer JR. External fixation of unstable metacarpal and phalangeal fractures. *J Hand Surg* 17B:151–155, 1992.

Rafael MM, Williams MD, Keifhaber TR, et al. Treatment of unstable dorsal proximal interphalangeal fracture/dislocations using a hemi-hamate autograft. *J Hand Surg* 28:856–865, 2003.

Sarris I, Goitz RJ, Sotereanos DG. Dynamic traction and minimal internal fixation for thumb and digital pilon fractures. *J Hand Surg* 29:39–43, 2004.

Schenck RR. Dynamic traction and early passive movement for fractures of the proximal interphalangeal joint. *J Hand Surg* 11A:850–858, 1986.

Stern PJ, Roman RJ, Kiefhaber TR, McDonough JJ. Pilon fractures of the proximal interphalangeal joint. *J Hand Surg* 16A:844–850, 1991.

Weiss AP, Hastings H II. Distal unicondylar fractures of the proximal phalanx. *J Hand Surg* 18A:594–599, 1993.

15 | Fractures and Dislocations of the Spine

Gbolahan O. Okubadejo   Brett A. Taylor
Lawrence G. Lenke   Keith H. Bridwell

Spinal trauma includes injuries occurring in the axial skeleton from the occipitocervical junction to the coccyx. The anatomic classification of spinal trauma is organized into upper cervical, subaxial cervical, thoracic, lumbar, and sacral. The pathophysiology of spinal trauma and the initial assessment of a suspected spinal injury are similar for all patients.

When a patient with a spinal injury is being examined, the key questions are as follows: What is the mechanism of injury? Are there other injuries, including life-threatening ones? What are the injured anatomic structures of the spine? Is there actual or impending neurologic damage? Can the spine function as a weight-bearing column? What is the best treatment method (operative or nonoperative) for the particular fracture? The most important decision initially is whether definitive management should be operative or nonoperative.

ANATOMY

The function of the spine as a support column is broken down into the four anatomic segments: cervical, thoracic, lumbar, and sacrococcygeal. Normally, these segments align in a linear fashion in the coronal or frontal plane. However, in the sagittal plane, there are approximately 25 degrees of cervical lordosis, 35 degrees of thoracic kyphosis, and approximately 50 degrees of lumbar lordosis, thereby allowing the skull to align directly over the midportion of the top of the sacrum.

The cross-sectional anatomy of the spine is organized into **three columns** (Fig. 15-1). The **anterior column** consists of the anterior longitudinal ligament, anterior half of the vertebral body, annulus fibrosus, and disc. The **middle column** consists of the posterior half of the vertebral body, annulus, disc, and posterior longitudinal ligament. The **posterior column** includes the facet joints, ligamentum flavum, posterior elements, and interconnecting ligaments.

The three-column theory of the spine produces a basic classification system of spinal injuries. Thus, spinal injuries are classified into four different categories depending on the specific column(s) injured: compression fractures, burst fractures, seat belt–type flexion-distraction injuries, and fracture-dislocations (Table 15-1). **Compression fractures** are characterized by failure of the anterior column under compression, with intact middle and posterior columns. When the anterior and middle columns fail under axial loading forces, a **burst fracture** is produced. Distraction of the middle and posterior column produces a seat belt type of **flexion-distraction** injury. This is also known as a Chance fracture. **Fracture-dislocations** are characterized by involvement of all three columns in compression, distraction, rotation, and/or shear.

Although the three-column theory of the spine provides an excellent model to describe the individual spinal segments injured, it is essential to determine the spine's overall structural stability. For example, compression injuries to the anterior and/or middle column may cause kyphosis. Because spinal injuries

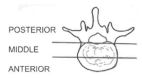

POSTERIOR

MIDDLE

ANTERIOR

FIG. 15-1 The three columns of the spine.

result from a combination of various forces acting on the spinal column—including compression, distraction, axial load, rotation, torsion, or shear—careful attention is paid to alignment in the coronal and sagittal planes to identify potential subluxation or dislocations of the spine.

Osseous Anatomy

The **cervical spine** comprises the first seven vertebrae and connects the skull to the thoracic spine. The cervical spine functions to protect the spinal cord and nerve roots while supporting the skull and allowing flexibility to position the head. Approximately half of neck flexion-extension occurs between the base of the skull and C1. Similarly, half of the rotation of the head on the neck occurs at the C1-C2 articulation. The remaining motions of flexion, extension, rotation, and side bending occur between the C2 and T1 articulations.

The atlas (C1) and the axis (C2) differ markedly in structure from the lower five cervical vertebrae (C3 through C7). The atlas is unique among vertebrae in that it has no vertebral body but rather a thick anterior arch with two bulky lateral masses and a thin posterior arch. The axis has the odontoid process or dens, which is the fused remnant of the body of the first cervical vertebra. The odontoid process sits cephalad on the body of C2 and rests just posterior to the anterior arch of the atlas, where it is held tightly by ligaments. The remaining lower cervical vertebrae (C3 through C7) have small vertebral bodies that are convex on the superior surface and concave on the inferior surface. Arising anterolaterally from the bodies are transverse processes that have both anterior and posterior tubercles. The foramen transversarium is located between the posterior tubercle and the lateral part of the vertebral body. The vertebral artery passes through this foramen, entering at C6 and exiting at C2. The exiting nerve roots pass just posterior to the vertebral arteries at the level of the disc space.

Posterior to the vertebral foramina are the lateral masses comprising that portion of bone between the superior and inferior facets. The lateral masses are important anatomic structures for the placement of screws in posterior plating procedures of the cervical spine. The cervical facet joints are oriented more in a horizontal than a vertical plane, with the superior facet sitting anterior to the inferior facet of the level above. This allows for a great amount of flexion and ex-

TABLE 15-1 Classification of Spinal Injuries

| | Columns injured | | |
Type of injury	Anterior	Middle	Posterior
I Compression fractures	Yes	No	No
II Burst fractures	Yes	Yes	No
III Flexion–distraction injuries	Yes/No	Yes	Yes
IV Fracture–dislocations	Yes	Yes	Yes

tension of the neck but limits side bending. The remainder of the posterior elements of the cervical spine include the lamina and spinous processes, which are posterior and medial to the facet joints and lateral masses.

There are 12 vertebrae of the **thoracic spine**. The differential features of thoracic vertebrae are the thin pedicles, which connect the vertebral bodies to the posterior elements; the transverse processes, which project superolaterally from the posterior part of the pedicle and are larger in size than the cervical transverse processes; and the ventral surface of the transverse process, which has a costal articulation. The thoracic spine is a more rigid column than the cervical or lumbar spine because of the rib cage. As in the cervical spine, the facets of the thoracic spine are oriented in the coronal plane, with the superior facet anterior to the inferior facet. At the thoracolumbar junction, the facet joints change gradually from a coronal to a more sagittal orientation.

The vertebrae of the **lumbar spine** are larger than the cervical or thoracic vertebrae. The pedicles are wider and broader, and they are usually able to accept bone screws. The facet joints are oriented sagittally, with the inferior facet of the segment above medial to the superior facet of the segment below. The transverse processes project straight laterally from the superior facets and are quite large. The posterior elements (lamina and spinous processes) are also larger in the lumbar spine.

The **sacrum and coccyx** are normally fused and attach the axial skeleton to the pelvis by sacroiliac articulation, the sacrotuberous ligaments, and sacrospinous ligaments.

Ligamentous Anatomy

The ligaments of the spinal column support the osseous structures. We distinguish between those supporting the anterior and middle columns and those stabilizing the posterior column. The stabilizers of the anterior and middle columns are the **anterior longitudinal ligament** and the **posterior longitudinal ligament**. These ligaments extend the entire length of the spine and insert on the vertebral bodies. They are the major stabilizers of the vertebral bodies and discs during flexion and extension. The anterior longitudinal ligament is closely attached to the intervertebral disc and has a ribbon-like structure. The posterior longitudinal ligament is widest in the upper cervical spine and narrows as it proceeds caudally. It thins over the vertebral bodies and thickens over the intervertebral discs.

The ligamentous structures stabilizing the posterior column include the **supraspinous ligament, the interspinous ligament, the facet joint capsule,** and **the ligamentum flavum**. The ligamentum flavum runs from the superior margin of the caudad lamina to the ventral surface of the cephalad lamina. There are right and left ligaments separated by a small fissure that merges with the interspinous ligaments posteriorly and medially and with the fibrous facet capsules laterally. The posterior ligamentous structures are stabilizers during flexion.

The ligamentous structures of the upper cervical spine are unique. The odontoid process is held snugly against the posterior wall of the anterior arch of the atlas by the **transverse ligament**. Additional stability is afforded by the **apical ligament** and the paired **alar ligaments**, which run superiorly from the odontoid process to the anterior rim of the foramen magnum. This allows rotation of C1 on C2 but prevents posterior translation of the dens within the ring of the atlas, which would place the spinal cord at risk.

The **intervertebral discs** are complex structures made up of an outer annulus fibrosus and an inner nucleus pulposus. The **annulus fibrosus** is a laminated structure consisting of collagen fibers that are oriented 30 degrees from horizontal. The inner layers are attached to the cartilaginous endplates, whereas the outer fibers are firmly secured to the osseous vertebral bodies. The annulus surrounds and contains the **nucleus pulposus**, a matrix of protein, glycosaminoglycans, and water. Injury to the intervertebral disc may not be obvious on conventional radiography, but it must be considered in evaluating overall spinal stability and potential neurologic compromise. Magnetic resonance imaging (MRI) allows direct visualization of the intervertebral disc.

BIOMECHANICS

In the sagittal projection, the spine is made up of three smooth curves, producing cervical lordosis, thoracic kyphosis, and lumbar lordosis, with a smooth transition between them. The center of gravity passes anterior to the midthoracic spine and just posterior to the midlumbar spine before intersecting the top portion of the sacrum. This implies that most of the spinal column experiences compressive forces anteriorly through the vertebral bodies and tensile forces through the posterior elements and ligaments.

The distribution of materials and their properties matches the function of the spine. The vertebral bodies are well equipped for handling compressive loads. A vertebral body consists mainly of trabecular bone, which is the primary weight-bearing component of the vertebral body in compression. Removal of a vertebral body's cortex reduces its strength by only 10%. The marrow contents of the vertebral body act as a hydraulic system when compressed. This viscoelastic property allows the vertebral body to absorb more energy.

Posteriorly, the major stabilizers of the spine are the ligamentous structures of the posterior column. These are predominantly made of collagen and are very strong when loaded in tension.

The intervertebral discs are important to the structural stability of the spine. The inner layers of the annulus and the nucleus transmit loads from vertebra to vertebra. With significant force application, the annular fibers fail, which can result in segmental instability and traumatic disc herniations.

The rib cage stabilizes the thoracic spine. This increased stability creates stress risers at the junction of the more mobile cervical spine above and lumbar spine below.

The criteria for determining traumatic **spinal instability** are controversial. The three-column concept of spinal anatomy provides a framework in which to consider specific anatomic areas of injury. Thus, when only one column is injured, the spine is usually stable. When two or three columns are injured, it is usually unstable (i.e., unable to function adequately as a support column and to protect the neural elements). This definition is applicable both acutely and chronically. Thus, in many situations, the question of spinal stability is unclear and rests on the interpretation of pertinent radiographs, the neurologic examination, and sound clinical judgment. It is, however, critical to identify clear instability quickly, as this will play a direct role in determining the treatment path undertaken.

Neurologic Injuries

Based on the anatomic location of the spinal injury, there are three categories of neurologic injury: those of the spinal cord, conus medullaris, and cauda

TABLE 15-2 Neurologic Examination of the Upper Extremity

Root	Motor	Sensory	Reflex
C4	Diaphragm	Top of shoulder	
C5	Elbow flexion (biceps)	Lateral arm	Biceps
C6	Wrist extensors (ECRL/ECRB)	Lateral forearm, thumb/index finger	Brachioradialis
C7	Elbow extension (triceps)	Middle finger	Triceps
C8	Finger flexors (FDP)	Medial forearm, ring/little finger	
T1	Finger abduction (interossei)	Posterior shoulder	

ECRL = extensor carpi radialis longus; ECRB = extensor carpi radialis brevis; FDP = flexor digitorum profundus.

equina. Injuries to the cervical and thoracic spine may directly affect the spinal cord or nerve roots (Table 15-2). The distal spinal cord is termed the *conus medullaris* and usually lies at the thoracolumbar junction at the pedicle level of L1. The sacral nuclei, which control bowel and bladder function, are located in the conus. The cauda equina consists of all lumbar and sacral roots below the conus (usually L2 and below). Injuries to the cauda equina are peripheral nerve root injuries; they have a better prognosis for return of function than do spinal cord or conus injuries.

Spinal cord injuries in the cervical or thoracic spine are designated as complete or incomplete. **Complete** lesions are characterized by total loss of motor, sensory, and reflex function below the level of injury. These injuries result in quadriplegia in the upper cervical spine and paraplegia in the thoracic spine. Complete spinal cord injuries of the cervical spine are described by the lowest level of cervical root function. This has implications for the patient's functional independence. A C3 quadriplegic is ventilator-dependent and without any function of the upper or lower extremities. Patients with C6 or below quadriplegia function independently.

Complete spinal cord injuries in the thoracic spine produce paraplegia. The location of the lesion is irrelevant to the functional outcome because the segmental thoracic nerve roots supply sensation only to the thorax and innervation to the intercostal muscles. However, a proximal thoracic paraplegic vs. a distal thoracic paraplegic is at increased risk for respiratory problems because of increased intercostal paralysis.

Incomplete spinal cord injuries are categorized into four types, based on the cross-sectional location of the injury in the spinal cord. These syndromes are anterior cord, posterior cord, central cord, and Brown-Séquard syndrome. In the **anterior cord syndrome**, the injury is to the anterior spinal cord, which contains the corticospinal motor tracts. This results in motor paralysis with preservation of deep pressure sensation and proprioception due to the intact posterior columns. The **posterior cord syndrome** is rare and results from damage to the posterior columns. This results in loss of proprioception and deep pressure sensation but in the maintenance of motor function due to the intact anterior motor columns. **Central cord syndrome** results from damage to the central gray matter and centrally oriented white matter tracts. In the cervical spine, the centrally oriented white matter tracts provide motor innervation to the upper extremities. As a result, the upper extremities will be more involved than the lower. In the thoracic region, a central cord injury affects the proximal musculature of the lower extremities more than the distal. In **Brown-Séquard syndrome**, half the cord is damaged in the coronal projection. Thus, there is ipsilateral motor paralysis, loss of position sense, and contralateral loss of pain and temperature sensation because the motor tracts and posterior columns decussate in the brainstem, whereas the sensory tracts decussate one to two levels above where they enter the spinal cord. Frequently, there is overlap between these syndromes.

The second group of neurologic injuries involves the **conus medullaris**. These injuries occur with trauma to the thoracolumbar junction and frequently involve elements of the lower spinal cord and cauda equina. Injuries at this level are very difficult to diagnose accurately in the acute setting, especially in the face of spinal shock. Because the conus medullaris usually ends at the level of the L1 pedicle, spinal injuries at this level may damage the upper motor neurons of the sacral cord or the lower motor neurons to the sacral or lumbar roots, which have already exited the spinal cord. Thus, it is not unusual to regain motor strength in the lower extremities, which are innervated by lumbar nerves, but yet continue to have absent bowel and bladder function because of a conus injury that has damaged sacral nerve root innervation to the bowel and bladder.

Cauda equina injuries occur with fractures or dislocations of the L2 level and below. The neurologic deficit may range from a single nerve root injury to a **cauda equina syndrome**, in which there is marked weakness of the lower extremities and involvement of the nerve roots supplying the bowel and bladder.

The decrease in spinal canal cross-sectional area following fracture or dislocation does not always correlate with the severity of neurologic injury or the prognosis for recovery, because the size of the canal and the presence of bone or disc material within it only reflect the final resting place of these fragments, not the magnitude of energy absorbed, the maximum displacement, or the trajectory of the displaced fragments. However, residual spinal canal compromise of greater than 50% or absolute spinal canal dimensions less than 10 to 13 mm indicate acute or impending neurologic dysfunction.

Decompression of the spinal canal in complete spinal cord injuries does little or nothing to improve neurologic outcome. Surgical decompression is recommended for incomplete spinal cord, conus, or cauda equina lesions. Significant improvement in neurologic outcome is possible, especially with cauda equina (lower motor neuron) lesions.

The incidence of penetrating spinal trauma from **gunshot wounds** is increasing. Rarely is the spinal column rendered unstable from a gunshot wound; however, neurologic injury is frequent. Cervical and thoracic-level injuries often produce quadriplegia or paraplegia, respectively. Similarly, injury to the cauda equina occurs with lumbar gunshot wounds. Most of the neural damage is secondary to the transference of kinetic energy to the neural tissues. Surgical removal of a bullet is rarely indicated except in an incomplete spinal cord or cauda equina lesion with a space-occupying fragment of bone or bullet identified. Because of the heat generated, these bullet wounds have a low infection rate except when they have traversed the colon prior to entering the spinal column. If the bullet is lodged in the spinal column or canal, this is one indication for its elective removal.

Diagnosis and Initial Management

The diagnosis and initial management of patients with spinal fractures and dislocations depend to a great degree on the area of the spine involved. Nevertheless, there are commonalities.

Patients with spinal injuries may have additional life-threatening injuries; therefore, initial priorities are to secure an airway, provide ventilation, and achieve hemodynamic stabilization.

Precautions for the stabilization of the entire spinal column begin at the accident site. Patients with a history of trauma to the head, neck, or back or conscious patients who report any neurologic symptoms are immobilized in a cervical collar with complete head and neck immobilization on a spine board until an appropriate evaluation can be performed. A history of the mechanism of injury and a detailed report of any neck or back pain and motor or sensory changes in the extremities are essential. Unconscious patients with major trauma are a more difficult challenge, and suspicion must remain high until a thorough examination for potential spinal injury is performed.

A thorough neurologic examination is performed as soon as possible. Neurologic examinations include a complete assessment of motor, sensory, and reflex function for both upper and lower extremities. Perianal sensation and a rectal examination are critical to determine the function of the sacral roots and sacral cord. Sacral sensory sparing or any trace of distal motor function implies possible return of function. Also, spinal shock for the first 24 to 48 h may have the appearance of a complete spinal cord injury in patients who will later be found to have sensory and motor function. The resolution of spinal shock is indicated by the return of the **bulbocavernosus reflex**. This is tested while a digital rectal examination is being performed. Pulling on the Foley catheter will result in contraction of the anal sphincter when the bulbocavernosus reflex is present. When the bulbocavernosus reflex returns in the face of a complete spinal cord injury, the chances are that the neurologic deficit will be permanent.

Radiographic Examination

Screening radiographs include anteroposterior and lateral views. In the setting of definite spinal injury, the entire spine should be visualized by plain radiography. On the lateral radiograph, one should examine the height of all the vertebral bodies and the intervening disc spaces. These heights should be fairly uniform and symmetrical. When the height of a vertebral body is decreased, an angular deformity (i.e., kyphosis) is produced on the lateral radiograph. The anterior and posterior vertebral body lines should align throughout the whole spine. With injury to the middle column (posterior vertebral body), retropulsion of bone into the spinal canal may be evident on the lateral view. The lateral radiograph also will show the posterior elements, including the facets, laminae, and spinous processes. A widened distance between the interspinous processes is indicative of distraction injury to the posterior column.

The anteroposterior radiograph of the spine is examined. Each vertebral body should sit directly on top of the one below, with symmetrical and evenly placed disc spaces between the bodies. The right and left borders of the vertebral bodies should be well aligned. The two round pedicular shadows of each vertebral body should be present and symmetrical. Widening of the interpedicular distance at one level may be indicative of a middle-column burst-type injury. Careful examination delineates the posterior elements of the spine. The posterior elements of a segment are somewhat distal to the corresponding vertebral body. The shadow of a spinous process is usually visible, allowing for comparison of the distance between spinous processes at each level. The transverse processes at each level are examined for fracture, as are the ribs in the thoracic spine, the sacrum, sacroiliac articulations, and iliac wings of the pelvis.

It is very important in patients with spinal trauma to not miss additional spinal injuries. Up to 10% of patients with spinal trauma at one site will have another injury to the spinal column at an adjoining or distant site. This is especially important in cervical or thoracic spine-injured patients who may have spinal cord injuries resulting in sensory loss to more distal areas of their thoracic and lumbar spine, adding to the difficulty of diagnosis of injuries in these areas.

In considering what further imaging one should obtain, it is generally accepted that a computed tomography (CT) scan should be performed when bone injury has been diagnosed. MRI is more controversial. Such scans in patients with neurologic deficits may further clarify injuries to the spinal cord, conus medullaris, or cauda equina. This modality also helps to identify hemorrhage or epidural hematoma. Finally, MRI can be useful in identifying a ligamentous lesion that has not been clearly demonstrated with x-rays and CT.

Initial Management

All patients are kept supine on a well-cushioned mattress and are log-rolled every 2 h to decrease pressure on sensitive areas. Antiembolism stockings are used to prevent deep vein thrombosis. Cardiac status and oxygen saturation are monitored continuously. A nasogastric tube is placed for the accompanying gastrointestinal ileus. A Foley catheter allows accurate determination of urine output and simplifies nursing care. Intravenous fluids maintain an adequate fluid volume. Complete blood counts are obtained at presentation and then several times in the early postinjury period. Intravenous pain medications are dictated by the patient's age, medical status, and amount of pain. Range-of-motion exercises of uninjured extremities are begun early in the hospital course.

The initial care of patients with cervical spine injury is somewhat different. Such patients with spinal malalignment, regardless of neurologic status, are placed in **skeletal-tong traction**. We use graphite Gardner-Wells tongs, which are MRI-compatible. They are placed one finger breadth above the earlobe in line with the external auditory canal. The skull bolts are finger-tightened until the pressure valve is released in the center of the bolt, indicating adequate force. The tongs are applied in the emergency room when spinal malalignment is identified. Approximately 5 lb per level of injury is slowly added to the traction apparatus under close neurologic and radiographic surveillance. Thus, a patient with a C4-C5 facet dislocation may require 25 lb of traction or more to reduce the malalignment. It is not uncommon to require anywhere from 50 to 100 lb of traction for dislocations of the lower cervical spine to accomplish reduction in large adults. Once reduction is achieved, a load of 10 to 15 lb is sufficient to maintain reduction. A lateral of the cervical spine radiograph ensures maintenance of proper alignment and should be repeated frequently, especially after returning from tests that require mobilization of the patient.

The pharmacologic treatment of acute spinal cord injury is administration of steroids in an attempt to diminish edema around the neural elements following injury. Such medication should be given to all cervical spine–injured patients with any neurologic deficit, patients with injuries to the thoracic spine and incomplete paraplegia, those with incomplete cauda equina lesions with neurologic deterioration, and patients who cannot immediately be taken to surgery. Methylprednisolone 30 mg/kg is administered as a loading dose intravenously over 1 h. A continuous intravenous drip of methylprednisolone at a dose of 5.4 mg/kg/h is continued for 24 h for patients who present within 3 h of injury. Patients presenting between 3 and 8 h after injury receive methylprednisolone for 48 h. No clear benefit from the use of steroids has been established for patients presenting 8 h or more following injury. Any neurologic deterioration while on methylprednisolone merits reconsideration of its use. The risk of this high-dose steroid regimen is gastrointestinal hemorrhage; therefore all patients are protected with H_2 antagonists such as cimetidine or ranitidine for a minimum of 72 h.

Spinal injuries are divided into four groups based on the involved segment: upper cervical, subaxial cervical, thoracic and lumbar, and sacral.

INJURIES OF THE UPPER CERVICAL SPINE (OCCIPUT TO C2)

Classification

Eight types of injuries of the upper cervical spine are encountered. The four most frequently seen are atlas fractures, atlantoaxial subluxations, odontoid fractures, and traumatic spondylolisthesis of the axis (C2 hangman's fractures). The four less common injuries are occipital condylar fractures, atlantooccipital dislocations, atlantoaxial rotary subluxations, and fractures of the C2 lateral mass.

Atlas fractures result from impaction of the occipital condyles on the arch of C1. This causes single or multiple fractures of the ring of C1, which usually splays apart and thus increases the space for the spinal cord; therefore neurologic injury is rare in such cases. There are four types of atlas fractures. The first two are stable injuries: isolated fractures of the anterior or posterior arch. Anterior arch fractures are usually avulsion injuries from the anterior portion of the ring. These injuries commonly occur with flexion and compression. Posterior arch fractures result from hyperextension, with compression of the posterior arch of C1 between the occiput and C2. The third type of atlas fracture is a lateral mass fracture. The fracture lines run anterior and posterior to the articular surface of the C1 lateral mass, with asymmetrical displacement of the lateral mass from the remainder of the vertebrae. This is best seen on an open-mouth odontoid view of the C1-C2 complex. The fourth type, burst fractures of the atlas (or Jefferson's fracture) classically has four fractures in the ring of C1: two in the anterior portion and two in the posterior ring. Potential instability of these fractures is best identified by examining the overhang of the C1 lateral masses on the C2 articular facets, as noted on the open-mouth odontoid view. Total lateral displacement on both sides of more than 6.9 mm indicates rupture of the transverse ligament with resultant atlantoaxial instability.

Atlantoaxial subluxation is secondary to rupture of the primary stabilizer of the atlantoaxial articulation, the transverse ligament. This produces atlantoaxial instability, which may place the spinal cord at risk. Thus potential complications from this injury include neurologic injury resulting from the odontoid compressing the upper cervical cord against the posterior arch of C1.

Identification of **odontoid process fractures** requires a high index of suspicion. Such must be ruled out in all patients with neck pain following a motor-vehicle accident and elderly patients involved in trivial trauma to the head and neck region. If there is significant anterior or, more commonly, posterior displacement of the odontoid process, spinal cord injury may result. The incidence of neurologic injury in such cases is approximately 10%. Odontoid fractures are further classified into three types, based on the anatomic level at which they occur (Fig. 15-2).

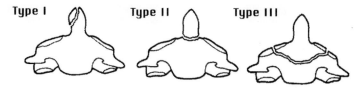

FIG. 15-2   The three types of odontoid fractures.

Type I fractures represent an avulsion fracture from the tip of the odontoid process, where the alar ligament inserts.

Type II fractures are the most common type of odontoid fracture and occur in the midportion of the dens proximal to the body of the axis. The limited blood supply and small cross-sectional cancellous surface area lead to a high incidence of nonunion. Other risk factors for nonunion are angulation, anterior or posterior displacement of more than 4 mm, and patient age greater than 40 years.

Type III injuries are those in which the fracture line extends into the vertebral body of C2. Because of the larger cross-sectional area and the presence of cancellous bone with a rich blood supply, these type III fractures consistently unite if they are adequately aligned (Fig. 15-3).

Traumatic spondylolisthesis of the axis, or hangman's fracture, is a bipedicle fracture with disruption of the disc and ligaments between C2 and C3, resulting most commonly from hyperextension and distraction. This fracture is named for the injury resulting from judicial hanging with a rope in the submental position.

Hangman's fractures are further classified based on the amount of displacement and angulation of the C2 body in relation to the posterior elements (Fig. 15-4A to D).

Type I injury is a fracture of the neural arch without angulation and with as much as 3 mm of anterior displacement of C2 on C3.

Type II fractures have anterior displacement greater than 3 mm or angulation of C2 on C3. These fractures usually result from hyperextension and axial load followed by severe flexion, which stretches the posterior annulus and disc and produces the anterior translation and angulation.

Type IIA injuries are a flexion-distraction variant of type II fractures. They demonstrate severe angulation of C2 on C3, with minimal displacement,

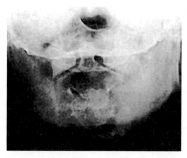

FIG. 15-3   An open-mouth view indicating a type III odontoid fracture.

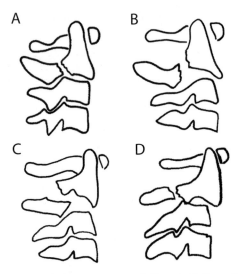

FIG.15-4   Hangman's fracture types: *A.* Type I. *B.* Type II. *C.* Type IIa. *D.* Type III.

apparently hinging on the anterior longitudinal ligament. It is important to recognize this type of hangman's fracture because the application of traction may distract the C2-C3 disc space and further displace the fracture.

Type III injuries are bipedicle fractures associated with unilateral or bilateral facet dislocations. These are serious, unstable injuries and often have neurologic sequelae.

Fractures of the **occipital condyles** result from combined axial loading and lateral bending. There are two types: avulsion fractures or comminuted compression fractures.

Atlantooccipital dislocations are rare injuries resulting from total disruption of all ligamentous structures between the occiput and the atlas. The mechanism of injury is usually extension or flexion. Death is usually immediate due to severe brainstem involvement with complete respiratory arrest.

Atlantoaxial rotary subluxation occurs most often secondary to vehicular accidents. The main difficulty is lack of early recognition.

Lateral mass fractures of the axis are the result of combined axial-loading and lateral-bending forces.

Associated Injuries

Associated injuries include compression of the spinal cord or cervical nerve roots, head injuries, and other fractures, particularly of the cervical spine. Fractures of the occipital condyles are associated with severe head trauma and are accompanied by cranial nerve palsies. Fifty percent of patients with a fracture of the posterior arch of the atlas have another cervical spine injury, the most common being a traumatic spondylolisthesis of the axis or a displaced odontoid fracture. A high index of suspicion and careful physical and radiographic examinations constitute the best method of finding associated injuries.

Diagnosis and Initial Management

Physical Examination

As should always be common practice, the primary survey is the first step prior to assessing for orthopedic injuries. Once issues with airway, breathing, and circulation have been addressed, the focus may then turn to orthopedic and neurologic concerns.

The patient has pain localized to the neck, and there may be a feeling of instability or fixed deformity. The initial assessment is performed as described.

Radiographic Examination

Initially, a cross-table lateral radiograph is obtained for all patients with suspected injuries of the cervical spine. This radiograph includes all seven cervical vertebrae and the C7-T1 junction. When this is not possible due to the interposition of the shoulders in patients with short necks, the patient's arms are pulled down to lower the shoulders or one arm is extended above the head while keeping the other arm at the side during the procedure (swimmer's view) (Fig. 15-5).

Additional required views include an anteroposterior view and an odontoid or open-mouth view, which details the C1-C2 articulation in the coronal plane (Fig. 15-3). Right or left oblique and voluntary flexion-extension views are obtained as indicated.

Four lines are essential to examine on the lateral radiograph: the anterior vertebral body line, the posterior vertebral body line, the spinal laminar line, and the line connecting the tips of the spinous processes. All of these landmarks should align in a smooth arc from C1 to T1 (Fig. 15-6). Any malalignment indicates potential vertebral subluxation or dislocation.

The soft tissue shadows on the lateral radiographs of the cervical spine represent the retropharyngeal and retrotracheal shadows. These soft tissue shadows are expanded by the hematoma associated with injury of the cervical spine and may be the only indication of subtle injuries. The soft tissue shadow should be no more than 6 mm from the anterior aspect of C2 and no more than 2 cm at the anterior edge of C6 (i.e., "**6 at 2 and 2 at 6**").

Fractures of the occipital condyles are difficult to visualize on plain radiographs and require axial CT for delineation.

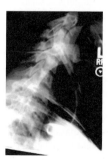

FIG. 15-5   Swimmer's view of cervical spine.

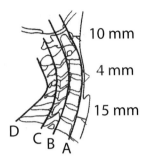

FIG. 15-6   Normal bony arcs and soft tissue shadows seen on the lateral view of the cervical spine: (*A*) anterior vertebral body line, (*B*) posterior vertebral body line, (*C*) laminar line, and (*D*) spinous process line.

Atlantooccipital dissociation is identified on the lateral radiograph of the cervical spine or lateral view of the skull, which profiles the atlantooccipital junction quite well. There is dissociation between the base of the occiput and the C1 arch and severe soft tissue swelling.

Fractures of the atlas are diagnosed on a lateral radiograph of the cervical spine and/or an open-mouth odontoid view. The lateral radiograph demonstrates fracture lines within the posterior arch of C1. The open-mouth view indicates splaying of the lateral masses of C1 on the articular surfaces of the axis. Axial CT is helpful in the evaluation.

Atlantoaxial subluxation due to disruption of the transverse ligament is best demonstrated on lateral flexion-extension views and is indicated by an increase in the atlantodental interval (ADI), which is normally less than 3.5 mm. This is measured from the posterior aspect of the anterior arch of C1 to the anterior aspect of the odontoid process (Fig. 15-7*A* and *B*). Angulation greater than 11 degrees is also indicative of instability. However, spasm of the spinal extensor muscles accompanying an acute injury may prevent adequate voluntary flexion-extension radiographs. Once this problem is recognized, an axial CT scan is obtained to ascertain whether instability is purely ligamentous or due to a bony avulsion.

Radiographs following atlantoaxial rotary subluxation are often reported as normal because it is difficult to obtain radiographs parallel to the plane of both C1 and C2 due to the accompanying torticollis. Open-mouth radiographs often help recognize this injury by demonstrating a "wink sign." This occurs because of the unilateral overlap of the lateral mass of C1 on C2. CT is helpful in describing the direction and rotation of C1 on C2.

Odontoid fractures are seen on radiographs of the lateral cervical spine or on an open-mouth view. Occasionally, three-dimensional CT reconstruction or conventional tomography may be necessary to identify and fully evaluate these fractures. Axial CT may miss the fracture line, as it is in the plane of the axial image.

Hangman's fractures are seen on the lateral radiograph. Lateral mass fractures with minimal comminution may require CT for identification.

MRI may be obtained for patients with spinal cord or nerve root injuries and also for evaluation of the intervertebral discs, annular structures, and posterior ligaments.

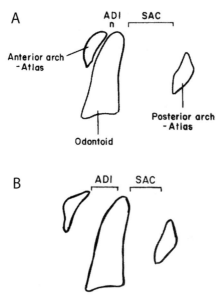

FIG. 15-7 Atlantoaxial relations. *A.* Normal relation of the atlas and dens seen on the lateral view. *B.* Atlantoaxial subluxation as indicated by an increase in the atlantodental interval (ADI).

Initial Management

Occipital condylar fractures are managed initially in a cervical orthosis. Fractures of the occipital condyles are generally stable injuries that can be treated with orthotic immobilization with a two-poster orthosis or a rigid Philadelphia collar. Most of these fractures heal uneventfully, although occasionally post-traumatic arthritis occurs, requiring posterior atlantooccipital fusion.

Traction is **contraindicated** following **atlantooccipital dislocation**. Even 5 lb may overdistract and stretch the brainstem, with catastrophic results. Initial treatment is application of a halo vest to maintain stability of the spine while attention is given to the patient's respiratory and neurologic status. Once the patient is stabilized, a fusion from the posterior occiput to the upper cervical spine is performed, with continued immobilization in a halo vest for approximately 3 months.

Initial management of type I, II, and III fractures of the atlas requires a rigid cervical orthosis. Jefferson's fractures are placed in traction.

Atlantoaxial subluxation and atlantoaxial rotary subluxation are managed initially with a cervical orthosis.

Type I odontoid fractures are managed with a cervical orthosis. Type II and III fractures are initially managed with cervical tong traction to reduce and/or maintain sagittal alignment.

Type I hangman's fracture is treated with a rigid cervical orthosis. Types II and IIA are managed with a halo vest. Type IIA injuries should not be treated with traction, as this may cause overdistraction and subsequent neurologic injury. The initial management of type III fractures is application of traction to reduce the facet dislocation. Reduction by closed means may not be possible because of the dissociation between the vertebral body and the posterior elements.

Definitive Management

Definitive management of fractures of the atlas is based on the type of fracture. Type I and II fractures may be managed in a cervical orthosis in a compliant patient, whereas type III injuries are managed with a halo vest. Type IV, or Jefferson's, fractures with a competent transverse ligament (less than 6.9-mm displacement of the lateral masses) are stable and are also managed with a halo vest. Jefferson's fractures with an incompetent transverse ligament (more than 6.9-mm displacement) are unstable and managed with extended cervical traction to reduce the splaying until the bone fragments are sticky. This is necessary because the halo vest cannot provide the axial distraction necessary to maintain fracture reduction. After preliminary healing, application of a halo vest for the remainder of the 3- to 4-month period allows complete healing. When a C1 fracture is presumed healed, voluntary lateral flexion-extension radiographs of the cervical spine are obtained to make sure that there is no significant atlantoaxial subluxation. If there is more than 3.5 mm of atlantoaxial subluxation in an adult, posterior C1-C2 fusion is performed with or without transarticular C1-C2 screw fixation. Fusion from the posterior occiput to C2 may also be performed. However, the range of motion of the neck would be compromised by this procedure.

Atlantoaxial subluxation due to bony avulsion of the transverse ligament is managed with a halo vest for 3 months. Purely ligamentous injuries are managed with a C1-C2 posterior fusion, possibly with C1-C2 transarticular screws.

Atlantoaxial rotary subluxation recognized within several weeks of injury is reduced with cervical traction. This may require up to 30 to 40 lb of traction to reduce the rotary dislocation. Often a "pop" is heard and felt at reduction. A halo vest is applied. Even with prolonged use of a halo vest, long-term stability may not be achieved because the C1-C2 facet joint is a saddle-type joint and depends on ligamentous restraint for stability.

Atlantoaxial arthrodesis is the treatment of choice for chronic instability and pain or for patients with an associated neurologic deficit. For chronic injuries, closed reduction through cervical traction is not possible; they are managed with open reduction and C1-C2 arthrodesis.

Type I odontoid fractures are stable injuries that are managed with an orthosis for symptomatic comfort. However, the type I avulsion injury is often associated with atlantooccipital dislocations; therefore this more serious injury must be ruled out. There are four types of definitive treatment for type II odontoid fractures: halo vest management of minimally displaced or angulated fractures followed by posterior C1-C2 arthrodesis if healing does not occur within 4 months; primary posterior C1-C2 arthrodesis as long as the posterior arch of C1 is intact; posterior C1-C2 transarticular facet screw fixation and fusion; and anterior screw fixation of the dens under biplanar fluoroscopy. The theoretical advantage of anterior screw fixation is that it does not require a C1-C2 fusion and thus preserves motion of the upper cervical spine. Provided that type III odontoid fractures are adequately reduced, halo vest immobilization for 3 months is the treatment of choice. When reduction is lost after halo vest placement, cervical traction for 3 to 4 weeks to allow early fracture healing be-

fore continuing with the halo vest is required, or reduction by traction and posterior C1-C2 fusion may be performed.

Type I hangman's fractures are stable injuries and are managed with a cervical orthosis for 3 months in compliant patients. Type II fractures displaced
less than 5 mm and minimally angulated are managed with a halo vest if reduction can be maintained. Fractures displaced more than 5 mm are managed
in cervical tong traction, with slight extension prior to application of the halo
vest, which will also need to be applied with neck extension. Traction is contraindicated for type IIA fractures. These fractures are managed with early
halo application under fluoroscopic guidance and with compression across the
fracture site for maintenance of reduction. Type III fractures are reduced open
when closed reduction is not possible, and posterior spinal fusion of C2-C3
is performed. Postoperatively, halo vest immobilization is maintained for
3 months in these cases.

Lateral mass fractures of the atlas are stable injuries that require only orthotic
immobilization. Occasionally, with late symptomatic facet degeneration, some
of these may require posterior fusion for pain relief.

Complications

The complication of high cervical fractures is bony or ligamentous instability.
Management is posterior fusion of the unstable segments. Failure to identify
an injury of the upper cervical spine is not an infrequent occurrence, especially in multiply traumatized patients. Fortunately, neurologic injury is rare in
these instances because of the large amount of space available for the spinal
cord in the upper cervical spine.

INJURIES TO THE SUBAXIAL CERVICAL SPINE

Although bone injuries are often the obvious manifestations of cervical spinal
trauma, it is essential to accurately identify ligamentous components of injury
to the subaxial cervical motion segments. It is often this ligamentous failure
that permits translation of the cervical motion segment, leading to severe neurologic damage. It is also well accepted that ligaments heal with scar tissue
that is weaker than the preinjured ligamentous structure, potentially resulting
in chronic instability.

An important difference between injuries of the upper and subaxial cervical
spine is the increased risk of cervical cord injuries in the lower cervical spine.
This is a reflection of two factors: the overall diminished size of the spinal
canal in the lower cervical spine and the increasing prevalence of injuries that
narrow rather than expand the canal. Thus, the immediate and long-term goals
for injuries in the lower cervical spine are to obtain and maintain spinal column
alignment so as to optimize the environment for the spinal cord and existing
nerve roots.

Classification

There are five types of injuries to the **subaxial cervical spine**: isolated posterior element fractures, minor avulsion and compression fractures, vertebral
body burst fractures, teardrop fractures, and facet injuries causing spinal
malalignment. These injuries occur through several mechanisms as classified
by Allen and colleagues: compressive flexion, vertical compression, distractive flexion, compressive extension, distractive extension, and lateral flexion.

Isolated posterior element fractures of the lamina, articular process, or spinous process may occur by a compression-extension sequence with impaction of the posterior elements on one another. Additional lesions include unilateral or bilateral laminar fractures and often contiguous posterior element fractures secondary to the impaction of the adjacent posterior elements.

Minor avulsion and compression fractures of the subaxial cervical spine include anterior compression or avulsion injuries of the vertebral body and combined anterior and posterior bone injuries with minimal displacement and angulation.

Vertebral body burst fractures are usually the result of axial loading injuries with different amounts of flexion possible, as in diving accidents. They involve the anterior and the middle columns, with the potential for bony retropulsion into the spinal canal.

Teardrop fractures of the subaxial cervical spine are a particular group of fractures with a high association of severe spinal cord injury and spinal instability. These injuries occur when the neck is in a flexed position, with axial compression as the main loading force. The inferior tip of the proximal vertebral body is driven down into the caudad body by compression and flexion. This produces the typical teardrop fragment on the anteroinferior aspect of the affected body. The true significance of this injury lies in the three-column instability pattern produced. The typical fracture line proceeds from superior to inferior and exits through the disc space, which is severely damaged. Damage to posterior-element ligaments and bones is characteristic of the teardrop injury. This produces a grossly unstable injury of all three spinal columns in which the entire vertebral body is retropulsed into the spinal canal, causing either partial or complete spinal cord injury.

Facet injuries are divided into fractures and ligamentous injuries. Both may allow segmental translation with subluxation or dislocation of the vertebral segments. The primary mechanism of injury is a posterior distraction force applied to the already flexed spine. This produces a spectrum of injury ranging from an interspinous ligament sprain to complete posterior ligamentous and facet joint failure, producing facet subluxation or dislocation. These injuries are further divided into unilateral and bilateral facet injuries. Thus, facet injuries are described as unilateral or bilateral facet fractures with or without subluxation, unilateral facet dislocations, perched facets, or bilateral facet fractures. Unilateral facet fractures or dislocations display a variety of neurologic injuries, ranging from a normal examination to single-root deficits or spinal cord syndromes. The increasing spectrum of distraction and flexion injuries produces the perched facet injury. This occurs with bilateral facet injuries causing perching of the inferior facet on the superior facet, with segmental kyphosis between the two affected vertebral body segments. Neurologic deficits are variable but most commonly include isolated root deficits. The most severe facet injury is bilateral facet dislocation. This is a purely ligamentous injury, with disruption of the entire posterior ligamentous complex, including the interspinous ligament, ligamentum flavum, both facet capsules, and, in severe cases, disruption of the posterior longitudinal ligament and intervertebral disc. This injury produces the highest incidence of neurologic deficit of any facet injury because of the loss of space available for the spinal cord as a result of vertebral translation (Fig. 15-8). The incidence of bilateral facet fractures associated with dislocations is extremely small. Both of these injuries predispose to rotational and translational instability.

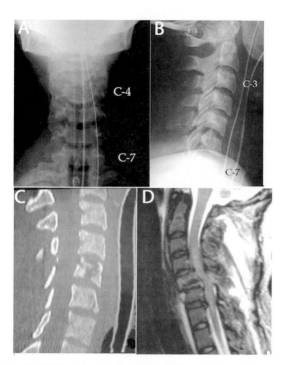

FIG. 15-8   C5-C6 fracture-dislocation. *A.* Anteroposterior radiograph. *B.* Lateral radiograph. *C.* Lateral CT scan. *D.* MRI study.

Diagnosis and Initial Management

Physical Examination

The primary sign of a subaxial inury to the cervical spine may be the associated neurologic deficit. Other than neck pain and a sense of instability, there may be no symptoms indicating a fracture without neurologic deficit. Patients with unilateral facet dislocation have a mild rotational deformity of the neck: the head is tilted and rotated to the contralateral side of the facet dislocation.

Radiographic Examination

A common, isolated posterior element fracture, the unilateral vertebral arch fracture, often is not evident on the initial lateral radiograph of the cervical spine. Oblique views or nonstandard views, such as a 20-degree oblique or pillar view, may be necessary to establish the diagnosis. When fracture of both an ipsilateral pedicle and lamina occurs, the articular process may rotate into the frontal plane and be viewed as a "transverse facet" on the anteroposterior radiographic view.

Vertebral body burst fractures involve the anterior and middle columns of the cervical spine. The lateral radiograph indicates compression of the anterior and middle columns, with retropulsion of the middle column posteriorly into the spinal canal. Burst fractures **always** require an axial CT or MRI examination to document the amount of middle-column retropulsion. As anterior compression approaches 50%, middle-column injuries or concomitant posterior ligamentous injuries must be considered. It is difficult to identify posterior ligamentous injuries in a patient with a burst fracture because voluntary flexion-extension views are unobtainable. Warnings include a widened distance between interspinous processes, fractured posterior elements including facet fractures, or sagittal MRI evidence of ligamentous damage.

Teardrop fractures are first suspected on the radiograph of the lateral cervical spine, which will show retrodisplacement of the cephalad vertebral body on the caudad and, possibly, the anteroinferior teardrop fragment. Fractures of posterior elements may also be noted on the lateral or the anteroposterior radiograph. CT or MRI through the involved segment also demonstrates the fractures and the diminished diameter of the spinal canal due to the significant retrolisthesis.

Facet dislocations are identified on the lateral radiograph. Unilateral dislocations are characterized by approximately 25% anterior olisthesis of the cephalad vertebra on the caudad vertebra; bilateral dislocations have 50% anterior olisthesis. Axial CT further defines the injury. Perched facets are diagnosed on the lateral radiograph by the increased distance between the spinous processes. An obvious segmental kyphosis is also seen between the involved vertebral bodies and anterior translation of the cephalad vertebral body on the caudad body.

Initial Management

Initial management of isolated fractures of the posterior elements and minor avulsion and compression fractures calls for a cervical orthosis.

Initial management of burst fractures with greater than 25% loss in height, retropulsion, or neurologic deficit involves cervical tong traction to stabilize the spinal segment and an attempt at indirect reduction of retropulsed fragments via ligamentotaxis, thereby decompressing the neural canal.

Initial management of teardrop fractures is the application of cervical tong traction to increase the spinal canal diameter by indirect reduction via ligamentotaxis.

Initial management of unilateral or bilateral facet injuries causing any spinal subluxation or dislocations, perched facets, or bilateral facet dislocations is cervical tong traction for reduction. The one caveat is that there is a small but significant incidence of disc herniation accompanying bilateral facet dislocations. In these patients, there is the potential that a closed reduction maneuver will retropulse the injured disc into the spinal canal and cause further neurologic compromise. The disc herniation is best identified by MRI but is suspected when the disc space at the level of dislocation is markedly decreased in height on the lateral radiograph. Therefore, in patients with a normal neurologic examination, reduction is performed in an incremental fashion, with careful attention to the sequence of neurologic examination and radiographic reduction.

MRI provides the best imaging of the soft tissue, discs, and ligaments following spinal trauma (Fig 15-8D). Although timing for obtaining MRI is controversial, many authors recommend first attempting closed reduction but stopping the reduction procedure for MRI if the patient's neurologic exam changes. This helps to rule out a herniated disc, which is present in up to 50% of patients after reduction. In an awake patient with a complete neurologic injury, reduction is attempted prior to obtaining an MRI examination. In an awake patient with an incomplete neurologic deficit, reduction is attempted as long as the neurologic examination does not deteriorate. MRI or, alternatively, cervical myelography may be performed if a patient's neurologic examination changes during the reduction maneuver. Treatment of a traumatic disc herniation associated with a facet dislocation is anterior discectomy and fusion preceding a single-level posterior instrumentation and fusion. Unilateral facet dislocation is often difficult or impossible to reduce with pure longitudinal cervical traction. These cases require a manual reduction maneuver after application of the appropriate amount of cervical traction. Manually turning the rotated head and chin toward the ipsilateral side of injury often produces a palpable clunk and feeling of reduction for the patient. This obviously must be done with careful neurologic monitoring and radiographic control. This reduction maneuver unlocks the dislocated facet and places it back into the normal position; that is, the superior facet sits anterior to the inferior facet. A prereduction MRI should be performed to determine whether a concomitant cervical disc herniation is present.

Associated Injuries

Associated injuries are identical to those of the upper cervical spine.

Definitive Management

Options for definitive treatment of injuries to the subaxial cervical spine include (1) orthotic immobilization with a sternal-occipital-mandibular immobilizer (SOMI) (Fig. 15-9A); (2) halo vest immobilization (Fig. 15-9B); (3) posterior fusion and stabilization using wires, cables, clamps and/or screws and plates; (4) anterior approaches for decompression and strut-graft fusion with or without plate and screw stabilization; and (5) a combination of these four treatment modalities. The two primary considerations for choosing a particular treatment plan include the presence of neural compression and actual or anticipated spinal instability.

Traditionally, posterior stainless steel wire constructs have provided adequate stabilization for fusion in the subaxial cervical spine by using spinous processes and/or facet wiring techniques. Sublaminar wire techniques are not

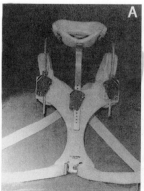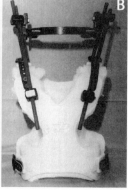

FIG. 15-9   *A.* SOMI orthosis. *B.* Halo vest.

recommended in the subaxial cervical spine following trauma because of the risk of iatrogenic neurologic injury. In addition, with the presence of injury to posterior bone elements, these wiring techniques may be impossible or must be extended to normal levels above and/or below the injury. Lateral mass plating techniques have been developed in an attempt to provide stabilization to areas with spinous process and laminar injuries but intact lateral masses. This is especially helpful if posterior bone elements are intact. This technique requires screw placement into the lateral masses, which poses some risk of neurologic and vascular complications associated with it; long-term results for this technique are not yet available.

The halo vest is often a useful modality in the management of injuries to the bones of the subaxial cervical spine. As a general rule, the more osseous the injury (i.e., the less ligamentous), the more useful the halo vest. Ligamentous injuries will heal with scar tissue in a halo, and this scar tissue will not maintain long-term spinal stability. For single-level or multilevel bone injuries, the halo vest is often the optimal treatment device. However, halo vest management poses the risk of many potential complications. The most commonly encountered complication is pin-tract infection, causing pin loosening. Thus, these patients must be followed closely when they are being treated on an outpatient basis.

The majority of isolated fractures of posterior elements are stable and not associated with a major neurologic deficit (except for isolated cervical root deficits). These injuries are managed in a SOMI. Occasionally, with multiple injuries spanning several segments, a halo vest provides better control of alignment.

Minor avulsion and compression fractures are managed in a cervical orthosis or halo vest.

The definitive management of cervical burst fractures is dependent on the loss of height of the vertebral body, retropulsion, neurologic status, kyphosis, and the presence of posterior-element injury. Fractures with less than 25% loss of height, minimal retropulsion, and kyphosis in a neurologically intact patient are managed in a halo vest for approximately 3 months. With increasing middle-column retropulsion, there is an increased likelihood of spinal cord injury. These patients are candidates for anterior decompression via corpectomy and strut-graft stabilization. If the posterior ligaments are intact, stability is maintained with an anterior strut graft and halo vest for approximately 3 months. An alternative to provide additional stability is an anterior cervical plate attached to the segments above and below the fractured vertebral body, thereby stabilizing the strut graft internally and possibly obviating the halo vest. In patients with vertebral body burst fractures and posterior ligamentous disruption, anterior strut grafting with anterior plate fixation cannot resist flexion forces; thus posterior stabilization is also necessary.

Definitive management of teardrop fractures is based on the extent of damage to bones, ligaments, and nerves. When there is significant compression of the spinal canal, anterior corpectomy of the retropulsed vertebral body is performed with autogenous iliac crest strut grafting. Application of an anterior cervical plate is an option to further stabilize these segments. Because of the instability of the posterior column, either halo vest placement (for posterior bone injuries) or posterior instrumentation and fusion is performed. Some studies have found an increased incidence of long-term progressive kyphosis with the use of halo immobilization for unstable teardrop fractures. These authors would thus recommend anterior corpectomy and plating for such injuries.

Unilateral facet fractures without subluxation are managed in a SOMI orthosis or halo vest for 3 months or until bone healing is noted. The residual rotatory instability of a facet fracture with subluxation may be uncontrolled in a halo vest; therefore these injuries may heal in a malunited rotated position, which can exacerbate a nerve root deficit. For those injuries in which reduction cannot be maintained with a halo vest, management is anterior cervical discectomy and fusion with anterior cervical plating in addition to a halo vest to provide reduction and stability for posterior column healing.

When closed reduction of a facet dislocation is successful, the patient's neurologic status and overall medical condition are monitored. When the patient is considered neurologically and medically stable, single-level posterior instrumentation with fusion is performed. Posterior wiring techniques are the traditional method of internal stabilization. Posterolateral mass plating techniques are also being used for internal stabilization of these injuries. With both of these techniques, patients are kept out of a halo, which aids in both pulmonary and psychological recovery. As an alternative, these patients may also be treated with an anterior discectomy, fusion, and plating technique followed by a cervical orthosis after 3 months. Bilateral facet fractures are approached anteriorly because the involvement of the posterior column precludes posterior instrumentation. Anterior cervical discectomy and fusion with or without anterior cervical plating is performed at the involved level (Fig. 15-10). Postoperative treatment with a halo vest may be necessary to immobilize the fractures of posterior elements.

Complications

Complications of burst fractures include progressive kyphosis with potential neurologic sequelae due to failure to diagnose a posterior ligamentous injury. In cases where there is greater than 50% loss of height of a vertebra in a neurologically intact patient, voluntary flexion-extension radiographs after healing of the compression fracture are necessary to rule out posterior ligamentous injury, which will result in chronic instability. Complications associated with the use of anterior strut grafts include anterior dislodgment with esophageal compression, posterior dislodgment with potential spinal cord compression, and breakage or nonunion of the strut graft.

Complications of teardrop fractures revolve around the difficulty of stabilizing unrecognized posterior ligamentous injuries. Management with anterior

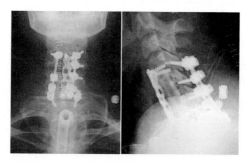

FIG. 15-10   Postoperative radiographic appearance of C5 corpectomy and fusion. *A.* Anteroposterior view. *B.* Lateral view.

corpectomy and strut graft in the face of posterior-column injury has resulted in graft dislodgment, late kyphotic deformities, and the need for reoperation even with postoperative halo vest treatment. Anterior and posterior surgical approaches with internal stabilization via plates anteriorly and posteriorly appear to stabilize these injuries maximally.

Complications of cervical facet injuries are the development of acute or chronic instability. This is frequently due to the inadequate treatment of ligamentous injuries in a halo, which will not produce long-term stability; failure to recognize a concomitant disc herniation in the presence of a facet subluxation or dislocation during the closed reduction maneuver; failure to anticipate rotational instability; and the use of interspinous wiring techniques that do not control rotational instabilities. Acute and chronic cervical instability has been quantified to be present when more than 3.5 mm of segmental translation or greater than 11 degrees of segmental angulation are present. Patients who have this degree of instability, even if asymptomatic, should be considered for posterior instrumentation and fusion.

INJURIES OF THE THORACIC AND LUMBAR SPINE

Fractures of the thoracic, thoracolumbar, and lumbar spine are classified into four general categories: compression fractures, burst fractures, flexion-distraction injuries (Chance fractures), and fracture-dislocations.

The most common and benign of thoracic and lumbar fractures are simple **compression fractures**. These typically are wedge-shaped fractures of a vertebral body involving only the anterior column (Fig. 15-11*A*). They occur after trivial trauma in elderly patients with osteoporosis or following more significant trauma in younger patients. They may be located in any part of the thoracic or lumbar spine, most frequently between T11 and L2. One should have a high suspicion for the presence of burst fracture if interpedicular widening is seen on an anteroposterior radiograph. CT scan can help to differentiate between the two by close inspection of the posterior vertebral column. Compression fractures can be unstable when the posterior ligamentous structures are disrupted. This may allow progressive vertebral wedging to occur, which would then manifest as increasing kyphosis over the long term and could eventually lead to significant functional impairment or neurologic compromise.

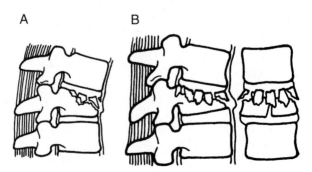

FIG. 15-11   *A.* Compression fracture of the lumbar spine. *B.* Burst fracture of the lumbar spine.

Burst fractures involve the anterior and middle columns with or without injury to the posterior column. The mechanism of injury is high-energy axial loading with slight flexion. The vertebral body literally explodes or "bursts," often resulting in retropulsion of the posterior vertebral body wall into the spinal canal (Fig. 15-11*B*). The proposed mechanism is vertebral endplate failure, with disc tissue being driven into the vertebral body.

Flexion-distraction injuries (Chance fractures) are three-column injuries with the fracture propagating through the posterior elements and pedicle and exiting through the vertebral body (Fig. 15-12*A*). These can also be completely ligamentous injuries, entering through the posterior ligaments and exiting through the disc space, or combined injuries to bones and ligaments (Fig. 15-12*B*). Chance fractures often occur during a head-on automobile collision in which the patient is wearing a lap belt without concomitant use of a shoulder belt. The mechanism of injury is acute flexion of the torso on the seat belt. During impact, the upper part of the body is accelerated anteriorly over the seat belt, producing a distraction force posteriorly around a fixed fulcrum just anterior to the abdomen. Intraabdominal damage has been reported in 45% of patients with this mechanism of injury.

Fracture-dislocations are the result of significant energy applied to the spine with a variety of forces—including flexion, distraction, extension, rotation, shear, and axial-loading components—producing spinal malalignment (Fig. 15-13). These injuries always involve all three columns of the spine and are extremely unstable. They have a marked propensity to cause profound neurologic injury.

Diagnosis and Initial Management

History and Physical Examination

The neurologic examination is critical in patients with thoracic and lumbar spinal injuries, particularly so in those with burst fractures. Clinically, patients may have tenderness to palpation over the affected posterior elements if these are also injured.

The diagnosis of flexion-distraction spinal injuries includes a high index of suspicion from the mechanism of injury, as noted previously. Often, these patients present to the emergency room with a seat-belt type of abrasion over the anterior abdominal wall. A tender, palpable gap may be present in examining the back, indicative of the distracted spinous processes. The incidence of neurologic complications in flexion-distraction injuries is low in patients without

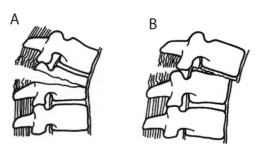

FIG. 15-12 *A.* Chance fracture of the lumbar spine. *B.* Dislocation of the lumbar spine.

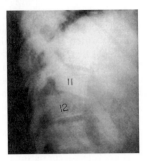

FIG. 15-13 Fracture-dislocation of T11 on T12.

an associated dislocation. Patients with fracture-dislocations often have multi-system injuries due to the violent nature of the trauma. Gross spinal malalignment may be obvious in examining the back, which may have a palpable step-off in the posterior spinal contour.

Radiographic Examination

The diagnosis of a compression fracture is normally made on routine lateral radiographs of the affected region of the spine. Typically, loss of anterior body height vs. posterior height is noted, depending on the amount of compression seen. Axial CT can reliably document an intact posterior vertebral body wall, thereby confirming an intact middle column and thus verifying an anterior compression injury.

The diagnosis of burst fracture is made on either plain radiographs or CT. Radiographic signs of a burst fracture include a widened interpedicular distance at the fracture level on the anteroposterior projection, vertebral body compression with segmental kyphosis, and retropulsion of the posterior cortex of the vertebral body on the lateral projection. The plain radiographs are also examined for subluxation or dislocation in the coronal or sagittal planes and for evidence of posterior-column injury (Fig. 15-14*A* and *B*). Axial CT demonstrates a break in the posterior cortical wall, with different degrees of spinal canal compression from retropulsed bone (Fig 15-14*C* and *D*). MRI should be obtained for patients with neurologic deficits.

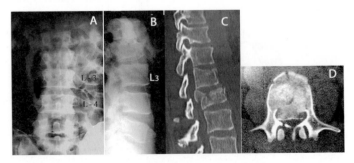

FIG. 15-14 Appearance of L2 burst fracture. *A.* Anteroposterior radiograph. *B.* Lateral radiograph. *C.* Lateral CT scan. *D.* Axial CT scan.

Plain radiographs are essential in the diagnosis of flexion-distraction injuries. The lateral radiograph indicates widening of the posterior column either within or between the bony elements and localized kyphosis. There are also different degrees of distraction of the middle column and thus either a fracture propagating through the pedicles or a widening of the posterior disc space. The anteroposterior radiograph indicates a widened interspinous distance, indicative of ligamentous posterior column injury, fracture through the spinous process lamina, or splayed posterior elements. If translational forces are present and sustained, ligamentous flexion-distraction injuries may progress to unilateral or bilateral facet subluxation or dislocation. Unilateral dislocation is characterized by anterior displacement of the superior vertebra on the inferior by 25% on the lateral radiograph. When displacement is 50% or greater, a bilateral facet dislocation is likely. CT scan helps to further elucidate the fracture pattern, and MRI should be considered for patients with ongoing neurologic deficit.

Plain radiographs indicate fracture-dislocations of the thoracic and lumbar spine in either the coronal or sagittal plane or both. Occasionally, thoracic subluxations are subtle and may involve only a slight lateral or anterior translation of one vertebral body on another. When subluxation proceeds to frank dislocation, the spinal malalignment is obvious on the lateral radiograph. CT is mandatory for these fractures in order to assess unrecognized fractures of posterior elements that may affect operative management. Axial CT often demonstrates two vertebral bodies in the same transaxial slice, indicating dislocation of a vertebral segment. The "empty-facet sign" is present when there is complete facet dislocation. Unlike the case in burst fractures, the middle column is often intact when the primary mechanism of injury is a shearing force. In this instance, compromise of the vertebral canal is secondary to the extreme vertebral malalignment rather than retropulsed bone. MRI should be obtained for patients with incomplete neurologic injuries.

Initial Management

The initial treatment of a patient with a spinal thoracic or lumbar fracture includes supine bed rest with log-rolling to minimize damage to pressure-dependent areas. A thorough systemic review for associated injuries is performed. It is essential to perform serial neurologic examinations on patients who are awaiting definitive treatment of fractures. Deterioration in the neurologic examination is an indication for emergent surgery. Steroids should be administered within the context of the guidelines previously mentioned.

Associated Injuries

Multisystem trauma—such as liver or spleen lacerations, aortic arch tears, and intraabdominal trauma—is often associated with high-energy thoracolumbar fractures. Some 45% of patients with flexion-distraction injuries have associated intraabdominal injuries. Conversely, 25% of patients with intraabdominal injuries from wearing lap belts have flexion-distraction spinal injuries. Patients with thoracic spinal injuries may also have concomitant rib fractures with hemothorax or pneumothorax.

Definitive Management

Definitive management of thoracic and lumbar compression fractures depends on the age of the patient, location of the injury, amount of compression deformity, and any evidence of posterior column distraction injury. Neurologic compromise and instability are also key determinants of surgical intervention. Elderly patients with multiple osteoporotic compression fractures of the spine are often treated symptomatically without immobilization. Concern for possible pathologic involvement with tumor or infection must be maintained in the elderly patient population. In younger patients, compression fractures with less than 50% loss of height are usually stable injuries that can be treated with a spinal orthosis for pain control during healing. For lesions in the thoracolumbar junction and lumbar spine, a hyperextension orthosis may be used in an attempt to limit the kyphosis that follows these injuries. In the majority of these patients, even with a well-molded hyperextension cast or orthosis, some settling occurs during the healing process; usually, however, it is of little significance as long as the middle and posterior columns are intact.

For patients with greater than 50% compression deformity, it is essential to rule out middle-column involvement and posterior-column distraction. Radiographs demonstrate a widened distance between intraspinous processes or fracture of a posterior element, and the sagittal MRI also may document a posterior ligamentous injury. These injuries may require surgery with posterior compression instrumentation and fusion with or without an anterior corpectomy and anterior fusion to prevent a progressive kyphosis and neurologic sequelae.

Definitive management of thoracic and lumbar burst fractures depends on the patient's neurologic status and age, the location of the fracture, degree of compromise of the spinal canal, involvement of posterior elements, coronal or sagittal subluxation, amount of segmental sagittal kyphosis, concomitant multisystem injuries, and body habitus. Methods of management are nonoperative bracing or casting or operative stabilization via anterior, posterior, or combined surgical approaches.

Burst fractures are managed **nonoperatively** when the patient is neurologically intact, there is minimal segmental kyphosis and bony retropulsion (less than 50% canal compromise), no coronal or sagittal subluxation, and no posterior-column involvement. A molded two-piece hyperextension spinal orthosis is applied. A thoracolumbar orthosis is usually maintained for a total of 12 weeks. Younger patients with kyphosis and a thin body habitus are managed with a hyperextension Risser cast to limit postinjury settling of the fracture. When L4 or L5 is fractured, a single thigh is incorporated into the cast or brace to increase control of sagittal alignment in the lower lumbar spine. The nonoperative treatment of lumbar burst fractures in neurologically intact patients with greater than 50% canal compromise is controversial. The majority of such injuries heal uneventfully without neurologic sequelae. The spinal canal remodels over time, thus increasing the space available for the neural elements. However, settling of the burst fracture usually results in an increase in segmental kyphosis.

Indications for **operative** management of a burst fracture in a **neurologically intact** or minimally involved patient are signs of instability—three-column injuries, subluxation in the coronal or sagittal plane, significant segmental sagittal kyphosis at the fracture site, progressive neurologic deficit, progressive kyphosis, or greater than 50% loss of vertebral height. Other considerations include concomitant injuries or body habitus that will not allow orthotic or cast treatment. Fractures of the thoracolumbar junction or upper lumbar spine are approached posteriorly, reduced, bone-grafted, and stabilized. The preservation of sagittal alignment and maintenance of motion segments are important and accomplished by using posterior pedicle screw fixation systems when the pedicles are of sufficient size. The recommended fusion levels for posterior-only procedures include instrumentation from two or three levels cephalad to the injury to two levels caudad. In cases where there is inadequate support from the anterior and middle columns, anterior corpectomy and strut grafting are performed as second-stage procedures. Significant burst fractures of the thoracic spine in the neurologically intact patient with anterior collapse and posterior-column injury are usually managed with combined anterior corpectomy and fusion, followed by posterior compression instrumentation and fusion to minimize the risk of further bone retropulsion and neurologic injury.

Operative management of burst fractures associated with **significant neurologic deficit** is individualized. The primary concern is decompression of the spinal canal. The **anterior approach** to the spine is the most thorough method of clearing it of retropulsed bone and disc material; it is the treatment of choice for this group of patients. It is important to note that a **posterior-only approach** as a means of obtaining indirect decompression and stabilization has also been shown to be effective. The surgical approach is dictated by the level of pathology: a thoracotomy for T1 to T10 fractures; a thoracoabdominal approach usually through the tenth rib for T11, T12, and L1 fractures; and a retroperitoneal flank approach below the diaphragm for L2 to L5 fractures. The intervertebral discs above and below the fracture are excised and a subtotal corpectomy of the injured vertebra is performed, leaving the anterior and deep cortex intact. As an alternative, a reach-around posterior approach can provide anterior decompression and strut grafting via a costotransversectomy or a far lateral lumbar approach.

Following spinal canal decompression, a strut graft or titanium mesh cage is placed from the inferior endplate of the cephalad vertebra to the superior endplate of the caudad vertebra. Success or failure of the surgery rests on the stability and healing of the graft more than on any instrumentation placed. Anterior instrumentation devices secure the strut graft and at times may act as a stand-alone device along with postoperative bracing. However, the spine may also be instrumented and fused posteriorly in a second stage with rods and hooks over the same levels as the anterior construct for further stabilization.

The spine is approached **posteriorly first** for **burst fractures with significant posterior-column disruption** or subluxation. The posterior instrumentation is used for reduction and restoration of sagittal plane alignment. At the same sitting, anterior corpectomy and strut-graft fusion are performed.

Definitive management of flexion-distraction injuries depends on the anatomic structures involved and the amount of displacement. Lesions occurring entirely through bone are managed in a hyperextension cast. This is particularly successful when the fracture line has propagated through the pedicles bilaterally. Injuries in which the fracture involves the pars interarticularis and pure soft tissue are managed operatively because the pars has very little cancellous bone, which means that fracture healing is less reliable; ligamentous healing does not result in adequate stability. It is important to identify traumatic disc disruptions and herniations prior to the surgical reduction of displaced posterior elements because posterior compression forces may displace herniated disc material into the spinal canal, causing neurologic injury. A short-segment fixation with pedicle screw instrumentation and fusion is performed via a posterior approach. A thoracolumbar orthosis is worn for 4 months postoperatively.

Definitive management of fracture-dislocations is posterior operative reduction, stabilization, and fusion. Thoracolumbar and lumbar injuries are instrumented with pedicle screw and rod constructs, limiting the number of distally instrumented and fused motion segments if possible. Postoperative bracing increases the fusion rate by protecting the instrumentation until fusion occurs.

The timing of operative reduction and stabilization is determined by the patient's neurologic status and overall medical condition. The primary indication for emergent operative reduction is a neurologically incomplete patient with a progressing neurologic deficit in the setting of radiographically determined canal compromise. Patients with complete spinal cord injuries are stabilized as soon as possible to decrease the duration of enforced bed rest. A patient with an incomplete neurologic injury that is improving is observed until improvement plateaus. The spine is then reduced and stabilized.

Complications

The most significant complication of compression fractures is progressive kyphosis resulting from settling of the vertebral body, unrecognized posterior-column ligamentous injuries, multiple contiguous compression fractures, and pathologic fractures. Neurologic abnormalities are not seen with typical compression fractures, which involve only the anterior column.

Complications of nonoperative management of burst fractures are residual segmental kyphosis, progressive kyphosis secondary to unrecognized posterior-column injury, and vertebral collapse due to settling. All these have a potential for increasing neurologic deficits. Complications of operative management of burst fractures are failure of instrumentation due to inadequate anterior-column reconstruction, vascular or neurologic injury during the surgical approach, and dislodgment of strut grafts. Pseudarthrosis is rare with either operative or nonoperative treatment.

Complications of flexion-distraction injuries are inadequate posterior-column reduction with orthosis for bone injuries, unrecognized ligamentous components of the injury, and rare traumatic disc herniations. These last may be retropulsed into the spinal canal by posterior compression forces during operative reduction.

Complications of fracture-dislocations of the spine are an increase in spinal deformity due to inadequate treatment in a spinal orthosis or a Charcot spinal arthropathy below a complete spinal cord injury.

SACRAL FRACTURES

Classification

Sacral fractures are classified anatomically into zones I, II, and III, using the Denis three-zone system.

Zone I fractures are lateral to the neural foramen. They are associated with a 6% rate of neurologic injury. Neurologic deficits result from superiorly displaced sacral fracture fragments compressing the L5 nerve root against the undersurface of the L5 transverse process. Zone I injuries also include various ligamentous avulsion injuries around the periphery of the sacrum. These account for 50% of sacral fractures.

Zone II fractures are longitudinal fractures through the sacral foramen. They are associated with a 28% incidence of neurologic deficits. The neurologic injury is usually characterized by S1 compression associated with sciatica. L5 is involved when fracture fragments are displaced superiorly; other sacral nerve roots can be involved if the fracture extends through these levels, causing displacement. Because these fractures are unilateral, incontinence is rare, but sensory changes over the involved dermatomes are common. Zone II fractures account for 34% of sacral fractures.

Zone III fractures occur least frequently, at 16%. These fractures involve the central canal and are associated with a high (57%) incidence of neurologic deficits, with loss of sphincter control, saddle anesthesia, and acute cauda equina symptoms. Transverse fractures occur as isolated injuries due to a flexion force imparted to the lower part of the sacrum and the coccyx. Below S4, there is little chance of a significant neurologic deficit because the sacral nerve roots have exited proximal to this area. Some 76% of these patients have impairment of bowel, bladder, or sexual function.

Another pattern of injury to this segment of the spine has recently been classified. These are injuries at the lumbosacral junction. Isler has classified them according to where the fracture line extends relative to the L5-S1 facet joint. Type A injuries are lateral to the facet joint, type B injuries extend through the L5-S1 facet, and type C injuries occur through the spinal canal. Types B and C are associated with instability and varying degrees of neurologic injury.

Diagnosis and Initial Management

History and Physical Examination

Sacral fractures are most frequently due to high-energy trauma. Physical findings are back and buttock pain, ecchymosis over the sacrum, and sacral pain on rectal examination. Specific low lumbar and sacral root neurologic deficits should prompt consideration of sacral fractures. The fifth lumbar root is often involved when it is trapped between the transverse process of L5 and the superiorly migrating fragment of the sacral ala. Evaluation of the Achilles and bulbocavernosus reflexes is mandatory in assessing sacral root function. Sacral fractures may result in anesthesia over the sacral dermatomes, impotence, and a flaccid bowel and bladder. Incontinence rarely occurs with unilateral root injury between S2 and S5. Decreased sensation is a more usual consequence. When there is doubt about the integrity of the structures innervated by the sacral segments, urodynamics can be helpful in assessing the motor function of the bladder.

Radiographic Examination

Radiographic documentation of sacral fractures is difficult because of the complex shape of the sacrum and pelvis. Fifty percent of sacral fractures without neurologic deficit are missed on initial examination. The initial radiographic examination includes lateral and anteroposterior, or Ferguson, projections. The Ferguson projection centers the proximally directed beam on the sacrum. Radiographic findings associated with sacral fractures are fractures of low lumbar transverse processes, asymmetrical sacral foramen, and irregular trabeculation of the lateral masses of the proximal sacral segments. CT is the most accurate method of evaluating sacral fractures. When the sacral segments are too osteopenic to produce reliable radiographic images, suspected fractures are identified on bone scan.

Initial Management

The focus of initial management of sacral fractures is pain relief. The patient is kept at bed rest and log-rolled from side to side until the pain subsides to the point where mobilization can be initiated, usually within 7 to 10 days. Contraindications to nonoperative management include fractures associated with soft tissue compromise, incomplete neurologic deficit with documented neural compression, and extensive disruption of the posterior lumbosacral ligaments.

Associated Injuries

These include multisystem and neurologic injuries associated with fractures of the sacrum.

Definitive Management

Isolated sacral fractures without fractures of the anterior pelvic ring or neurologic deficits are stable and do not require treatment beyond relief of symptoms. After the initial period of bed rest, the patient is mobilized with avoidance of weight bearing on the affected side for 4 to 8 weeks and then with weight bearing as tolerated. It may take up to 2 to 4 months for a fracture of the posterior pelvic ring to heal completely. Sacral fractures that present as elements of a pelvic injury are managed to reestablish the pelvic ring. The goals of surgery are neurologic decompression where applicable and establishment of stability. Percutaneous and open techniques are designed to obtain stabilization.

Complications

Complications of sacral fractures are chronic pain secondary to sacroiliac arthritis or change of alignment of the sacrum and loss of voluntary control of bowel and bladder. Sacroiliac arthritis is managed with arthrodesis.

Neurologic deficits associated with zone II injuries are managed with observation, because many of these injuries are neuropraxias that will resolve spontaneously. Symptoms that persist beyond 6 to 8 weeks may benefit from foraminal decompression. Deficits associated with zone III injuries should undergo aggressive radiologic examination to identify the cause of the neurologic injury, because early posterior decompression may result in the return of bowel and bladder control and reversal of foot drop. Late decompression is often complicated by epidural fibrosis and minimal return of function.

SELECTED READINGS

Allen GL, Ferguson RL, Lehmann TR, O'Brien RP. A mechanistic classification of closed, indirect fractures and dislocations of the lower cervical spine. *Spine* 7:1–27, 1982.

Bohlmann HH. Acute fractures and dislocations of the cervical spine: an analysis of 300 hospitalized patients and review of the literature. *J Bone Joint Surg* 61A:1141, 1979.

Bohlmann HH. Treatment of fractures and dislocations of the thoracic and lumbar spine: current concepts review. *J Bone Joint Surg* 67A:165–169, 1985.

Bracken MB, Shephard M, Holford T, et al. Administration of methylprednisolone for 24 or 48 hours or tirilazad mesylate for 48 hours in the treatment of acute spinal cord injury. Results of the Third National Acute Spinal Cord Injury Randomized Controlled Trial. National Acute Spinal Cord Injury Study. *JAMA* 277(20):1597–1604, 1997.

Clark CR, White AA III. Fractures of the dens. A multicenter study. *J Bone Joint Surg* 67A:1340, 1985.

Denis F. The 3-column spine and its significance in the classification of acute thoracolumbar spinal injuries. *Spine* 8:817–831, 1983.

Eismont FJ, Currier BL, McGuire RA. Cervical spine and spinal cord injuries: recognition and treatment. AAOS *Instr Course Lect* 53:341–358, 2004.

Rizzolo SJ, Cotler JM. Unstable cervical spine injuries: specific treatment approaches. *J Am Acad Orthop Surg* 1:57–66, 1993.

Vaccaro AR, An HS, Lin S, et al. Noncontiguous injuries of the spine. *J Spinal Disord* 5:320–329, 1992.

Vaccaro AR, Kim DH, Brodke DS, et al. Diagnosis and management of thoracolumbar spine fractures. *J Bone Joint Surg* 85A:359–373, 2003.

Vaccaro AR, Kim DH, Brodke DS, et al. Diagnosis and management of sacral spine fractures. *J Bone Joint Surg* 86A:375–385, 2004.

Fractures and Dislocations of the Pelvic Ring and Acetabulum

D. Kevin Scheid

This chapter reviews fractures and dislocations of the pelvic ring and acetabulum and dislocations of the hip.

ANATOMY OF THE PELVIC RING

The bony pelvic ring consists of two innominate bones (hemipelvis) and the sacrum, which are held together by an intricate ligamentous network. Each innominate bone consists of three parts: ilium, ischium, and pubis, which fuse at the acetabulum on skeletal maturity. The **anterior column**, or iliopubic column, includes the anterior wall of the acetabulum, the anterior ilium, and the superior pubic ramus (Fig. 16-1*A*). The **posterior column**, or ilioischial column, includes the posterior wall of the acetabulum and extends from the postero-inferior ilium at the greater sciatic notch to the ischial tuberosity (Fig. 16-1*B*). Specific landmarks on the anterior column that are helpful during surgery include the anterosuperior iliac spine, anteroinferior iliac spine, iliopubic line, iliopubic eminence, and pubic tubercle. Landmarks on the posterior column include the greater sciatic notch, lesser sciatic notch, ischial spine, and ischial tuberosity.

Each innominate bone articulates with the sacrum posteriorly at the sacroiliac joints. The joints are covered with hyaline cartilage on the sacral side and fibrocartilage on the iliac side. All sacroiliac joint stability is derived from **interosseous , posterior sacroiliac, and anterior sacroiliac ligament complexes** (Fig. 16-2). The anterior pelvic ring is joined at the cartilage-covered pubic symphysis and is held by an enveloping fibroligamentous complex. Two additional (sacroischial) ligaments, the sacrospinous and sacrotuberous, confer stability to the pelvic ring. Together, these ligament complexes resist vertical and rotational forces on each hemipelvis. The pelvic brim divides the upper (false pelvis) and lower (true pelvis).

Vascular, neurologic, and genitourinary structures lie within and along the inner pelvis, making them susceptible to injury during pelvic disruption. The **common iliac artery** gives rise to the **internal iliac and external iliac arteries**. The **superior and inferior gluteal, vesical, and lumbosacral arteries** all arise from the internal iliac artery. The **sacral venous plexus** is particularly susceptible to injury with pelvic ring disruption and is difficult to control or embolize.

The **lumbosacral plexus**, which includes the fourth and fifth lumbar and sacral nerve roots, lies along the anterior sacrum. The sciatic, gluteal, and splanchnic nerves arise from this plexus. The obturator nerve runs along and below the pelvic brim to exit the obturator foramen.

The bladder, urethra, vagina, and rectum are all susceptible to being punctured or torn by bony spicules, shear forces, and compression.

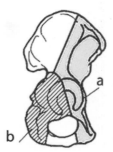

FIG. 16-1   Anterior (*a*) and posterior (*b*) columns of the pelvis.

FRACTURES AND DISLOCATIONS OF THE PELVIC RING

Classification

Pelvic fractures have previously been classified according to the presumed mechanism of injury as lateral compression, anteroposterior compression, vertical shear, and complex fractures. The more useful AO classification of Tile is based solely on pelvic stability and therefore better dictates the needed treatment.

Type A fractures are stable both vertically and rotationally. They do not truly disrupt the pelvic ring, as do **type B** and **type C** fractures. An iliac wing fracture involving the crest that does not disrupt the integrity of the pelvic ring or an isolated transverse fracture of the sacrum are examples of type A fractures. Avulsions of the ischeal tuberosity or iliac spines are also type A injuries.

Type B fractures are vertically stable but rotationally unstable. They include many lateral compression and anteroposterior compression injuries. The hemipelvis is disrupted rotationally, causing both anterior and posterior ring injuries. Although these injuries can be quite severe and cause gross **rotational** instability to the hemipelvis, the hemipelvis is not **vertically** unstable and will not displace vertically because of the partially intact posterior ligamentous structures. The two common subgroups of type B injuries include the "open-book" (B1) injury, with anterior pelvic ring disruption and disruption of the **anterior** sacroiliac ligaments. The hemipelvis is unstable to **external** rotation but vertically stable because of intact **posterior** sacroiliac ligaments

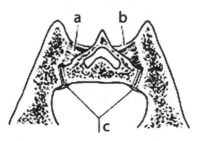

FIG. 16-2   Transverse section through sacroiliac joints. (*a*) Interosseous ligaments, (*b*) posterior sacroiliac ligaments, (*c*) anterior sacroiliac ligaments.

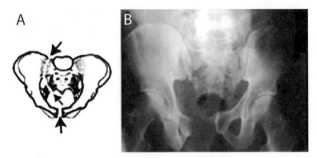

FIG. 16-3   *A.* B1 injury with disruption of the anterior ring and anterior sacroiliac ligament. The posterior sacroiliac ligaments remain intact, providing vertical stability. *B.* AP view of the pelvis with a typical B1 injury.

(Fig. 16-3*A* and *B*). The second most common subgroup of type B injuries comprises those unstable to **internal** rotation; they include the "lateral compression" (type B2) injuries. The internally rotated hemipelvis disrupts the **posterior** sacroiliac ligaments and crushes the anterior ring (pubic rami). The anterior sacroiliac ligaments and sacrospinous and sacrotuberous ligaments remain intact. The rotating hemipelvis frequently crushes the anterior sacrum or sacral ala. The intact ligaments keep the hemipelvis vertically stable. The disrupted anterior ring and posterior sacroiliac ligaments cause internal rotational instability (Fig. 16-4*A* to *D*).

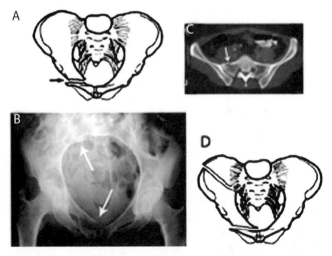

FIG. 16-4   *A.* B2 injury with disruption of the anterior ring and posterior sacroiliac ligament. The anterior sacroiliac, sacrospinous, and sacrotuberous ligaments remain intact, providing vertical stability. *B.* Inlet view of the pelvis with internal rotation of the right hemipelvis. Fractures of the right ramus and right sacral ala are seen. *C.* CT scan showing buckle fracture of the anterior sacral ala. *D.* B2 injury with fracture of the ilium posteriorly.

Type C fractures are both **vertically** and **rotationally** unstable. Like type B injuries, the anterior and posterior pelvic ring is disrupted. Unlike type B injuries, sufficient disruption of bones or ligaments has occurred to allow the hemipelvis to displace vertically. The posterior injury can involve the sacrum, sacroiliac joint (Fig. 16-5*D*), posterior ilium, or any combination thereof. The anterior injury can involve the pubic symphysis or ischial and pubic rami (Fig. 16-5*A* to *C*). Because of the combined injuries to bones and ligaments, these fracture-dislocations will migrate vertically due to the pull of the torso muscles.

Diagnosis and Initial Management

History and Physical Examination

There is always a history of significant trauma. A rapid initial physical examination includes inspection for pelvic, abdominal, and perineal bruising; digital inspection for rectal or vaginal tears, indicating an open fracture; blood at the urethral meatus, indicating possible urethral tear; pelvic asymmetry; iliac crest mobility; lower extremity malrotation; and leg-length discrepancy. There is also a focused neurologic and vascular examination of the lower extremities.

Radiographic Examination

An anteroposterior pelvic film usually raises suspicion of a pelvic ring disruption. Inlet and outlet views and computed tomography (CT) scans define the posterior injury and thus possible instability of the pelvic ring. If the result is equivocal, suspected instability is documented fluoroscopically by examination under anesthesia.

vertical displacement—all SI ligaments ruptured

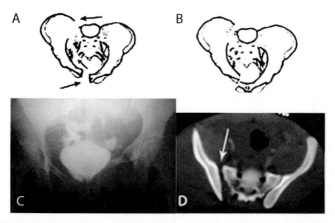

FIG. 16-5 *A.* C-type injuries showing vertical instability of the hemipelvis. The anterior injury can involve the symphysis or *(B)* the ischial and pubic rami. *C.* Cystogram showing rupture of the bladder with dye extravasation. *D.* The posterior injury can involve the posterior ilium, sacroiliac joint, or sacrum.

Initial Management

Hemodynamically stable patients are closely monitored. Hemodynamic instability is a life-threatening emergency. Hemodynamically unstable patients may be placed in medical antishock trousers (MAST) to increase peripheral vascular resistance and decrease motion of the fracture by direct pressure. Use of the MAST suit for other than initial transport and stabilization is not indicated because of complications secondary to prolonged inflation. A bed sheet tied circumferentially around the pelvis may decrease venous bleeding in type B1 and C injuries. Immediate intervention for the bleeding pelvis after removal of the MAST suit is rapid reduction and external fixation to tamponade bleeding vessels. Anterior ring stabilization alone will usually suffice to tamponade retroperitoneal hemorrhage, even if there is vertical instability; however, skeletal traction is added to prevent vertical migration of the hemipelvis until definitive posterior fixation is done. If bleeding persists, as indicated by continued hemodynamic instability, CT of the pelvis with contrast may demonstrate a hematoma consistent with active bleeding. Selective arterial embolization can be attempted to control hemorrhage and restore hemodynamic stability. Indications for emergent open control of hemorrhage or for packing are rare: open fracture and inability to control hemorrhage, major vessel disruption uncontrollable by embolization, and lifesaving hemipelvectomy.

Associated Injuries

Pelvic fractures are frequently associated with vascular and genitourinary system injuries. Type B1 injuries, unstable in external rotation, have a greater incidence of associated vascular injuries than do type B2 injuries, unstable to internal rotation. **Vascular injuries** are life-threatening and must be managed aggressively. Rapid evaluation is required to rule out thoracic, intraperitoneal, or external bleeding and to direct management of the patient in extremis toward the retroperitoneum and the pelvic fracture. The hypovolemic patient with an unstable pelvic ring fracture is assumed to have significant retroperitoneal hemorrhage due to injury of the sacral venous plexus, bleeding due to bone fracture, and major or minor arterial injuries.

Genitourinary injury is suspected with any pelvic fracture and is more common in type B2 injuries. Blood at the urethral meatus, fractures of the ischial and pubic rami, and a floating prostate on rectal examination indicate urethral injury. A retrograde urethrogram determines the presence of a urethral tear prior to catheterization of the bladder. A cystogram determines whether the bladder is intact (Fig. 16-5*C*).

Definitive Management

The goal of early management is stabilization of the unstable pelvis. This is most frequently accomplished by application of an anterior external fixator.

In **rotationally unstable (type B)** fractures, only anterior ring stability is required to convert an unstable pelvic ring to a stable structure. Displaced or grossly unstable lateral compression (type B2) fractures require anterior ring stabilization only. Often, an external fixator is used to externally rotate and reduce the internally rotated hemipelvis. Open-book (type B1) injuries with instability on stress views greater than 2.5 cm of symphysis dissociation or gross radiographic and clinical instability also warrant stabilization of the anterior pelvic ring (Fig. 16-6*A* and *B*). In equivocal cases, examination with imaging

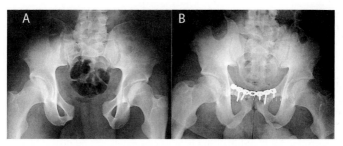

FIG. 16-6   *A* and *B*. Open-book injury to the pelvis treated with reduction and plating. (*Courtesy of Robert F. Hall, Jr., M.D.*)

under general anesthesia will assess the degree of rotational instability. An external fixator or pubic symphysis plate is sufficient to internally rotate and stabilize the externally rotated hemipelvis.

In **vertically unstable** fractures, anterior and posterior stabilization is required.

Anterior stabilization is accomplished as in type B injuries. Relative indications for internal fixation of the disrupted symphysis pubis or fractures of pubic rami include exposure of the area for laparotomy or bladder repair or when external fixator pins would violate a planned acetabular surgical incision, thereby increasing the chance of postoperative infection. The **technique of external fixation** follows many of the guidelines set forth for external fixator use in long bones. Two to three pins at least 5 mm in diameter are placed in each hemipelvis. Increased pin spacing improves stability. External fixator systems that do not require parallel pin placement allow individual angling of pins for optimal positioning. The shape of the iliac wing makes it a challenge to insert the pins between the two cortical tables. Pins are placed through small horizontal incisions over the iliac crest. The starting point for the first pin is 2 cm posterior to the anterosuperior iliac spine. The second pin is inserted in the broad iliac tubercle 6 to 10 cm posterior to the first pin. A drill hole is made in the cortex of the crest only, and pins are inserted by hand with a T-handled chuck. Imaging can be used with tangential views to ensure that the pins remain between the cortical tables. Directing each pin toward the rectum offers an initial three-dimensional mental landmark for pin placement within the cortical tables. Maximal pin depth, with the tips of the pins ending in the ilium just above the acetabulum, affords the greatest stability and longevity of the pin. Rotation of the fluoroscope in different directions allows tangential views of each pin, verifying placement between the cortical tables. A simple quadrilateral frame is attached to the pins, the pelvis reduced by manipulation under fluoroscopy, and the frame tightened to hold the reduction.

The **technique of open reduction and internal fixation** of the anterior pelvic ring calls for a horizontal Pfannenstiel or vertical laparotomy incision. Two anterior plates oriented at 90 degrees to each other are considered more stable than a single plate. A Foley catheter in the bladder not only decompresses the bladder but also serves as an easily palpable landmark for bladder location.

There are no external fixator constructs or any form of anterior internal fixation that would, alone, provide enough stability to maintain reduction of a vertically unstable fracture. Therefore, when vertical instability is present, the posterior ring must be stabilized. This can be done acutely in a stable patient or delayed until the patient has stabilized. Traction should be employed if posterior fixation is delayed. Various **techniques of posterior fixation** have evolved, and their use depends on the location of the posterior injury and the surgeon's experience. **Posterior iliac fractures** are stabilized by using standard plating techniques. Lag screws compress the fracture, and a neutralization plate is applied. The approach is anterior through an iliac crest incision, exposing the inner table, or posterior, with the patient in a lateral decubitus or prone position. Exposure of the more lateral iliac fracture is easier through an inner pelvic approach. Posterior iliac fractures are more easily exposed through a posterior approach, especially in obese patients.

Sacroiliac joint stabilization is most commonly accomplished by image-guided, percutaneously placed iliosacral screws. In experienced hands, one and usually two screws placed into S1 or S1 and S2 are sufficient. Anterior iliosacral plating can also be done if it offers advantages in a given case. Sacral bars are rarely used.

The majority of patients presenting for delayed posterior fixation have had an external fixator placed on admission or during resuscitation. The external fixator may have to be detached to allow mobility of the hemipelvis for anatomic reduction. After anatomic posterior reduction is obtained, the fixator is resecured.

Anterior sacroiliac joint fixation with two- or three-hole plates has been used successfully for many years. Stability of fixation is increased by the use of two plates. This is important when there is room for only one screw on the sacral side due to the proximity of the L5 nerve root. Occasionally, the sacroiliac joint is approached posteriorly. A **posterior approach** is most commonly employed when a large iliac fragment is present and is attached to the sacrum by the iliolumbar and iliosacral ligaments. Direct exposure of this fragment facilitates its reduction and fixation.

The advantage of **percutaneous iliosacral lag screws** is the direct fixation of the ilium to the sacrum. The disadvantages are potential iatrogenic neurologic injury from screw penetration into the sacral foramina or spinal canal and violation of the sacroiliac joint itself with the screws. Two large-diameter cannulated screws are inserted from the posterolateral ilium into the S1 body or sacral ala. Washers or small plates are used to prevent migration of the screw head through the ilium as the screw is tightened. The technique requires clear visualization by using image intensification. The patient's position must allow enough under-table clearance to obtain appropriate inlet, outlet, and lateral views with the fluoroscope. When there is inadequate visualization of the sacral foramina on the outlet view because of obesity or bowel gas, alternative methods of fixation are considered, or the procedure is delayed until the bowel is well prepped. On the inlet view, the pin is angled slightly anteriorly to pass through the vestibule of the sacral ala at a perpendicular angle (see the article by Carlson and Scheid in the "Selected Readings" at the end of this chapter). The tip of the guide pin is placed in the anterior third of the S1 body to maintain the maximal distance between it and the sacral spinal canal. On the outlet view, the guide pin should be angled slightly cephalad, ending in the upper half of the S1 body. A final check with a true lateral view ensures accurate guide-pin placement.

Sacral fractures are stabilized in situ by using the percutaneous iliosacral screw technique described for sacroiliac joints. Problems unique to sacral fractures are loss of foraminal landmarks secondary to the fracture pattern and crushing of interposed nerves between bone fragments while the screws are being tightened. When anatomic reduction of the sacral fracture is not achieved by closed methods, a combination of posterior open reduction and percutaneous screw placement is used. The patient is positioned prone and the sacrum is exposed through a posterior longitudinal incision. The fracture is reduced and nerves are decompressed. With the help of fluoroscopy, percutaneous iliosacral screws are placed. Even with a direct approach to the sacrum or sacroiliac joint posteriorly, exposure of the outer posterior ilium is not required to place percutaneous screws. This will help prevent posterior wound breakdown.

Complications

Complications include posttraumatic arthritis of the sacroiliac joint; symptomatic malunion, resulting in leg-length discrepancy; malrotation; and neurologic symptoms due to inflammation and entrapment of lumbar and sacral nerve roots. **Arthritis** of the sacroiliac joint is managed conservatively initially and with arthrodesis if necessary. Symptomatic **malunion** is managed with a shoe lift and gait modification. Occasionally, a correctional osteotomy is indicated. **Neuritis** is managed with nonsteroidal anti-inflammatory drugs, neuroleptics, and occasionally nerve decompression.

ACETABULAR FRACTURES

Classification

The anatomic classification of acetabular fractures was published by Judet et al. in 1964 and refined by Letournel in 1981. Acetabular fractures are classified into five **simple** and five **associated** fractures.

Simple Fractures

Posterior-wall fractures represent posterior dislocations of the femoral head. They involve different amounts of the posterior rim of the acetabulum. Sciatic nerve injury and marginal impaction of the remaining intact posterior wall are common (Fig. 16-7*A*). A frequent mistake is classifying a large fracture of the posterior wall as a fracture of the posterior column.

Posterior-column fractures by definition require disruption of the ilioischial line on the anteroposterior pelvic view. They include the ischial portion of the bone and often involve a disruption of the obturator foramen (Fig. 16-7*B*).

Anterior-wall fractures are rare. They involve different portions of the anterior rim or half of the acetabulum. The fracture does not involve the inferior pubic ramus (Fig. 16-8*A*).

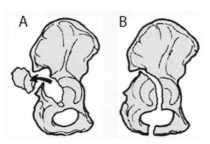

FIG. 16-7 *A.* Posterior-wall fracture. *B.* Posterior-column fracture.

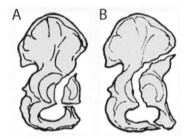

FIG. 16-8   *A.* Anterior-wall fracture. *B.* Anterior-column fracture.

Anterior-column fractures are characterized by disruption of the ilio-pectineal line. Low column fractures involve the inferior acetabulum and include disruption of the inferior pubic ramus. Superior fractures involve different parts of the anterior half of the ilium (Fig. 16-8*B*).

Transverse fractures divide the hemipelvis into superior and inferior halves. The line can traverse the articular surface at any level, and the obturator foramen is intact (Fig. 16-9*A* and *B*).

Associated Fractures

Fractures of both the **posterior column and posterior wall** represent a dislocation of the hip with an associated posterior-column fracture. There is a break in the obturator foramen (Fig. 16-10).

T-shaped fractures are transverse with an associated vertical fracture into the obturator foramen and out through the inferior ramus (Fig. 16-11).

Fractures of the **anterior wall or column with posterior hemitransverse,** as the name implies, combines an anterior-wall or anterior-column fracture with the posterior half of a transverse fracture (Fig. 16-12).

Both-column fractures are diagnosed more often than they occur. A true both-column fracture has no articular surface attached to the **intact** portion of the ilium, which remains attached to the sacrum (Fig. 16-13).

Transverse with posterior-wall fractures usually do not involve a break in the obturator foramen (Fig. 16-14).

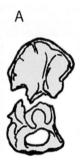
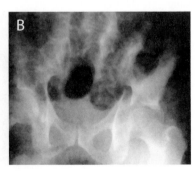

FIG. 16-9   *A* and *B.* Drawing and radiograph of transverse acetabular fracture.

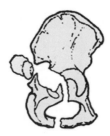

FIG. 16-10   Posterior-column–posterior-wall fracture.

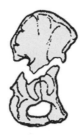

FIG. 16-11   T-shaped fracture.

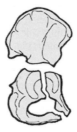

FIG. 16-12   Anterior-wall or -column fracture with a posterior hemitransverse fracture.

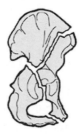

FIG. 16-13   Both-column fracture.

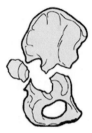

FIG. 16-14   Transverse with posterior-wall fracture.

Diagnosis and Initial Management

History and Physical Examination

There is always a history of significant injury. The patient has pain localized to the hip. The leg may be rotated and shortened. Motion of the hip elicits severe pain. A partial or complete sciatic nerve injury may exist.

Radiographic Examination

Radiographic evaluation is important for preoperative planning. Virtually all fractures can be classified with an anteroposterior pelvic film and two oblique views. Although both column outlines can be seen on the anteroposterior view (Fig. 16-15*A*), the two oblique, or Judet, views at 45 degrees best display the individual columns. The **iliac oblique** view is taken with the fractured side tilted down or away from the x-ray tube. This view profiles the ilium and best displays the posterior column of the affected side (Fig. 16-15*B*). The **obturator oblique** view, taken with the fractured side tilted up toward the tube, best displays the outline of the anterior column (Fig. 16-15*C*). CT provides additional information not easily found on plain films, including undisplaced fragments of the ilium or impacted segmental fragments of the acetabulum. The shortcomings of axial CT include the inability to determine dome step-off and difficulty in classification without comparison to plain films. Three-dimensional CT scans are accurate representations of the fracture but usually provide little additional information.

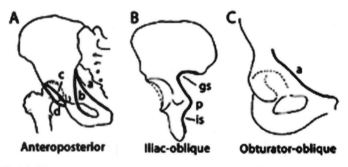

FIG. 16-15   *A.* Anteroposterior view of the hemipelvis. *B.* Iliac oblique projection. *C.* Obturator oblique projection.

Initial Management

Like pelvic ring injuries, acetabular fractures frequently occur with injuries to other organ systems. During resuscitation, an anteroposterior pelvic film will show most acetabular pathology. When hemodynamic stability is achieved, Judet views and a CT scan are usually obtained to determine whether traction is necessary. Distal femoral skeletal traction is applied: 20 to 30 lb of skeletal traction will suffice to partially reduce the femoral head and disimpact the joint.

A dislocated femoral head is reduced as though there were no acetabular fracture. If necessary, skeletal traction is applied while the reduction is held manually. Open reduction is necessary for the rare irreducible dislocation.

Associated Injuries

Associated injuries of the femoral head, pelvis, genitourinary system, and sciatic nerve occur frequently. Unfortunately, the best acetabular reconstruction may have a poor result because the **articular surface of the femoral head is damaged**. Some of this damage can occur after injury as the subluxed head articulates with the edges of fractured bone. For this reason, the patient is placed in skeletal traction until it is determined that the fracture is undisplaced and that there are no intraarticular fragments. A concomitant **pelvic ring** injury complicates the preoperative planning. **Genitourinary** injuries are less frequent than with pelvic ring disruptions. **Sciatic nerve** contusion with selective injury to the peroneal section of the nerve is common in fractures of the posterior column and wall. Local soft tissues are frequently compromised and are carefully inspected before determining the timing of surgery and the approach.

Definitive Management

Goals of surgery include reduction of the articular surface, removal of debris from the joint, and stable fixation, which will allow non-weight-bearing ambulation and range of motion. The primary relative indication for nonoperative management is a congruous joint that is stable without traction. Fractures of the posterior wall that involve up to half of the posterior articular surface may be stable. If posterior stability is documented, nonoperative management is considered. However, if the fragment is large enough to obtain stable fixation, internal fixation will decrease the chance of late loss of reduction. Very low transverse T-shaped and anterior-column fractures can be managed nonoperatively if the weight-bearing portion of the joint is stable and congruous.

Surgical approaches are divided into two categories: limited and extensile. The term *limited* implies visualization of one column. The term *extensile* implies exposure of part or all of both columns through one incision. Occasionally, two limited incisions are used to achieve exposure of both columns. The approach used depends on the type of fracture and the surgeon's experience.

The **limited** approaches are the Kocher–Langenbeck and ilioinguinal approaches. The **Kocher–Langenbeck** approach exposes the posterior column and posterior half of the superior dome. Fractures that can be exposed through this approach include those of the posterior wall, posterior column, and associated posterior column–posterior wall (Fig. 16-16*A* and *B*). Transverse fractures alone and transverse fractures including the posterior wall can be reduced and stabilized with this approach if the anterior fracture does not require fixation or if it can be stabilized with a percutaneous lag screw.

The **ilioinguinal** approach affords exposure of the anterior column from inside the pelvis. Exposure from the anterior sacroiliac joint around the inner

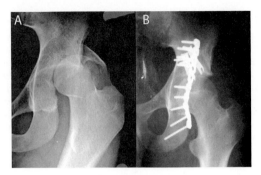

FIG. 16-16   *A and B.* Posterior wall fracture-dislocation of the hip treated by open reduction and internal fixation. (*Courtesy of Robert F. Hall, Jr., M.D.*)

pelvic brim and down to the pubic symphysis is possible. This exposure is demanding but extremely valuable for certain fractures. Fractures routinely exposed through this approach include anterior-wall and anterior-column fractures. As in the case of the Kocher–Langenbeck approach, other fractures can be stabilized through this approach including transverse, anterior column with posterior hemitransverse, and occasionally both-column fractures. When the ilioinguinal approach is used for a transverse or associated fracture, the posterior fracture must either not require fixation or be secured with an image-guided posterior-column lag screw.

The two **extensile** approaches are the triradiate and the extended iliofemoral. The advantage of these approaches is that they expose both columns as well as the articular surface. The disadvantage is the increased soft tissue dissection and resultant propensity for heterotopic bone formation.

The **triradiate** approach combines the posterior Kocher–Langenbeck approach with an anterior limb designed to expose the inferior half of the ilium and the proximal half of the anterior column.

The **extended iliofemoral** approach, like the triradiate approach, provides exposure of the two columns but also affords greater exposure of the proximal half of the ilium.

The indication for an extensile approach is a fracture that cannot be satisfactorily reduced and stabilized via a limited approach. The more recently described Stoppa approach (midline abdominal) can be used to obtain increased direct exposure of the quadrilateral surface of the acetabulum.

A CT scan has been recommended to assess the adequacy of the fracture reduction, as plain radiographs are felt to be inadequate for the assessment of anything beyond the general contour of the acetabulum and posterior wall. A delay of more than 12 h between the injury and reduction of the dislocation, severe intraarticular comminution with involvement of the weight-bearing dome, and a residual fracture gap are some of the factors predictive of an unsatisfactory clinical result, as seen in about 30% of patients with this injury.

Complications

Complications of acetabular fractures are similar to those of hip dislocation and are covered under "Dislocations of the Hip," below.

DISLOCATIONS OF THE HIP

Classification

Dislocations of the hip are classified according to the location of the femoral head as being posterior, anterior, or obturator (inferior). **Posterior** dislocations are by far the most common type. The mechanism of injury is an axial load applied to the flexed adducted hip, as would occur when the knee strikes a dashboard.

Anterior and obturator dislocations are caused by hyperabduction of the hip. The greater trochanter impinges on the acetabular rim and levers the head out of the acetabulum. Extension and external rotation force the hip anteriorly, resulting in an anterior dislocation. Flexion and internal rotation force the hip inferiorly, resulting in an obturator dislocation.

Associated Injuries

Multisystem injuries, sciatic nerve injury, and fracture of the femur, knee, acetabulum, femoral head, and neck are associated with hip dislocations. Multisystem injuries reflect the high-energy trauma required to dislocate a hip. The presence of injuries to other systems is determined by adhering to the assessment guidelines outlined in Chap. 1. Sciatic nerve injury follows posterior dislocation of the hip and occurs when the femoral head impacts and stretches the nerve. The injury is almost always a neurapraxia and is manifest by partial loss of function, most frequently peroneal nerve function. The most accurate method of determining whether the femoral head and acetabulum are fractured is CT. Fractures about the knee are ruled out by a focused examination and radiographs.

Diagnosis and Initial Management

History and Physical Examination

The patient has severe pain. When the hip is dislocated posteriorly, there is a history of significant trauma. The leg is shortened. The hip is flexed approximately 30 degrees and internally rotated. Anterior dislocations are often the result of less significant trauma and are characterized by external rotation and different degrees of abduction. Obturator dislocations are caused by significant trauma and are characterized by at least 45 degrees of fixed abduction of the hip.

Radiographic Examination

The diagnosis is confirmed by an anteroposterior radiograph of the pelvis. Spot anteroposterior and lateral radiographs of the hip are also obtained to evaluate the femoral head and acetabulum. Radiographs of the femoral neck, femoral diaphysis, and knee are examined to rule out fracture. After reduction, new films are obtained to assess whether the reduction is concentric. In equivocal cases, a CT scan is obtained.

Initial Management

Initial management is reduction. The patient is sedated. Posterior dislocations are reduced by flexing the patient's knee, applying traction in line with the femur, and adducting the hip. Anterior and obturator dislocations are reduced by pulling in line with the femur while an assistant pulls the thigh laterally. For anterior dislocations, the hip is also rotated internally. Straight traction is safe in the reduction of hip dislocations. Internal and external rotation must be performed very gently because of the risk of fracturing the femoral neck. If reduction is not possible with intravenous sedation, the patient is anesthetized in the operating room, and reduction with the aid of fluoroscopy is performed. Interposition of the capsule and external rotators in the acetabulum may prevent closed reduction, necessitating open reduction.

Definitive Management

Definitive management is skeletal traction until a CT scan has ruled out any intraarticular fragments. Initial weight bearing is started and gradually increased over 6 weeks. Surgical intervention is necessary for irreducible dislocations and to debride the joint when the reduction is not concentric. If the dislocation is posterior, very little posterior dissection is necessary once the gluteus maximus has been split. The acetabulum is cleared of debris and the femoral head is reduced. Care is taken to preserve the posterior blood supply. Postoperative management is as described under "Initial Management," above.

Complications

Complications of acetabular fractures and hip dislocation are posttraumatic arthritis, heterotopic ossification, avascular necrosis, and instability. **Arthritis** is characterized clinically by pain with motion and radiographically by loss of joint space and formation of osteophytes. Management is conservative, with nonsteroidal anti-inflammatory drugs. If conservative management fails, patients are considered for arthroplasty.

Heterotopic ossification is more common following an extensile surgical approach and when there is concomitant head injury. Indocin decreases the severity of heterotopic ossification and is administered to patients who are not threatened by a prolonged bleeding time. Once heterotopic ossification has been diagnosed, passive range-of-motion exercises are stopped for a minimum of 8 weeks, or until the bone mass shows radiographic signs of maturing. The position of the hip is determined. If it is not in a position of function (i.e., 0 degrees of abduction, 10 to 20 degrees of flexion, and neutral rotation), the patient is placed in skeletal traction to improve the alignment, because there is a high probability of ankylosis. The bone mass may be excised after it matures. Maturity is indicated by normal serum alkaline phosphatase levels and a cold bone scan. More recent evidence suggests that earlier excision may be safe. **Avascular necrosis** of the femoral head is rare after acetabular fracture or hip dislocation. Its diagnosis and management are covered in Chap. 17. **Chronic instability** is extremely rare after dislocation without fracture; it has been successfully managed with imbrication of the posterior capsule of the hip joint. If there are no signs of posttraumatic arthritis, chronic instability after acetabular fracture is managed with reduction, stabilization, and bone grafting of the nonunion. If there is arthritis, an arthroplasty or arthrodesis is performed.

SELECTED READINGS

Fractures and Dislocations of the Pelvis

Bucholz RW. The pathological anatomy of Malgaigne fracture–dislocations of the pelvis. *J Bone Joint Surg* 63A:400–404, 1981.

Carlson DA, Scheid DK. Safe placement of S1 and S2 iliosacral screws. *J Orthop Trauma* 14(4):264–269, 2000.

Chen AL, Wolinsky PR, Tejwani NC. Hypogastric artery disruption associated with acetabular fracture: a report of two cases. *J Bone Joint Surg* 85A:333–338, 2003.

Hanson PB, Milne JC, Chapman MW. Open fractures of the pelvis: review of 43 cases. *J Bone Joint Surg* 73B:325–329, 1991.

Moreno C, Moore EE, Rosenberger A, Cleveland HC. Hemorrhage associated with major pelvic fracture: a multispecialty challenge. *J Trauma* 26:987–993, 1986.

Acetabular Fractures

Judet R, Judet J, Letournel E. Fractures of the acetabulum: classification and surgical approaches for open reduction: preliminary report. *J Bone Joint Surg* 46A:1615, 1964.

Letournel E, Judet R. *Fractures of the Acetabulum*. Berlin: Springer-Verlag, 1993.

Matta J, Anderson L, Epstein H, Hendricks P. Fractures of the acetabulum: a retrospective analysis. *Clin Orthop* 205:230–240, 1986.

Moed BR, Carr SE, Gruson KI, et al. Computed tomographic assessment of fractures of the posterior wall of the acetabulum after operative treatment. *J Bone Joint Surg* 85A:512–522, 2003.

Dislocations of the Hip

Epstein HC. *Traumatic Dislocations of the Hip*. Baltimore: Williams & Wilkins, 1980.

17 | Intracapsular Fractures of the Proximal Femur

Arsen M. Pankovich   John A. Elstrom

The "unsolved" fracture remains a significant clinical problem, although much has been done to solve it. This chapter presents the anatomy of the proximal femur, including its inner architecture and vascular supply, etiology and mechanism of injury, initial management, diagnosis, definitive treatment, complications, and some future avenues. The major categories of fracture in this area are low-energy fractures of the femoral neck, high-energy fractures of the femoral neck, and fractures of the femoral head.

ANATOMY

Gross Anatomy

The femoral head and neck extend proximally from the intertrochanteric line anteriorly and from the intertrochanteric crest posteriorly (Fig. 17-1). The femoral head forms an ovoid depression, the fovea capitis, just distal and posterior to the medial border. The ligamentum teres is attached to the fovea capitis.

The joint capsule is attached proximally to the acetabular edge, distally to the intertrochanteric line anteriorly, and posteriorly to the neck surface about 1 to 1.5 cm proximal to the intertrochanteric crest. A number of nutrient canals are present on the surface of the neck and at the junction with the head. Retinacula, the ascending fibrous bands that extend over the neck surface, contain blood vessels and are covered by synovium.

Blood Supply

The blood supply to the femoral neck and head is derived from the extracapsular arterial ring situated at the base of the femoral neck (Fig. 17-2). The anterior and posterior parts of the arterial ring are derived from the lateral and medial circumflex arteries, respectively.

Ascending cervical arteries, from the arterial ring, perforate the capsule and become retinacular vessels. Usually there are three to eight posterosuperior arteries that supply the femoral head and one to three inferoposterior arteries that supply the metaphyseal neck; there are only a few arteries on the anterior surface of the neck. The artery of the ligamentum teres, a branch of the obturator or medial circumflex artery, supplies the bone around the fovea capitis and often is not patent in elderly individuals; thus its contribution to the blood supply of the femoral head is not significant. Blood supply to the femoral neck is also derived from the ascending nutrient femoral vessels.

Bone Structure

The structure of the femoral neck and head consists of cancellous bone. A rather thin cortex covers the neck anteriorly and posteriorly and dense bone forms calcar femorale, which extends from below the femoral head and inferior surface of the neck to the proximal medial wall of the shaft. The dense structure of calcar femorale is the result of osseous response to the stress

264

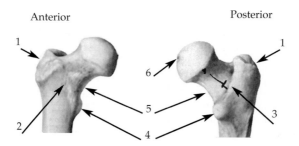

FIG. 17-1   The osseous proximal femur. (1) Greater trochanter. (2) Inter-trochanteric line. (3) Intertrochanteric crest. (4) Lesser trochanter. (5) Femoral neck and calcar femorale. (6) Fovea capitis.

forces, which pass through it from the pelvis to the femoral shaft. A thin sub-chondral plate covers the cancellous bone of the femoral head, and its surface is covered with the hyaline articular cartilage. No blood vessels penetrate the subchondral plate, and the articular cartilage receives its nutrition from the joint fluid.

Anatomic sections and radiographs of the proximal femur show a trabecular pattern that follows the mechanical principles and corresponds to the mathematical analytic predictions made by Koch (Fig. 17-3).

Medial compressive and lateral tensile trabeculae exist and essentially cross each other perpendicularly (Fig. 17-4). Thinning of these trabeculae and a decline in their number reflect the degree of osteoporosis in the femoral head and neck.

Garden concluded that pinning along the compressive and tensile trabeculae would create a stable fixation configuration. His fixation system did not prove his theoretical conclusions in osteoporotic bone, although no system has worked well in bone so affected. Singh had advanced an index of osteoporosis

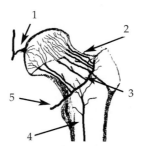

FIG. 17-2   The vascular supply of the proximal femur. (1) Artery of the ligamentum teres from obturator artery. (2) Ascending cervical arteries, which become retinacular vessels. (3) Arterial ring (posterior view). (4) Femoral nutrient vessels. (5) Medial femoral circumflex artery.

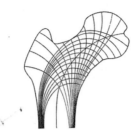

FIG. 17-3   Koch's mathematical model of the trabecular architecture of the upper femur in response to stress loading.

based on the changes and decrease in number of trabeculae in the femoral head and neck, but actual staging on the contralateral side is often difficult when the quality of the x-ray images is not adequate.

Central Axis and Alignment Index

The angle formed by the central axes of the femoral neck and shaft, an antero-posterior central index, usually greater in children, is about 125 to 140 degrees in an anteroposterior plane, and the neck is anteriorly oriented (anteverted) about 10 to 15 degrees in the lateral plane (Fig. 17-5). The alignment index (Garden) is not always easily determined (and its lines drawn) because of the fan-shaped distribution of the trabeculae.

LOW-ENERGY FRACTURES OF THE FEMORAL NECK

Etiology

Hip fractures occur more often in women than in men. Although it has been established that osteoporosis develops earlier in white women than in men or individuals of other races and that it might predispose to hip fractures, osteo-porosis alone does not cause a fracture. Yet low bone density is often present in those elderly women who sustain these fractures. Clearly, a fall to the hip in the vicinity of the greater trochanter produces a force strong enough to cause a fracture. External rotation of the extremity during the fall causes compression of

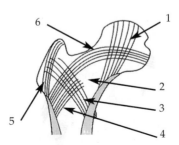

FIG. 17-4   Distribution and patterns of trabeculae in the upper part of the femur. (1) Principal compression group. (2) Ward triangle. (3) Secondary compression group. (4) Secondary tensile group. (5) Greater trochanteric tensile group. (6) Principal tensile group.

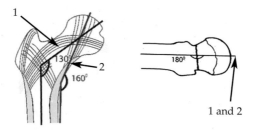

FIG. 17-5   (1) Central axis, (2) alignment index.

the posterior surface of the femoral neck on the lip of the acetabulum, causing a fracture, often comminuted. Other contributing factors have been implicated, such as inactivity with loss of muscle mass, muscle weakness, and loss of body fat; whereas normally, muscle and body fat absorb some of the applied energy and thus decrease the impact on bone. Conditions that can decrease bone density, such as improper diet and alcohol intake, and those that might cause weakness, dizziness, and malaise—such as dehydration, a syncopal episode, or a chronic disease—would predispose a person to a fall. These fractures occur mostly at home as the patient is standing or walking. A frequently posed question as to which came first, a fracture of the femoral neck that led to a fall or a fall that led to a fracture, has not been clearly answered, although a fracture preceding a fall, an indirect mechanism, would probably be a rare event. However, some authors believe that the incidence of such indirect fractures is higher than suspected, since the cyclic stressing of the osteoporotic femoral neck can cause a stress fracture that then leads to a complete indirect fracture and results in a fall. In such cases patients report pain and discomfort in the hip area prior to a fall.

Classification

In determining fracture type, three criteria should be applied:

1. Location of the fracture. This is usually described as subcapital, transcervical, or basicervical (Fig. 17-6).
2. Inclination of the fracture line to the horizontal plane—the Pauwels' classification system. It defines stability of the fracture as follows: type I is

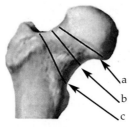

FIG. 17-6   Fracture zones: (*a*) subcapital, (*b*) transcervical, (*c*) basicervical.

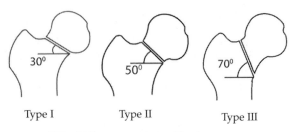

FIG. 17-7   Pauwels' classification system.

inclined about 30 degrees, type II is inclined about 50 degrees, and type III is inclined about 70 degrees. The angle of inclination (Fig. 17-7) is of clinical importance, as an angle below 30 to 40 degrees is essentially perpendicular to the primary compression trabeculae, thus compressing the fracture fragments and producing stability at the fracture site. When the angle of inclination is about 70 degrees, somewhat in the direction of the tensile trabeculae, shearing forces acting on the fragments lead to instability at the fracture site.

3. Relation of the fracture fragments—Garden classification system: type I is incomplete and impacted; type II is complete and undisplaced; type III is complete and partially displaced but with an intact posterior retinacular ligament; and type IV is completely displaced with disruption of all retinacular vessels (Fig. 17-8).

The relation of the fragments and their contact is important for stability at the fracture site, since impacted fractures, often in various degrees of valgus, promote compression and stability. Completely displaced fractures, on the other hand, often have comminution of the posterior neck, creating an unstable fracture even after internal fixation; they have a potential for nonunion and

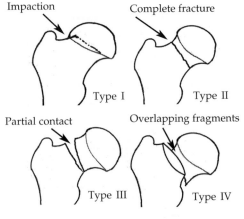

FIG. 17-8   Garden's classification system.

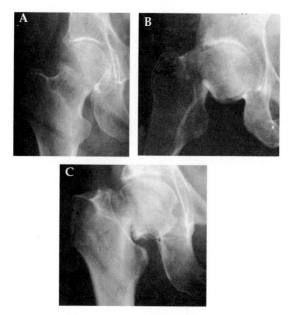

FIG. 17-9 *A.* Garden type I or AO-OTA type B1. *B.* Garden type III. *C.* Garden type IV.

loss of blood supply to the head. This last sets the stage for the development of avascular necrosis.

Garden used these criteria in his classification and was of the opinion that the various types of femoral neck fractures represent only different stages of the injury (Fig. 17-9).

The stable, impacted valgus fracture has been classified by the Association for Osteosynthesis–Orthopaedic Trauma Association (AO-OTA) as type B1 (Fig. 17-9*A*).

The completely displaced fracture with head in varus position has been classified by AO-OTA as type B3 (Fig. 17-10*A*).

The completely displaced fracture in the transcervical region with a vertical (steep) fracture line has been classified by AO-OTA as type B2 (Fig. 17-10*B*).

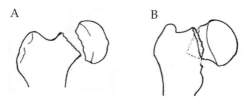

FIG. 17-10 *A.* AO-OTA varus-vertical type B3. *B.* Varus-adduction type B2.

DIAGNOSIS AND INITIAL MANAGEMENT

History and Physical Examination

There is usually a history of a fall. The main complaint is of groin pain, particularly when the extremity is moved. Shortening in external rotation of the involved extremity might be present, though not always pronounced. Palpation below the inguinum elicits pain. Examination of the circulatory and neurologic status is mandatory, as cardiovascular syncopy or initial stroke could have caused the fall. Other cardiovascular, pulmonary, and genitourinary problems are evaluated.

Radiographic Examination

An anteroposterior radiograph of the pelvis and anteroposterior and lateral radiographs of the hip are obtained.

Initial Management

The medical situation is evaluated and appropriate laboratory tests obtained. These usually include an electrocardiogram, chest radiograph, complete blood count, chemistries, and urinalysis. If a fracture was detected on the radiographs, Buck's traction is applied with a pillow under the knee for displaced fractures, or positional sand bags can be used. Protection of the sacral area and the heels, common sites of decubiti, is required. Patients with undisplaced fractures should be turned carefully. The patient's medical condition should be as optimal as possible for surgery; confounding medical problems can take 24 to 48 h to be stabilized. This is the responsibility of the medical consultant.

If there is concern that an occult fracture of the femoral neck might exist in spite of negative radiographs, further testing is mandatory. This usually means that the patient has groin pain and some pain on motion of the hip. An immediate magnetic resonance imaging (MRI) or computed tomography (CT) scan of the hip will most likely detect a fracture (Fig. 17-11A and B). Bone

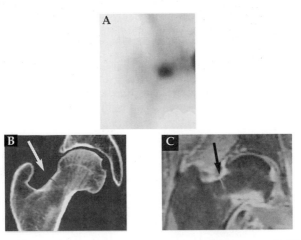

FIG. 17-11   Imaging of the suspected fracture. *A.* Bone scan. *B.* CT scan. *C.* MRI of the same hip.

scan is often positive only when done 2 to 3 days after injury (Fig. 17-11*C*). It is important to avoid missing the occult femoral neck fracture, as displacement of a fracture that could have been treated by simple hip pinning is an embarrassment for the surgeon.

It has recently been reported that femoral nerve block significantly improves pain control and decreases the need for analgesic injections. This also facilitates the patient's mobility in bed and nursing care.

HISTORICAL PERSPECTIVE IN TREATMENT

Fractures of the femoral neck must have been known to occur for ages, yet it was only in 1823 that Cooper described the associated anatomic findings and physical signs, noting the common nonunion at the neck and avascular necrosis of the femoral head. After x-rays were introduced as a diagnostic tool at the beginning of the twentieth century, the diagnosis was readily made and the first classifications described.

Treatment was bed rest, with all its attendant problems. Whitman described treatment in a spica cast and the still high mortality. Cotton tried to convert displaced fractures into an impacted type by striking the padded greater trochanter with a mallet, but the results did not improve much, as bed rest and spica casting were still disastrous. Leadbetter described a less traumatic reduction maneuver.

Internal fixation of fractures of the the femoral neck, though attempted previously, was established in the 1930s when Smith-Petersen introduced a triflanged nail. Subsequently, the originally solid nail was cannulated to allow for use of a guide wire (Johansson), a side plate was added (Thornton), and the nail and side plate were combined in a single device (Jewett). Massie and Pugh sliding-nail plates and several similar designs of sliding-screw plate systems have been marketed at various times. A number of threaded pins were also introduced (Moore, Knowles, Gouffon, Deyerle, AO/ASIF cancellous screws 6.5 mm in diameter, Asnis cannulated screws, and the Garden long threaded screw system).

Another milestone was reached when prosthetic replacement devices were designed and introduced in the treatment of displaced femoral neck fractures. Independently, the Judet brothers in France produced an acrylic prosthesis; then Moore, and soon thereafter Thomson, in the United States, described prostheses made of stainless steel. Since then, a bipolar prosthesis with a second gliding and bearing surface was introduced by Bateman in Canada and total hip replacement by Charnley in England.

TREATMENT OF LOW-ENERGY FRACTURES

The treatment of femoral neck fractures is surgical. Prolonged recumbency, particularly in frail patients of marginal health, leads to cardiopulmonary complications, thromboembolic incidents, and the development of decubiti. Surgical treatment should be considered a semiemergent procedure. Medical stabilization of a sick patient must be carried out prior to surgery. Following surgery, patients have less pain and their mobility is facilitated. They can ambulate with a walker and bear some weight.

Surgical methods involve either pinning or hemiarthroplasty, although total hip replacement is also occasionally indicated.

PINNING

Surgical Technique

Percutaneously or through a small incision, two to four pins are introduced laterally at the base of the trochanter and, under the control of an image intensifier, inserted through the femoral neck into the femoral head (Fig. 17-12).

Anatomic Reduction

In a large series of hip pinnings of displaced fractures, it was shown that anatomic reduction of the fracture along with a type of fixation that provides stability at the fracture site was essential to healing. Inserted pins or screws should be parallel in order to allow for further impaction of the head on the neck if resorption occurs at the fracture site. The densest bone in the femoral head is subchondral, and screws should penetrate to within 5 mm of the subchondral plate. A displaced fracture of the femoral neck can be reduced with traction and slight external rotation using a fracture table and an image intensifier, then internally rotating the limb to bring the femoral neck into alignment with the femoral head. Occasionally, a medially directed force at the greater trochanter will be beneficial in impacting the femoral head in slight valgus. An acceptable reduction finds the femoral head in no more than 20 degrees of valgus (or an AP central axis of 150 degrees). An anterior angulation of more than 20 degrees should also not be accepted. Excessive valgus often leads to avascular necrosis, and excessive apex anterior angulation often leads to nonunion. If a satisfactory reduction cannot be obtained, open reduction through a Watson-Jones approach or hemiarthroplasty should be carried out.

Complications

Avascular necrosis of the femoral head is a common complication, although it is not caused by pinning. Garden and others have observed that excessive valgus in impacted fractures is often associated with and presumably a cause of avascular necrosis. Proximity of the retinacular vessels to the surface of

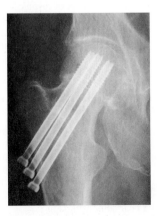

FIG. 17-12   Pinning of an impacted fracture of the femoral neck with cancellous screws.

the neck makes them vulnerable, and they can be severed by fracture fragments. Yet even in completely displaced fractures (Garden type IV), at least some retinacular vessels, though compressed and under tension, might retain their patency and restore the blood supply following reduction of the fracture and pinning.

Penetration of pins into the hip joint or cutting out of the head is often seen after pinning of displaced neck fractures, particularly when bone is osteoporotic. Likewise, nonunion may develop. Hemiarthroplasty and total hip replacement are ways of treating these complications.

HEMIARTHROPLASTY AND TOTAL HIP REPLACEMENT

Implants

A unipolar implant is a single-piece unit or a modular system that allows for the components (head, neck, and stem); it is selected to fit the size of an individual patient and, if necessary, can be converted to a total hip without changing the stem. A bipolar prosthesis has an interposing cup with an inner plastic (polyethylene) bearing and gliding surface; it is snapped onto a metallic head. Its outer metallic surface fits the acetabulum (Fig. 17-13).

Technique

Through a posterior or anterolateral incision, the hip capsule is exposed and opened. The femoral head is extirpated, the femoral neck appropriately trimmed, and the medullary canal reamed for the stem of the prosthesis. The size of the components is determined and they are inserted (cemented or not).

Complications

This procedure is definitive and without the problems of nonunion and avascular necrosis. The number of reoperations when compared to pinning is significantly less. However, the exposure is larger, the procedure lasts longer, the blood loss is greater, and bone cement, a toxic material, is used. Perioperative complications are more numerous and include blood replacement,

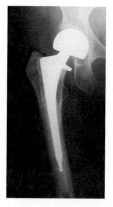

FIG. 17-13   Cemented bipolar prosthesis.

cardiopulmonary complications, thromboembolic incidents, posterior prosthetic dislocation following the posterior capsular approach, deep infection, periarticular calcification, and myositis ossificans; all of these are more common than after pinning. Osteoarthritis and protrusio acetabuli can develop from prosthetic pressure on the acetabular cartilage after unipolar and bipolar replacements.

INDICATIONS IN TREATMENT OF FEMORAL NECK FRACTURES

The primary indications for pinning of the femoral neck fracture are impacted and nondisplaced fractures (Garden types I and II) and displaced fractures (Garden types III and IV) in younger individuals and older patients with normal bone density. In fractures with more advanced osteoporosis and comminution of bone, when internal fixation is desirable, a sliding hip screw-plate system has been recommended in order to provide stability at the fracture site. Insertion of an antirotation screw is indicated in such cases. Historically, the Deyerle plate-multipin system had the same rationale. Primary indications for unipolar or bipolar hemiarthroplasty and femoral neck fractures or displaced fractures (Garden types III and IV) exist in elderly patients with osteoporotic bone whose life expectancy is relatively limited (5 to 10 years) and who probably would not need further surgery due to failure of the implant. It is concluded from meta-analysis that internal fixation and arthroplasty provide similar pain relief and functional outcome. Internal fixation provides a significantly higher number of revision operations. Arthroplasty is a longer procedure with greater blood loss and thus higher perioperative morbidity; it significantly increases the risk of infection and possibly causes a higher rate of mortality. Failures of pinning of displaced fractures of the femoral neck (Garden types III and IV) are likely due to comminution of the posterior wall of the neck, a condition found to be present in 70% of such cases.

The primary indication for total hip replacement in femoral neck fractures is preexisting arthritis or other underlying acetabular pathology, such as Paget's disease. Another situation that is gaining acceptance is a displaced fracture in a patient with good health whose life expectancy is at least 5 to 10 years, as such a patient needs a device that would not fail during their remaining years. Cementing of the femoral stem is the preferred method in osteopenic bone.

Complications

Mortality at 1 year for a patient with a femoral neck fracture approaches 30%. Infection can be managed by a two-stage revision with removal of components and implantation of antibiotic beads and intravenous antibiotics. If the hip has been pinned, the femoral head will usually have to be removed; if a prosthetic replacement has been performed, the prosthesis, along with any other foreign material such as cement, will have to be removed. Subsequent reconstructive procedures are usually required.

FUTURE AVENUES

Recent developments in hip replacement include minimally invasive surgery (MIS). Three approaches appear best suited for elective procedures: a modified Smith-Peterson and Watson-Jones approach and a two-incision approach (Berger) in which an anterior minimal incision is combined with reaming of the femoral canal through a separate supratrochanteric incision for passage of flexible reamers under imaging control. Although used mostly electively in patients with hip arthritis, MIS procedures are even more suitable for small-framed, frail patients with femoral neck fractures. The procedures are felt to be less traumatic to the soft tissues and perioperative medical complications are fewer, so early discharge of the patient is possible.

Reinforcement at the fracture site in the femoral neck has been studied in the laboratory and in clinical settings. Calcium phosphate cement (Norian SRS) has been useful in dentistry and in the treatment of fractures of the distal radius. Further research will hopefully produce better material and surgical techniques, as reinforcement of osteoporotic and comminuted femoral head and neck fractures seems a logical use.

HIGH-ENERGY FRACTURES OF THE FEMORAL NECK

Typically, the patient is a younger individual involved in a high-energy trauma. Accompanying multisystem injuries are common.

Classification

Five types have been recognized: type I, undisplaced neck fractures; type II, simple displaced neck fractures; type III, comminuted displaced neck fractures; type IV, fractures with associated fracture of the acetabulum or femur (Fig. 17-14); and type V, neck fractures that occur or are recognized during antegrade nailing of the femoral shaft fractures.

Diagnosis and Initial Management

A high degree of suspicion is necessary to detect femoral neck fractures in cases of high-energy injuries of the pelvis and femur. Routine plain hip radiographs are indicated and, if necessary, MRI and CT studies, since early diagnosis of an undisplaced fracture is important to prevent subsequent displacement, particularly during antegrade nailing of a femoral shaft fracture. Skeletal traction preoperatively must take into account that discontinuity of the femur prevents traction at the fracture site in the neck.

Definitive Management

Salvage of the femoral head is the primary consideration. Type I (undisplaced) fractures are stabilized with percutaneous cannulated screws. Type II (simple displaced) fractures are reduced closed. If there is any doubt as to the adequacy of reduction, open reduction through a Watson-Jones approach is indicated.

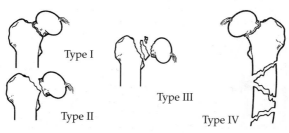

FIG. 17-14 Classification of high-energy fractures of the femoral neck.

Percutaneous cannulated screws or a compression screw-plate are used for fixation. Type III (comminuted) fractures are exposed through a posterolateral approach with the patient in the lateral decubitus position. The neck is reduced and stabilized with a compression screw and side plate. Bone grafting of the posterior neck is indicated. In type IV fractures associated with fracture of the acetabulum or femur, stabilization of the fractured femoral neck is the primary goal. If there is a posterior fracture of the acetabulum or hip dislocation, the femoral neck is approached posterolaterally. A femoral neck fracture with dislocation of the femoral head from the acetabulum may require hip replacement if there is significant displacement and the retinacular vessels are torn. In ipsilateral neck and femoral shaft fractures, fixation of the neck is done first and stabilization of the femur is accomplished by retrograde nailing or plating through a minimal incision if possible. In type V injuries, after the neck fracture is recognized during antegrade nailing, an attempt at neck fixation is made around the rod or through reconstruction holes if present. If the reduction is not perfect or fixation could not be obtained, the femoral nail is removed, the neck pinned, and the femur fixed by retrograde nailing or by means of a plate. In younger patients, it is recommended that closed or open reduction with capsulotomy be accomplished within 8 h in hopes of reducing the incidence of avascular necrosis.

Complications

Common complications are nonunion of the neck and avascular necrosis of the head. Treatment of these complications is controversial and difficult. Renailing and grafting and a variety of osteotomies have been utilized, with unpredictable results. Theoretically, core decompression and a free pedicle bone graft are of value in the management of avascular necrosis if done before arthritic changes occur. Often, the only choice is bipolar hemiarthroplasty or total hip replacement.

STRESS OR FATIGUE FRACTURES

Two types have been described by Devas, each corresponding to the primary tensile or compressive trabeculae. In the transverse (tensile) type, the initial infraction is in the superior cortex of the neck, with a tendency toward complete fracture and displacement. In the compression type, the bone adjacent to the calcar is the site of initial infraction, without a complete cortical calcar break, and it is noted on x-rays as a dense area of callus formation; the fracture is stable and shows minimal tendency toward displacement. It is felt by most surgeons that internal fixation by two or three pins or screws is indicated in order to eliminate groin pain and the possibility of progression into a complete or a displaced fracture.

FRACTURES OF THE FEMORAL HEAD

Classification

The third type of intracapsular fracture of the femur is fracture of the femoral head. These fractures are invariably associated with a dislocation of the hip joint. They are classified into four types. In type I, the fracture is below the fovea capitis. In type II, the fracture line extends above the fovea capitis. Type III and IV fractures are type I or type II injuries associated with fracture of

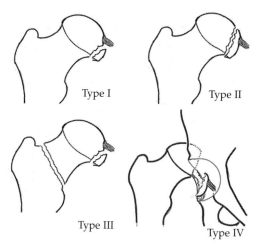

FIG. 17-15   Pipkin classification of fracture types of the femoral head.

the femoral neck or the acetabular rim, respectively (Fig. 17-15). Associated injuries to the knee and sciatic nerve or other systems are common.

Diagnosis

The physical findings are those of posterior dislocation of the hip. The hip is flexed and adducted and the extremity shortened. Rarely, the hip will be dislocated anteriorly with a fracture of the superior portion of the femoral head.

Radiographic Examination

Anterior and lateral radiographs of the hip indicate a dislocation with a retained fragment of the femoral head in the acetabulum. Computed tomography confirms the exact diagnosis.

Management

Initial management is reduction of the dislocation. Type I, II, and IV fractures are reduced closed. Type III fractures are reduced under anesthesia and an attempt is made to monitor the progress of the reduction fluoroscopically. Closed reduction should be terminated and open reduction performed if the femoral neck fracture starts to displace. Even if the dislocation can be reduced without displacing the fracture, immediate internal fixation of the femoral neck should be undertaken.

Definitive management is surgical. Type I fractures can be treated arthroscopically by removal of the loose fragment, as it is usually small and from a non-weight-bearing portion of the femoral head. Open excision of the fragment is another option. A number of different situations may exist. If there has been a failure of closed reduction and the hip dislocation is posterior, it should be reduced through a posterior surgical approach. CT is helpful in identifying the presence and location of intraarticular fragments as well as femoral neck or acetabular fractures associated with type III and IV injuries. Since reduction and internal fixation of fractures of the femoral head and neck through a posterior approach is problematic, it is sometimes useful to place the patient on a fracture table in the lateral position and apply skeletal traction through the distal femur so that an anterior approach can be undertaken simultaneously. Another alternative would be a delayed anterior approach with the patient supine, using a femoral distractor. If a small femoral head fragment is going to be excised following closed reduction, a preoperative CT scan is helpful in determining the approach. Anterior and inferior fragments should be approached anteriorly or preferably arthroscopically.

Type II fractures are managed by combined arthroscopic fragment repositioning and screw fixation under fluoroscopic control. An open anterior exposure of the hip joint allows a fracture fragment to be repositioned and fixed with cancellous lag screws inserted from the superior aspect of the neck. Reduction and fixation are indicated for persistent fracture displacement greater than 1 mm.

Type III fractures are reduced under anesthesia with fluoroscopic control and immediately fixed. Open reduction with internal fixation of the femoral neck fracture (and, if possible, the femoral head fracture) is safer as the risk of displacing the femoral neck fracture is reduced.

Type IV fractures often require open reduction and internal fixation of the acetabular fracture combined with excision or fixation of the femoral head fragment. An example of a complex fracture-dislocation is presented (Fig. 17-16).

Complications

Long-term complications include posttraumatic arthrosis and avascular necrosis. Heterotopic ossification may be treated prophylactically with indomethacin three times a day.

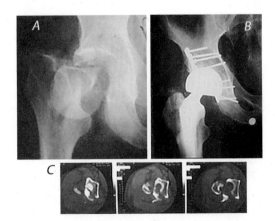

FIG. 17-16   A complex fracture-dislocation of the hip. *A*. Initial radiograph shows fracture of the femoral neck, dislocated femoral head rotated laterally, and a fracture of the acetabulum. *B*. CT scan shows described lesions. *C*. Postoperative radiograph shows a cemented bipolar prosthesis reduced into the anatomically reduced and fixed acetabulum.

Prognosis

Type I femoral head fractures do well with closed reduction followed by 4 weeks of traction. Patients who have fragment excision do not seem to do as well. These injuries are usually not treated by open reduction and internal fixation.

Patients with type II fractures treated by open reduction and internal fixation (which would require a division of the ligamentum teres) seem to do as well as those treated by closed reduction and traction if fracture displacement does not exceed 1 mm.

Type III and IV fractures and anterior fracture-dislocations have the poorest prognosis, with a high incidence of complications requiring hip arthroplasty.

SELECTED READINGS

Bhandari M, Devereaux PJ, Swiontkowski MF, et al. Internal fixation compared with arthroplasty for displaced fractures of the femoral neck. A meta-analysis. *J Bone Joint Surg* 85A:1673–1681, 2003.

Butler JE. Pipkin type II fracture of the femoral head. *J Bone Joint Surg* 63A:1292–1296, 1981.

Cassidy C, Jupiter JB, Cohen M, et al. Norian SRS cement compared with conventional fixation in distal radial fractures. A randomized study. *J Bone Joint Surg* 85A:2127–2137, 2003.

Eriksson F, Mattsson P, Larsson S. The effect of augumentation with resorbable or conventional bone cement on the holding strength for femoral neck fracture devices. *J Orthop Trauma* 16:302–310, 2002.

Garden RS. Reduction and fixation of subcapital fractures of the femur. *Orthop Clin North Am* 5:683–712, 1974.

Heim M, Adunski A, Chechick A. Nonoperative treatment of intracapsular fractures of the proximal femur. *Clin Orthop* 399:35–41, 2002.

Kenzora JE, McCarthy RE, Lowell JD, Sledge CB. Hip fracture mortality. Relation to age, treatment, preoperative illness, time of surgery, and complications. *Clin Orthop* 186:45–56, 1984.

Koch JC. The laws of bone architecture. *Am J Anat* 21:177–298, 1917.

Koval KJ, Zuckerman JD. Hip fractures: I. Overview and evaluation and treatment of femoral-neck fractures. *J Am Acad Orthop Surg* 2:141–149, 1994.

Koval KJ, Zuckerman JD. *Hip Fractures. A Practical Guide to Management.* New York: Springer-Verlag, 2000.

Lee BPH, Berry DJ, Harmsen WS, Sim FH. Total hip arthroplasty for the treatment of an acute fracture of the femoral neck. Long-term results. *J Bone Joint Surg* 85A:1673–1681, 2003.

Lestrange NR. The Bateman UPF prosthesis: A 48-month experience. *Orthopedics* 2:373–377, 1979.

Peljovich AE, Patterson BM. Ipsilateral femoral neck and shaft fractures. *J Am Acad Orthop Surg* 6:106–113, 1998.

Pipkin G. Treatment of grade IV fracture-dislocation of the hip. *J Bone Joint Surg* 39A:1027–1042, 1957.

Rizzo PF, Gould ES, Lyden JP, Asnis SE. Diagnosis of occult fractures about the hip. Magnetic resonance imaging compared with bone-scanning. *J Bone Joint Surg* 75A:395–401, 1993.

Scheck M. The significance of posterior comminution in femoral neck fractures. *Clin Orthop* 152:138–142, 1980.

Singh M, Nagrath AR, Maini PS. Changes in trabecular pattern of the upper end of the femur as an index of osteoporosis. *J Bone Joint Surg* 52A:457–467, 1970.

Soreide O, Lillestol J, Alho A, Hvidsten K. Acetabular protrusion following endoprosthetic hip surgery: a multifactorial study. *Acta Orthop Scand* 51:943–948, 1980.

Swiontkowski MF, Winquist RA, Hansen ST. Fractures of the femoral neck in patients between the ages of twelve and forty-nine years. *J Bone Joint Surg* 66A:837–846, 1984.

Zuckerman JD, Skovron ML, Koval KJ, et al. Postoperative complications and mortality associated with operative delay in older patients who have a fracture of the hip. *J Bone Joint Surg* 77A:1551–1556, 1995.

18 | Extracapsular Fractures of the Proximal Femur

Enes M. Kanlic   Miguel A. Pirela-Cruz

This chapter covers the fractures of the trochanteric area of the proximal segment of the femur, often referred to as extracapsular fractures, and the fractures of the subtrochanteric area of the diaphyseal segment of the femur.

Pertinent anatomy is discussed and a classification presented. Diagnosis, initial and final management, associated injuries, and complications are described.

ANATOMY

The proximal extent of the trochanteric segment of the femur is the intertrochanteric line anteriorly and the intertrochanteric crest posteriorly. The distal extent of the trochanteric segment is the lesser trochanter. The calcar is a thick plate of bone underlying the lesser trochanter. As the calcar extends proximally, it coalesces into the cortex of the posteromedial surface of the femoral neck. Avulsion of the lesser trochanter with a major part of the calcar creates a bone defect and makes the fracture unstable.

The neck-shaft angle of the femur in adults is approximately 125 degrees. The femoral neck is anteverted with respect to the transepicondylar axis by about 10 to 15 degrees (in Asian populations up to 30 degrees). The center of the femoral head is positioned 1 to 1.5 cm anterior to the axis of the femoral shaft as seen on the lateral radiograph. The femoral shaft is bowed primarily anteriorly and slightly laterally, which is of importance in adapting the fixation devices.

The trochanteric area is formed mostly of cancellous bone with numerous muscle attachments, particularly in the region of the greater trochanter. The vascular supply of the trochanteric area is abundant and its healing potential excellent. The subtrochanteric area is formed of cortical bone and also has a good blood supply, which may be damaged by the injury or at a surgical intervention.

CLASSIFICATION

It is common to discuss fractures located in the proximal 5 cm of the diaphyseal segment of the femur—the subtrochanteric fractures—together with the fractures of the trochanteric area. Subtrochanteric fractures behave biomechanically essentially the same as unstable fractures of the trochanteric area; thus they are treated in the same way. They behave differently than the fractures of the rest of the diaphyseal segment, considering mechanical forces acting on the fracture site. The contribution of the lateral cortex of the trochanteric area to the stability of a fracture in this area must be considered in determining different fracture types (Fig. 18-1).

In deciding to which segment or area of the proximal femur a particular fracture belongs, it is important to find **the center of the fracture**. The term *center* means what it says. However, while the center of a simple fracture is apparent, the center of a wedge fracture lies where the wedge is the broadest; the center of a complex fracture is usually identifiable only after the fracture has been reduced. Thus the center of the fracture determines its anatomic area, even if it extends to areas above or below.

281

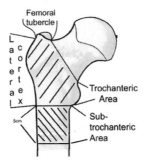

FIG. 18-1   Trochanteric and subtrochanteric areas of the proximal segment of the femur.

Some clarification of the terminology used by the Association for Osteosynthesis–Orthopaedic Trauma Association (AO-OTA) in this classification is needed. The word *petrochanteric* is commonly used in the German literature. It originates from the Latin word *per*, which means "through." It could be confusing if the term were mistakenly understood to mean peritrochanteric, as that would place the fracture in a location peripheral to the trochanteric area. The term *petrochanteric fracture* as used by AO-OTA designates fractures that do not cross the lateral cortex of the trochanteric area but extend only from the femoral tubercle to the lesser trochanter. On the other hand, **intertrochanteric fractures** involve the lateral cortex and extend to the medial cortex. The designations *per-* and *intertrochanteric fracture* indicate the precise locations of the three fracture types.

Terminology in the English literature most often designates all fractures of the trochanteric area as intertrochanteric fractures.

The classification created by Evans (1949) is well known and recognized as practical. This classification is the basis of every other classification and is still very useful. Five types are described (Fig. 18-2). Evans raised the concept of stability in trochanteric fractures.

It is important to recognize the degree of stability of a fracture from its anatomic configuration and consequent biomechanical behavior. These factors are then applied to deciding on the type of fixation device that would provide the optimal degree of fixation.

Trochanteric Fractures

Stable fracture configurations (Evans types A and B) are those with the posteromedial cortex intact or minimally comminuted; the postreduction configuration in these two types is mechanically stable and allows for use of a variety of fixation devices. **Unstable fracture configurations** (Evans types C and D) have extensive posteromedial comminution, bone-to-bone contact cannot be achieved fully, and the fracture site is mechanically unstable. In type C fractures, the *lateral cortex* is mostly intact, and although the postreduction configuration is unstable mechanically, many surgeons still use extramedullary fixation devices. In type D fractures, the lateral cortex is clearly violated, the instability is bicortical and therefore more difficult to control, and intramedullary devices are most effective.

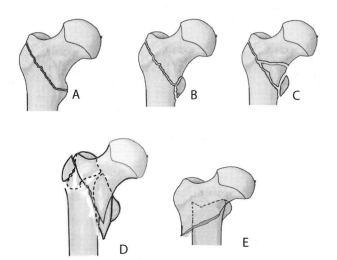

FIG. 18-2   Evans classification of trochanteric fractures.

In fractures with reverse obliquity (Evans type E), the main fracture line is essentially parallel to the femoral neck axis and traverses the lateral cortex. Thse fractures are unstable even when comminution is absent because there is a tendency for medial displacement of the distal fragment. These fractures appear to be a transitional type to the subtrochanteric fractures.

Subtrochanteric fractures comprise a category of their own, although anatomically the subtrochanteric area is considered a proximal end of the femoral diaphysis. These fractures are *unstable* because of a relatively small fracture contact area and from the significant forces exerted over the short off-set proximal segment (head, neck, and trochanteric areas) on the narrow distal diaphyseal segment. All fracture configurations are unstable, as they are exposed to the same loads, and all are suitable for the same fixation methods, mainly with intramedullary devices.

Subtrochanteric fractures are subdivided, like other shaft fractures, into simple, wedge, and complex fracture configurations (Fig. 18-3).

PATHOPHYSIOLOGY

Muscle pull on the fracture fragments of the proximal femur causes typical deformities. The degree of deformity varies and depends on the degree of injury. The gluteus medius and minimus muscles, which insert into the femoral tubercle, abduct the proximal segment. The gluteus maximus muscle inserts with its deep portion into the gluteal tuberosity of the femur (the lateral extension of the linea aspera); it extends and externally rotates the distal fragment. The iliopsoas muscle pulls the lesser trochanter and flexes and externally rotates the proximal fragment if the fracture line is below the lesser trochanter; if the fracture line is above the lesser trochanter, the pulls of the iliopsoas and of the gluteus maximus tend to be in balance. Sometimes the lesser trochanter is avulsed and it is only pulled anteriorly and proximally. The femoral shaft is pulled medially by the tight adductor muscles (Fig. 18-4).

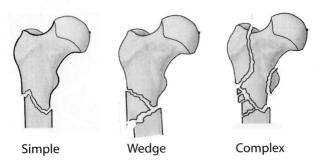

Simple   Wedge   Complex

FIG. 18-3   Subtrochanteric fractures.

Koch (1917) showed that compression stress exceeds 1200 lb/in. in the medial subtrochanteric area and that lateral stresses are 20% less. Those forces must be resisted by an "implant–broken bone" construct in order to achieve healing in the position obtained at surgery.

Osteoporosis is common in the elderly population, particularly in caucasian women. The diminished structural strength of the proximal segment of the femur makes it susceptible to fracture, even by low-energy trauma, like a simple fall at the ground level.

ASSOCIATED INJURIES

The most frequently associated injuries in the elderly are due to the patient's osteoporosis in other areas of the body. They are sustained at the same time

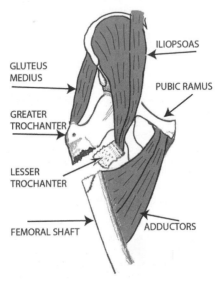

FIG. 18-4   Pull of the muscles in a subtrochanteric fracture with a proximal fracture extension and resulting deformity.

as the trochanteric fracture. The patient must be carefully examined for any signs of wrist fracture or head injury. Radiographs of the femur and knee in addition to those of the pelvis are routinely obtained.

DIAGNOSIS AND INITIAL MANAGEMENT

History and Physical Examination

There is pain in the groin area and inability to bear weight. Usually there is a history of a minor fall in the elderly or high-energy trauma in younger individuals. The injured leg is externally rotated, with the lateral edge of the foot often touching the surface of the bed. In addition, there is shortening of the extremity. Occasionally, there is ecchymosis of the proximal thigh.

Radiographic Examination

The clinical diagnosis is confirmed by the radiographic examination. Anteroposterior radiographs of the "distal" pelvis (iliac crests are less important than the proximal femurs) are most useful. The contralateral hip should be internally rotated 20 degrees to profile the femoral neck for length and angle templating and to estimate the degree of osteoporosis (Singh index). Lateral radiographs centered on the injured hip will help to determine the fracture configuration, especially the degree of posteromedial comminution. The lateral projection is obtained with the patient in the Danelius–Miller position (the patient lies supine on the table with the uninjured hip flexed; thus a cross-table lateral view is obtained). The film cassette is placed on the side of the injured hip and the x-ray beam directed from the opposite side.

If the radiographs of a painful hip after an injury are inconclusive, magnetic resonance imaging or computed tomography will confirm or rule out a fracture. Bone scan is informative only 48 to 72 h after the injury. The same observations apply to fractures of the femoral neck, as outlined in Chap. 17 (see Fig. 17-11).

Initial Management

Early stabilization of the fracture allows mobilization of the patient and minimizes the incidence of problems associated with prolonged recumbency (e.g., cardiopulmonary problems, urinary tract infections, thromboembolic incidents, and decubiti).

The patient is made as comfortable as possible by administering analgesics and supporting the injured extremity with pillows.

Frequently these patients have multisystem problems and must be optimized by a medical consultant with the goal of early surgery, preferably within 48 h of the injury.

NONOPERATIVE MANAGEMENT

Patients who were wheelchair- or bed-bound before their fractures occurred usually need surgical fixation to facilitate their care. Yet there are patients who will require nonoperative management, in particular when local chronic decubiti and edema are present; this is also the case for paraplegic or hemiplegic patients and patients with contractures that might make fixation impossible. These patients must be moved out of bed to either in a chair or a wheelchair immediately and then as often as tolerated; when in bed, they should be moved from side to side at 2-h intervals. Liberal use of analgesics should be made so that these patients can remain as comfortable as possible.

Patients who were ambulatory prior to the injury but are at high risk for surgery (recent myocardial infarct, recent stroke, and others) may have to be managed conservatively. Skeletal traction for a period of 2 to 3 months is indicated in such cases in order to maintain alignment and length of the extremity until the fracture has healed. Once the immediate postinjury pain has been controlled, patients should be allowed periods out of traction and out of bed, mostly in a reclining chair. As with other recumbent, usually older patients, they should be regularly rolled from side to side while in bed. Respiratory toilet and antithrombotic measures should be instituted immediately after the injury.

Although complications during conservative treatment are frequent, their incidence will be decreased and patients' care more manageable when the proposed treatment protocol is rigorously enforced. Ultimately, the result is often gratifying, since trochanteric fractures have a high healing potential. This is not the case with subtrochanteric fractures.

SURGICAL MANAGEMENT

The definitive management for the vast majority of the extracapsular fractures of the proximal femur is operative reduction and stabilization by internal fixation. The most important factors affecting the outcome are the patient's age and general health, the configuration of the fracture, and the degree of osteoporosis. The surgeon controls the quality of reduction and the stability of fixation. Goals of the reduction are to obtain, if possible, bone-to-bone contact along the medial cortex, to realign the fracture fragments, and in particular to avoid varus angulation.

Surgical Methods and Indications

Two basic types of implants are used to stabilize trochanteric and subtrochanteric fractures: extramedullary and intramedullary devices.

Extramedullary Devices

Implants. These devices are either single or two-part units. A variety of devices are available.

The **sliding compression screw-plate** (SCSP) and a more advanced **dynamic hip screw** (DHS) allow controlled collapse and impaction of the fracture fragments.

Technique. The fracture is reduced on a traction table under C-arm control. Usual maneuvers are external rotation, traction, and internal rotation followed by abduction. The lateral femur, distal to the level of the lesser trochanter, is approached through a 3- to 4-in. incision. Posterior fracture sagging, as seen on the lateral view, is controlled by pushing up with a hand or a crutch to allow insertion of a guidewire, which is driven into the femoral neck and head at an appropriate angle and under x-ray imaging control. A lag screw is introduced after reaming and taping. In stable fractures, three bicortical screws are sufficient to fasten the side plate to the femur and a barrel over the lag screw.

Important aspects of the technique are as follows:

1. The screw tip of a lag screw should reach to within 0.5 to 1 cm of the subchondral bone, as seen on the anteroposterior and lateral views (center-

center), in order to prevent a cut-out; the cancellous bone is denser in that part of the femoral head.

2. Two-thirds of the barrel should be occupied by the lag screw to prevent disengagement or bending of the lag screw inside the barrel.
3. A short barrel should be used only for a lag screw shorter than 80 mm to provide enough space for sliding.
4. Traction should be released intraoperatively (before side-plate fixation with screws) to allow for impaction and assess the amount of shortening that would occur.

Indications. These devices are used to fix trochanteric fractures with stable configurations (Fig. 18-5; left hip) and for some unstable fracture configurations with an intact lateral cortex.

Complications. If the device is applied in a fracture with a broken lateral cortex, through or close to the fracture site, and in fractures with reverse obliquity, uncontrolled sliding can occur and cause further instability. As a result, the lag screw may cut out (Fig. 18-6), which would necessitate a revision surgery, often in form of an arthroplasty.

With 95-degree fixed-angle devices, a blade plate or more commonly a dynamic condylar screw (DCS) is used in unstable trochanteric and subtrochanteric fractures or in situations where it is impossible to use an intramedullary device (Fig. 18-7). A period of toe-touch weight bearing is necessary in order to allow the fracture to heal in the fixed position. Only younger patients can withstand the long surgical procedure required, with a longer incision, more extensive soft tissue dissection, and greater loss of blood. They would also be able to protect the fixed fracture sites by long periods without weight bearing. Significant expertise is necessary to obtain good reduction, place the blade or a lag screw in the inferior part of the head (at a 95-degree angle), and attach it correctly to the shaft, thus bridging the fracture site. More recently, the procedure has become less extensive by use of a minimally invasive surgical

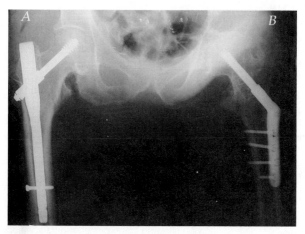

FIG. 18-5 Two fixation devices used in trochanteric fractures. *A.* A short IMHS device. *B.* A DHS device.

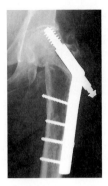

FIG. 18-6   Fracture with a reverse obliquity that caused uncontrolled collapse and cutout of the lag screw, resulting in nonunion.

(MIS) technique. Obviously, this surgical refinement had placed greater technical demands on the operating surgeon.

Intramedullary Devices

These devices consist of a short (15 to 21 cm) or long intramedullary nail, with a wide body (around 17 mm) proximally angled at 4 to 5 degrees of valgus. The distal part is narrower (11 to 13 mm), and has a dynamic slot or one to two holes for the locking screws. The lag screw is introduced through the wide proximal body and has a sliding capability. Rotation is prevented through a blocker positioned above the screw. The lag screw's threads must be in the center of the femoral head, as shown in Fig. 18-5 (the right hip).

The upper part of the nail is a mechanical barrier and prevents uncontrollable lateral sliding of the head-neck fragment or medial sliding of the shaft in frac-

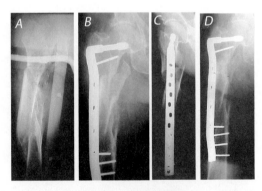

FIG. 18-7   A simple oblique subtrochanteric fracture in the femur with a malunited shaft fracture. It would be impossible to pass the nail through the obliterated and distorted femoral canal. *A.* Initial AP radiograph. *B.* Postoperative AP radiograph after application of a DCS device utilizing the MIS technique. *C.* A lateral postoperative radiograph showing some posterior displacement of the distal fragment to accommodate the plate at the malunion site. *D.* After 14 weeks, the fracture had healed.

tures with a break in the lateral cortex. In fixing unstable fractures with intramedullary devices as opposed to extramedullary devices, load shearing and positioning close to the weight-bearing axis of the femur is biomechanically advantageous. Intramedullary devices are applied by a minimally invasive percutaneous technique (bridging osteosynthesis), the nail being introduced by hand. A smaller screw is inserted through the distal locking slot or hole, which is positioned at a distance from the tip of the nail in order to prevent the development of a stress fracture.

Implants.   The **intramedullary hip screw** (IMHS), or **cephalomedullary nail,** uses the femoral tubercle at the greater trochanter as the entry portal. Fractures of the greater trochanter and the piriformis fossa do not affect the nail's ability to maintain a good apposition between the main proximal and distal fragments. A centrally positioned lag screw cores out bone 1 cm in diameter. Two screws in the proximal part of the cephalomedullary nail provide somewhat better rotational control and cause less damage to the cancellous bone in the head-neck area, particularly when this is osteoporotic (Fig. 18-8). The disadvantage of using two smaller lag screws is that it is harder to introduce them, and if the angle of insertion is not perfect, penetration outside of the femoral head can occur.

Indications.   If the fracture line does not extend more than 1 to 2 cm distal to the lesser trochanter, a short nail will provide adequate and safe fixation. If there is doubt in the case of stable fractures and all unstable fractures, a long nail reaching the distal femoral metaphysis is the implant of choice.

Many surgeons routinely use a long intramedullary nail in all unstable fractures, regardless of the distal extension of the fracture. Some surgeons do not even lock the nail distally, considering fixation achieved by nail passage through the reamed femoral isthmus.

Complications in the use of intramedullary nailing devices have included periprosthetic fracture when shorter nails of older type were used. In some cases there was a more distal extension of the fracture than initially recognized, which was later displaced at surgery. Forceful hammering of the nail has been

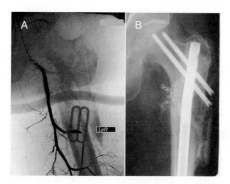

FIG. 18-8   *A.* A high-energy subtrochanteric fracture with a proximal extension; the sharp edge of the distal fragment had injured the profunda femoris artery, with consequent compartment syndrome. The radiograph shows coils used to stop the arterial bleeding. *B.* After cephalomedullary IMHS fixation the fracture healed.

described as responsible for creating a fracture. Locking screws of a larger diameter inserted through a hole close to the tip of the nail have caused a stress riser area; this has been coupled with the built-in 10-degree valgus in older-type nails, which tended to transfer the load to the tip of the nail by leaning to the lateral cortex. With regard to long nails, cases have been described where the tip of the straight nail penetrated the anterior cortex of the femur due to a more pronounced anterior femoral bow. In the newer devices, the shape of the stem has been improved.

A reconstruction nail (centromedullary) is inserted through the piriformis fossa, which must be intact if good alignment is to be acheived. The primary indication for use of a reconstruction nail is a fracture of the femoral shaft as well as a subtrochanteric fracture without proximal extension.

Special Considerations

Young patients need near anatomic reduction and stable fixation for good biomechanics and long-lasting full function. They are able to withstand more complex, open procedures, which last longer and involve a greater loss of blood. In these cases, application of 95-degree fixed-angled devices is indicated.

Postoperatively, these younger patients should be able to protect their reconstruction with toe-touch weight bearing for a few months until the fracture has healed.

Elderly patients need a stable implant–bone construct that will allow for immediate full weight bearing. Slight shortening, abductors' weakness, or mild malrotation are less troublesome to an older, less active patient. Percutaneous application of an IMHS device in unstable fracture configurations is clearly indicated.

SUMMARY OF INDICATIONS FOR USE OF VARIOUS FIXATION DEVICES

Various devices are indicated for fracture fixation; the choice of device is determined by the fracture configuration and the quality of bone.

Stable fractures are fixed with DHS devices or with a short IMHS device.
Unstable fractures with an intact lateral cortex are fixed as follows:

1. IMHS with a short nail if the fracture does not extend more than 1 to 2 cm distal to the lesser trochanter; otherwise a long nail is used.
2. A DHS device with reconstruction of the major posteromedial defect with an anteroposterior lag screw or with cerclage wires.

Unstable fractures with a fractured lateral cortex; these include fractures with reverse obliquity and subtrochanteric fractures with or without extensions:

1. A long IMHS
2. A 95-degree fixed-angle device
3. A dynamic condylar screw, blade plate, or proximal femoral locking plate

For patients with extreme osteoporosis, low healing potential, or significant comminution, one of the following:

1. Cemented (calcar-replacing) hemiarthroplasty
2. Total hip arthroplasty if the acetabulum is abnormal and the patient is fit for surgery (Fig. 18-9)

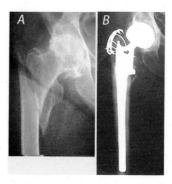

FIG. 18-9   *A.* An unstable pertrochanteric fracture and a severe coxarthrosis in an 84-year-old homebound woman. *B.* A cemented bipolar hemiarthroplasty allowed immediate weight bearing and produced a good functional result.

COMPLICATIONS

Loss of proximal fixation after cutting out of the lag screw of any device is the most common complication (4 to 20%). The most common causes are imperfect central positioning of the lag screw, varus malalignment at the time of surgery, and poor bone quality. For young patients a revision procedure is necessary; for older patients conversion to arthroplasty is usually done.

Peri-implant fractures distal to the tip of a short IMHS device (gamma nail) were often reported in the past. When a fracture occurs, the short nail must be replaced by a long one that reaches the distal metaphyseal area. Recently, a proximal 10-degree valgus angulation of the nail was replaced by a 4-degree angulation, a dynamic slot was positioned further proximally for insertion of a single smaller screw for distal locking, and a technique for insertion of the nail without hammering was introduced. As a result, these devices have become safer for general use.

Nonunion.   The incidence of nonunion has been reported at less than 2% for trochanteric fractures and up to 20% for subtrochanteric fractures. Nonunion in a younger patient is treated by repeated fixation, which includes exchange nailing and bone grafting, or in an older patient by arthroplasty.

Infection.   The incidence of infection has been reported at 0.15 to 15%. It is more common after open reduction and internal fixation than after percutaneous procedures. Implants that provide stability are left in place, after the area is debrided locally and deep cultures are obtained, until the fracture has healed. Antibiotics, based on the sensitivities of the pathogenic organisms, are administered as long as necessary to control local spread of infection and sepsis. Once the fracture has healed, the implants are removed; the area is debrided of avascular, often infected soft tissues and necrotic bone; and appropriate antibiotics are administered for at least 6 weeks. Local recurrences of infection, even years later, sometimes occur and require further surgical and medical management.

ISOLATED FRACTURES OF THE TROCHANTERS

Isolated fractures of the greater trochanter are the result of a direct blow or avulsion. It is important not to overlook a possible associated per- or intertrochanteric fracture. When it is minimally displaced, the fracture will heal without treatment. If displaced, nonunion frequently develops, but it is usually asymptomatic, affecting only a part of the gluteus medius insertion. In a younger individual, internal fixation of a larger displaced fragment is indicated in order to prevent or treat pain and limp.

Isolated fractures of the lesser trochanter are rare. They are the result of an avulsion by the iliopsoas tendon, often occurring in adolescents. In an elderly patient, lysis and avulsion usually signify a metastatic lesion, which requires additional studies to establish the diagnosis.

SELECTED READINGS

Ahrengart L, Tornkvist H, Fornander P, et al. A randomized study of the compression hip screw and gamma nail in 426 fractures. *Clin Orthop* 401:209–222, 2002.

Baumgaertner MR, Solberg BD. Awareness of tip-apex distance reduces failure of fixation of trochanteric fractures of the hip. *J Bone Joint Surg Am* 79:969–971, 1997.

Haentjens P, Cateleyn PP, De Boeck H, et al. Treatment of unstable intertrochanteric and subtrochanteric fractures in elderly patients: primary bipolar arthroplasty compared with internal fixation. *J Bone Joint Surg* 71A:1214, 1989.

Haidukewych GJ, Berry DJ. Hip arthroplasty for salvage of failed treatment of intertrochanteric hip fractures. *J Bone Joint Surg Am* 85A(5):899–904, 2003.

Hersovici D Jr, Pistel WL, Sanders RW. Evaluation and treatment of high subtrochanteric femur fractures. *Am J Orthop* 29(9 suppl):27–33, 2000.

Koval KJ, Skovron ML, Aharonoff GB, et al. Ambulatory ability after hip fracture. A prospective study in geriatric patients. *Clin Orthop* 310:150–159, 1995.

Koval KJ, Zuckerman JD. *Hip Fractures. A Practical Guide to Management.* New York: Springer-Verlag, 2000.

Saudan M, Lubbeke A, Sadowski C, et al. Pertrochanteric fractures: is there an advantage to an intramedullary nail? A randomized, prospective study of 206 patients comparing the dynamic hip screw and proximal femoral nail. *J Orthop Trauma* 16(6): 386–393, 2002.

19 | Fractures of the Femoral Shaft

Arsen M. Pankovich   *Kenneth A. Davenport*

ANATOMY

The femoral diaphysis is the tubular section of the femur that spans the region between the intertrochanteric and supracondylar areas. The important anatomic features of the femoral diaphysis are its shape, vascular supply, surrounding muscles, and neighboring neurovascular structures.

The femur has an **anterior bow** that varies widely but averages 12 to 15 degrees. Posteriorly, the cortex thickens into a ridge called the **linea aspera**, which is the origin of the medial and lateral intermuscular septa.

The **blood supply** is via endosteal and periosteal vessels. Endosteal vessels originate from nutrient arteries, which enter the proximal third of the femur via foramina in the linea aspera. These nutrient arteries arise from the vessels supplying the surrounding muscles. Following fracture, the periosteal vessels become the dominant vascular supply.

The muscles of the thigh are separated by the three intramuscular septa: medial, lateral, and posterior, forming the three thigh compartments (Fig. 19-1). The **anterior (quadriceps) compartment** is the largest and contains the quadriceps femoris muscle, iliopsoas muscle, femoral artery and vein, and femoral nerve in the upper part and saphenous nerve in the middle part. The **medial (adductor) compartment** contains the hip adductor muscles and the profunda femoris artery, which gives off three perforating arteries and is accompanied by a vein. The **posterior (hamstring) compartment** contains the three knee flexor muscles—biceps femoris, semitendinosus, and semimembranosus—the sciatic nerve, and many branches of the perforating arteries.

Unopposed action of the muscles results in the displacement of fragments, which is predictable depending on the level of the fracture. In fractures proximal to the isthmus of the medullary canal, the proximal fragment is abducted (gluteus), flexed, and externally rotated (iliopsoas). In fractures distal to the isthmus, the proximal fragment is in varus (adductors) and angulated posteriorly (quadriceps and gastrocnemius).

The main neurovascular structures of the thigh are the sciatic nerve, femoral nerve, femoral artery, and profunda femoris artery. The **sciatic nerve** is cushioned from the femur by muscles; therefore it is seldom injured in association with fractures of the femur. The femoral nerve innervates the quadriceps femoris muscle and gives off three branches: the medial and intermediate cutaneous and saphenous nerves. The femoral artery enters the posterior compartment of the thigh from the medial compartment via the adductor hiatus, or Hunter's canal, located just proximal to the distal metaphyseal flare of the femur. The artery is tethered by the intermuscular septum, and a fracture at this level may injure the vessel. The profunda femoris artery usually gives off three perforating arteries prior to ending proximal to the knee. Some branches of the perforating arteries perforate through the lateral intermuscular septum, where they terminate in the vastus lateralis. This is of clinical importance, since these branches may be cut during the surgical approach to the femur and then retract beneath the lateral intermuscular septum, thus causing uncontrolled bleeding.

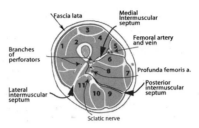

FIG. 19-1   Midthigh cross section showing the anterior, medial, and posterior compartments: (1) Vastus lateralis. (2) Vastus intermedius. (3) Rectus femoris. (4) Vastus medialis. (5) Sartorius. (6) Adductor longus. (7) Gracilis. (8) Adductor magnus. (9) Semimembranosus. (10) Semitendinosus. (11) Biceps femoris.

CLASSIFICATION

Fractures of the femoral diaphysis are classified according to location and stability. The location is defined as being in the proximal, middle, or distal third. Fractures of the proximal third are subtrochanteric fractures, while those of the distal third merge with supracondylar fractures.

In classifying fractures of the femoral diaphysis, the concept of fracture **stability** was used in determining treatment options. Stability was defined in terms of the percentage of the circumference of the cortex that is intact and the obliquity of the fracture line as indicators of fracture stability following intramedullary nailing. Fractures with at least 50% of the cortex intact and having an obliquity of less than 30 degrees are relatively stable in regard to length and rotation. The Winquist and Hanson and the Association for Osteosynthesis–Orthopaedic Trauma Association (AO-OTA) classifications are the two most commonly used schemes.

In a modified Winquist–Hanson system, five types are recognized (Fig. 19-2):

Type A fractures are simple transverse or short oblique fractures with no comminution.

Type B fractures may have some comminution, but they still have intact cortical contact between the proximal and distal fragments of at least 50%. A

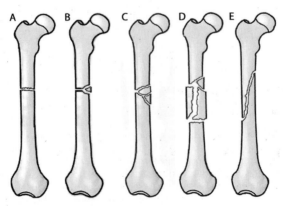

FIG. 19-2   Classification of diaphyseal fractures of the femur.

fracture with a butterfly fragment representing less than 25% would be an [AQ3] example of a type B fracture.

Type C fractures have cortical comminution or a large butterfly fragment involving more than 50% of the cortex, thus leaving cortical contact of less than 50% between the proximal and distal fragments.

Type D fractures have segmental comminution.

Type E fractures are long and oblique.

Stable fractures are types A and B, while types C, D, and E are unstable.

The AO-OTA classification recognizes simple fractures (type A, which includes spiral, short oblique, and transverse subtypes), wedge fractures (type B, with a variety of subtypes based on patterns of butterfly fragments), and complex fractures (type C, which are segmental and comminuted). Additional fracture subtypes are recognized by their position along the diaphysis.

DIAGNOSIS AND INITIAL MANAGEMENT

History and Physical Examination

A history of injury, pain, swelling, and obvious deformity is present.

Radiographic Examination

Anteroposterior and lateral radiographs are obtained and examined to rule out undisplaced comminution. Radiographs of the knee and pelvis will allow diagnosis of associated injuries, in particular ipsilateral fractures of the femoral neck, intertrochanteric fractures, or hip dislocations, which are missed in 30% of the patients who present with them. Radiographs of the contralateral femur provide useful information on femoral length and canal diameter.

Initial Management

Initial management makes patients as comfortable as possible and optimizes their condition for surgery. If surgery is to be preformed within 12 h of admission, 5 to 10 lb of skin traction is applied with the thigh resting on a pillow. When surgery is expected to be delayed, 10 to 20 lb of skeletal traction is applied via a tibial pin. The hip and knee are flexed 30 degrees, and the calf is supported in a sling. Radiographs are obtained in traction and traction is adjusted accordingly. For nailing, the fracture is ideally aligned and distracted 0.5 cm. Fractures of the femoral shaft should be stabilized within 24 h whenever possible. In the polytrauma patient, femoral fracture fixation improves mobility, decreases pulmonary complications, allows better care of other injuries, decreases infection rates, and thus reduces mortality rates. Benefits in both the polytrauma group and the isolated femoral fracture group include decreased length of hospital stay and a reduced cost of care.

Associated Injuries

Neurovascular injuries and compartment syndrome of the thigh and buttock are ruled out by a focused examination of the injured extremity. Vascular and nerve injuries are rare in closed fractures of the femoral shaft. With penetrating trauma, a vascular injury should be suspected even when pulses are normal; in these cases Doppler-assisted pulse pressures should be measured. When the ankle-brachial index is less than 0.9 after the fracture is reduced or stabilized, an arteriogram is warranted. The neurologic status of the extremity, including the presence or absence of nerve injuries, should be documented on admission and followed during the course of treatment. Nerve injuries must be identified prior to treatment as they may result from traction applied during operative stabilization. Injuries secondary to traction usually resolve spontaneously.

Compartment syndrome occurs rarely in the thigh. Risk factors for developing a compartment syndrome include coagulopathy, vascular injury, hypotension, external pressure on the thigh, treatment with a mast suit, and multiple injuries. The diagnosis is made on clinical examination and is confirmed with the measurement of compartment pressures greater than 40 mmHg, particularly when this condition is suspected in unconscious patients. The diagnosis of a compartment syndrome often indicates a poor prognosis with regard to mortality and morbidity, especially when it develops in the patient with multiple injuries. Following fasciotomy, a high infection rate is noted in those patients who survive. Renal failure and hyperkalemia can occur secondary to muscle necrosis and must be treated aggressively.

Skeletal injuries associated with fractures of the femoral diaphysis are fracture of the **femoral neck, intertrochanteric fracture, hip dislocation, pelvic ring injury**, and fractures and **ligamentous injuries around the knee**. The presence of an associated fracture is determined by close examination of radiographs of the knee, hip, and pelvis. The knee is carefully examined for evidence of soft tissue injuries, with the physician looking for an effusion, pain with palpation, palpation for defects in the extensor mechanism, by stressing the medial and lateral collateral ligaments, and testing anteroposterior stability to rule out rupture of a cruciate ligament. When it is not possible to rule out ligamentous injury, the patient is reexamined following fracture fixation, preferably while still under anesthesia.

Historical Treatment Perspective

The earliest treatment of femoral shaft fractures consisted of various methods of applying traction or of immobilizing the injured extremity. Examples of such treatment date back to ancient Egypt. A variety of materials were used in attempts to immobilize the fracture, while traction consisted of different types of skin traction. Closed reductions and subsequent treatment were based solely on gross anatomic alignment. Treatment remained unchanged until the mid-1800s, when Mathysen rediscovered the use of gauze bandages impregnated with plaster of Paris. This became the forerunner of modern-day casting material. Later on, the development of radiography allowed for more accurate diagnosis and fracture alignment.

The next major improvement in fracture care involved the use of skeletal traction to replace skin traction techniques, such as Buck's extension traction, developed during the American Civil War. Steinmann, Bohler, and Kirschner developed the methods and pins that, with some modifications, have been in use since the 1930s. The other major improvement was the Thomas ring splint, which made it easier to transfer patients and improved home care. Later changes in traction techniques included the development of the Bohler-Braun frame, the Pearson attachment, 90-90 traction, roller traction, and traction followed by cast bracing. Cast bracing dates back to the late 1800s, as used by Smith in Philadelphia, and its resurgence was championed by Sarmiento in the 1970s. It still has indications for use as a primary treatment or can be used in conjunction with skeletal traction in selected cases.

The use of external fixation in the treatment of femoral fractures dates to the 1930s. As a treatment form it was felt to lie somewhere between skeletal traction and open reduction with internal fixation. The use of external fixation increased steadily during this time and came into even wider use with the start of World War II. It was felt to be an ideal technique for early stabilization under battlefront conditions. Later, after World War II, it was avoided because of unacceptable results secondary to a high rate of chronic pin-tract infection and nonunion. This was later recognized to be due to design flaws. Modifications in technique, design, and materials (such as those seen in the Hoffmann fixator) resulted in a resurgence of use, becoming at one point the treatment of choice for certain types of injuries incurred during the Vietnam War. Although still used, external fixation has extremely limited indications for femoral fractures.

Reports of attempts at open reduction and plating of femoral fractures date back to the early 1900s. It was not until the 1960s, however, that this became a viable technique. The credit belongs to the AO group, with their developments of suitable implants and surgical techniques for successful use. Continued modifications in technique and the design of implants have led to improved outcomes, but because of mechanical considerations and open methods of implantation, results generally are inferior to those of intramedullary nailing.

Hey-Groves made the first attempts at intramedullary nailing in the early 1900s. Complications caused it to be abandoned until 1940, when Kuntscher, in Germany, reported using intramedullary nails to fix femoral fractures. Having developed a rigid nail and the technique for nail insertion to stabilize femoral fractures, he came to be seen as the father of intramedullary fixation. Prisoners of war returning to the United States from Germany who had fractures fixed with these methods showed excellent results. This resulted in an increasing trend toward operative treatment of femoral fractures. Modifications in nail design and operative technique followed. Changes in nail design have encompassed nail geometry (cloverleaf, open, closed, and solid), materials, and means of proximal and distal fixation.

Screws, bolts, blades, and deployable fins (Brooker-Wills nail) have all been used to provide fixation. Flexible intramedullary nails such as Rush rods and Ender pins were also used with varying degrees of success. Since the development of the portable fluoroscopy unit, closed methods of insertion have become the accepted norm, with nails being placed retrograde or antegrade. Studies now show intramedullary nailing to be the treatment of choice because of the uniformly good results being noted.

Techniques continue to be developed, the most recent being femoral plating by minimally invasive surgery (MIS) methods, which combine aspects of plating and nailing techniques.

Definitive Management

Fractures of the femoral diaphysis are managed with open reduction and plating, reduction and application of an external fixator, or closed reduction and intramedullary nailing. Skeletal traction, generally used to provide interim treatment, is occasionally used for definitive treatment when the patient is not a candidate for surgical intervention.

Plating

Relative indications for **plating** are inability (usually due to other injuries) to place the patient on the fracture table, a grade III open fracture, fractures around other implants (e.g., the femoral stem of a prosthesis), an associated fracture of the femoral neck or an intercondylar fracture of the distal femur, and obliteration of the medullary canal (usually due to a previous fracture).

Plate fixation restores continuity of the cortex while stress shielding the fracture site and the cortex to which it is attached. While stability at the fracture site is conducive to healing, whether by primary haversian healing across the fracture ends when fragments are in contact and compressed or by consolidation of a grafted area, delayed union may develop when a gap is present. Stress shielding of the underlying bone can cause disuse atrophy and cancellization of the cortex, with resultant bone fragility. Furthermore, fixation of a fracture is accomplished through an open procedure, which can cause local devascularization, again a possible reason for delayed healing. Other disadvantages of plating are a higher risk of infection compared to intramedullary nailing, prolonged avoidance of weight bearing postoperatively, increased rate of nonunion with secondary loss of fixation, and an elevated risk for refracture following plate removal.

Surgical exposure is via a lateral approach through the interval between the vastus lateralis and the lateral intermuscular septum. The vastus lateralis is elevated from the femur, keeping soft tissue stripping to minimum. Fracture fragments are identified and anatomically reduced. A broad dynamic compression plate is placed on the lateral cortex, anterior to the linea aspera. Fixation of 8 to 10 cortices proximal and distal to the fracture site is required. Medial cortical defects are grafted to stimulate healing and decrease the incidence of plate failure from prolonged healing time. Postoperatively, motion of the hip and knee is encouraged. Strict avoidance of weight bearing is maintained until bony trabeculae cross the fracture or the bone consolidates on the side opposite the plate, often taking 10 to 12 weeks from the time of surgery.

MIS plating techniques for the femur have recently been developed. Indications are distal metaphyseal injuries, subtrochanteric fractures, open fractures with vascular injury, comminuted fractures in children, and fractures in severely injured individuals with compromised pulmonary function. In principle, it is an extramedullary splint that bridges the gap of a comminuted fracture while being fixed to the main fracture fragments. This provides enough stability to allow the fracture to heal while decreasing periosteal stripping, bone devascularization, disturbance of the fracture hematoma, and further soft tissue injury.

Preoperative planning is essential to determine implant size and position of screws. The procedure is done on a radiolucent or fracture table. A reduction is obtained with longitudinal traction and manipulation, occasionally requiring the use of a femoral distractor or skeletal traction. Proximal and distal incisions are made after a precontoured plate is positioned against the skin parallel to the fracture once it has been reduced. Fluoroscopy is used to confirm this position. Incisions are carried down to the submuscular-periosteal interval and the chosen plate is then inserted above the periosteum and pushed to the opposite end of the femur. The plate is temporarily fixed at one end. A final reduction is then obtained and the other end is fixed to the bone. Final adjustments can be made at this time, following which, final screws are placed. Three to four screws are placed in the proximal and distal fragments, maximizing the spread of the screws at both ends. Postoperatively, patients start on range-of-motion exercises and toe-touch ambulation with progression of weight bearing when indicated by healing on follow-up radiographs.

External Fixation

The indication for **external fixation** is an open fracture with contamination. The purpose is to provide temporary fixation when conclusive fixation must be delayed. It is a quick procedure; it stabilizes the fracture without placing a foreign body in a contaminated wound, and it allows access to the wound. The disadvantages are lack of firm stability; the pins placed through the lateral muscles of the thigh "tack" them to the femur, often resulting in loss of knee motion; there is also a high incidence of nonunion.

At surgery, the fracture is reduced through the open wound after an adequate debridement of the open injury is performed. A lateral frame is applied with two to four half pins being placed proximal and distal to the fracture region. A **hybrid frame** may be used, with a ring being placed in the knee region with half pins placed lateral and proximal. The postoperative management is tailored to the patient. Generally, toe-touch weight bearing is maintained until the fracture has healed. Knee and hip motion is encouraged. After the soft tissues have healed, bone grafting can be done in order to enhance healing. The fixator can be removed and replaced with an intramedullary nail if there have been no signs of infection at the fracture or the pin sites.

Intramedullary Nailing

The majority of fractures of the femoral diaphysis are managed with intramedullary nailing. The advantages of this technique are fixation utilizing closed methods, which avoids further soft tissue injury while providing stable alignment. Mechanically, an intramedullary nail allows optimal loading of the fracture site, functioning as a load-sharing device that minimizes stress shielding. The intramedullary position of a nail results in a low bending moment while promoting bending strength and rigidity. The result is a union rate approaching 99%, an infection rate of less than 1% in closed fractures, and shortening or malunion occurring in less than 2% of the cases.

Nails are inserted either through the proximal femur and driven distally [i.e., antegrade nailing (Fig. 19-3)] or through the distal femur and driven proximally [i.e., retrograde nailing (Fig. 19-4)]. Antegrade nails are rigid, while

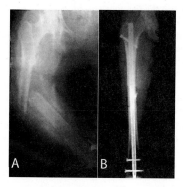

FIG. 19-3 *A.* Fracture of the femoral diaphysis. A type B fracture with comminution involving less than 50% of the cortex. This fracture was open with a grade II soft tissue injury. *B.* Stabilization with a reamed antegrade statically locked nail.

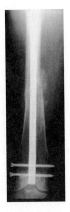

FIG. 19-4   Stabilization with a reamed rigid retrograde nail.

retrograde nails may be rigid or flexible. Rigid nails may be used with or without reaming. Flexible nails are inserted without reaming.

Type A and B fractures of the femoral diaphysis are managed with either type of intramedullary nail, with rigid nails being statically or dynamically locked. Type C, D, and E fractures of the femoral diaphysis are managed with rigid statically locked nails placed antegrade or retrograde.

Flexible intramedullary nailing of the femur involves the use of Rush or Ender nails. The indications for flexible nailing are limited and are confined to skeletally immature individuals, those cases where the femoral canal is small (less than 8 mm), and in the exceptional circumstance where soft tissue or concomitant injuries prevent the use of standard approaches for rigid nail placement. Flexible nailing of the femoral diaphysis is performed with the patient supine on the fracture table, with fluoroscopic control, and by inserting the nails through the portals on both sides of the distal femur. Postoperatively, knee flexion is encouraged when incisional pain allows, and full weight bearing is encouraged when the fracture pattern is stable.

Rigid intramedullary nailing is done antegrade or retrograde. In both approaches, static or dynamic fixation is obtained using the same biomechical principles; only the entry portals differ. The indications for antegrade nailing are type A to E fractures that occur just below the lesser trochanter down to within 7 cm of the knee joint. Relative indications for retrograde nailing include fractures of the distal third of the femoral shaft, ipsilateral femoral neck and shaft fractures, fractures in the obese patient (ease of nail insertion), floating knee, bilateral femur fractures, fractures above a total knee, acetabular or pelvic fractures, and femoral fractures in the pregnant patient (avoiding radiation to the fetus). Contraindications are systemic or local infection, open growth plates, a narrow intramedullary canal, or a preexisting deformity of the femur.

Antegrade nailing technique. The patient is placed on a fracture table. After the fracture is reduced under fluoroscopic control, the hip is adducted and a guidewire inserted through the piriformis fossa or into the trochanter, depending on the nail design, and driven across the reduced fracture. It is important that the guidewire be positioned appropriately for the type of nail being inserted. Attempting to insert a nail that is poorly aligned in the proximal canal can lead to blowout at the fracture site in hard bone, which can resist corrective centering forces at the base of the femoral neck. The femur is sequentially reamed in 1- and then 0.5-mm increments until an adequate size of canal is obtained. A nail of the appropriate size (usually 1.5 to 2 mm smaller than the last reamer) is driven across the fracture. In type A and B fractures, the nail can be locked dynamically: screws are placed proximally, not distally. This construct, however, can fail to control rotation. In treating type A and B fractures in the distal third of the femur, the nail is locked distally to prevent angular and/or rotational deformities. In type C, D, and E fractures (Fig. 19-5), the nail is locked statically, screws being placed proximally and distally. In fractures with the potential for shortening, care must be taken that the femur is pulled out to length by adequately scanning the fracture with the image intensifier to obtain a comprehensive view of all components on one image before distal locking is accomplished. Distal locking is facilitated on a fracture table and is done by the freehand technique of Dr. Robert Hall, Jr., using a ring forceps and a radiolucent drill. Postoperatively, patients with stable fractures are allowed to bear weight as tolerated. Patients with statically locked nails initially may bear 50% of their weight on the injured side; as radiographic healing progresses, weight bearing is advanced as tolerated. If radiographic signs of healing are delayed, full weight bearing is delayed.

Retrograde nailing technique.   Patient positioning for this procedure is supine on a radiolucent table with the knee on a bolster to obtain 45 to 60 degrees of knee flexion. Retrograde nailing is accomplished through the intercondylar notch, utilizing a medial parapatellar approach or by splitting the patellar tendon. The entry point is located anterior to the attachments of the posterior cruciate ligament and is in line with the long axis of the femur. A starting hole is made and enlarged with a cannulated drill. A guidewire is passed across the fracture site and sequential reaming is performed. The nail is inserted over the guidewire. Proximally, it should reach the level of the lesser trochanter, and the distal end is buried under the articular cartilage. Distal locking is done with

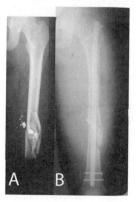

FIG. 19-5   Stabilization of a type C fracture resulting from a gunshot with an antegrade statically locked nail. (*Courtesy of Prahlad Pyati, M.D.*)

a drill-guide attachment to the nail, and proximal locking is done freehand in the anteroposterior plane with the help of the image intensifier.

Complications of Intramedullary Nailing

Complications specific to antegrade nailing are occasional thigh pain, trochanteric pain, or pain in the incision area. These do not always respond to nail removal. In addition, hetertopic ossification may occur and Trendelenburg gait patterns maybe present. Fractures of the femoral neck may occur during nail insertion; more commonly, however, they preexist and are overlooked on the initial evaluation.

Retrograde vs. antegrade nailing has shown an increased complication rate in regard to rotational deformity and shortening. Rotational deformities are often missed with intramedullary nailing of any type. They are the direct result of incorrect rotational alignment when the patient is positioned for surgery. Special care should be taken to check for correct rotational alignment prior to removing the patient from the operating room table. Fixation failures with intramedullary nailing can result from breakage of the intramedullary nail or breakage/failure of the transfixion screws. Breakage of a nail is the result of fatigue, which occurs with a nonunion. The late breakage of transfixation screws also implies a nonunion; when it occurs early, it signifies excessive early weight bearing. The failure of transfixation screws in terms of bone purchase is seen in osteoporotic bone or with poor insertion technique.

Complications of Femoral Fractures

These include malunion, nonunion, and infection.

Rotational and angular malunion (varus or valgus, seen in particular with fractures distal to the femoral isthmus) is managed by osteotomy and realignment and stabilization of the femur with a statically locked nail or plate. Fractures that have healed with significant shortening pose a difficult problem that is best prevented. Significant shortening is defined as shortening greater than 3 cm or when a gait disturbance or back pain is not relieved by a shoe lift. Management options include lengthening the involved femur, lengthening of the ipsilateral tibia, or shortening of the contralateral femur. Lengthening of the involved femur is the most attractive option because it corrects the deformity completely. It is achieved by applying an external fixator, osteotomizing the femur, and lengthening the femur incrementally by 1 mm per day. This procedure requires exceptional compliance on the part of the patient. Lengthening of the tibia is a simpler procedure, but the patient's knees will then be at different levels. Shortening of the contralateral femur is done closed; it has the lowest morbidity but results in overall loss of height.

Nonunion is managed by stabilizing the fracture fragments and using appropriate bone-grafting techniques, although occasionally grafting can be performed without revising the original fixation. When a nonunion follows intramedullary nailing, simple exchange nailing after reaming of the femoral canal is generally effective. Although intramedullary nails are usually the best means of stabilization, plating is occasionally indicated (e.g., if there is a fragment of broken nail in the canal that cannot be retrieved, when there is a segmental defect that requires exposure for extensive bone grafting, or in cases where an osteotomy will be needed to correct a deformity. In the rare case, compression can be applied to a hypertrophic nonunion by use of an external fixator.

Infection is managed with debridement, appropriate antibiotics, and treatment of the surrounding soft tissue. When there is an associated nonunion, it must be dealt with first, attempting to heal the fracture or at least ensure its stability; then the infectious process can be dealt with. If an internal fixation device is providing stability, it is usually left in place and fracture healing is obtained with cancellous bone grafting after the infection is under control. The assistance of an infectious disease specialist is essential. If the internal fixation device is not providing stability, its removal and external fixation should be carried out.

SELECTED READINGS

Brumback RJ, Reilly JP, Poka A, et al. Intramedullary nailing of femoral shaft fractures. Part I: Decision-making errors with interlocking fixation. *J Bone Joint Surg* 70A: 1441–1452, 1988.

Kanlic EM, Anglen JO, Smith DG, et al. Advantages of submuscular bridge plating for complex pediatric femur. *Clin Orthop* 426:244–251, 2004.

Kempf I, Grosse A, Beck G. Closed locked intramedullary nailing. its application to comminuted fractures of the femur. *J Bone Joint Surg* 67A:709–719, 1985.

Nowotarski PJ, Turen CH, Brumback RJ, Scarboro JM. Conversion of external fixation to intramedullary nailing for fractures of the shaft of the femur in multiply injured patients. *J Bone Joint Surg* 82A:781–788, 2000.

Pankovich AM, Goldflies ML, Pearson RL. Closed Ender nailing of femoral shaft fractures. *J Bone Joint Surg* 61A:222–232, 1979.

Schwartz JT, Brumback RJ, Lakatos R, et al. Acute compartment syndrome of the thigh. *J Bone Joint Surg* 71A:392–400, 1989.

Winquist RA, Hanson ST Jr, Clawson DK. Comminuted fractures of the femoral shaft treated by intramedullary nailing. *J Bone Joint Surg* 66A:529–539, 1984.

Wolinsky P, Tejwani N, Richmond JH, et al. Controversies in intramedullary nailing of femoral shaft fractures. *J Bone Joint Surg* 83A:1404–1415, 2001.

20 | Fractures of the Distal Femur

Robert C. Schenck, Jr.   James P. Stannard

This chapter reviews fractures of the distal femur, including supracondylar fractures of the distal metaphysis and intracondylar and condylar fractures of the articular surface of the distal femur.

ANATOMY

The knee is a compound joint consisting of a sellar joint between the trochlea of the femur and the patella and two condylar joints between the condyles of the femur and the tibial plateaus.

The distal femur consists of condyles and epicondyles. Medial and lateral condyles form the articular surface. They are narrower anteriorly, resulting in a trapezoidal shape of the distal femur. The medial condyle projects further distally than the lateral condyle. As a result, the **distal femur is in 7 degrees of valgus in relation to the femoral shaft**. The lateral condyle projects farther anteriorly (preventing lateral patellar subluxation) and posteriorly than the medial condyle. The epicondyles are small prominences on the outer portion of the condyles that serve as the origin for the respective medial and lateral collateral ligaments. The distal and posterior surfaces of both condyles are convex and articulate with the corresponding tibial plateau. The anterior surface of the distal femur (trochlea) is the coalescence of medial and lateral condyles. Its concave surface corresponds to the articular surface of the patella.

Classification

The Orthopedic Trauma Association (OTA/AO) classification of distal femur fractures is similar to the classification of other periarticular fractures. These fractures are divided into extraarticular fractures (type A), unicondylar fractures (type B), and bicondylar fractures (type C). These three types of fractures are further divided by level of comminution of the metaphysis or articular surface (subtypes 1 to 3) (Fig. 20-1).

Associated Injuries

Injuries associated with supracondylar fractures of the femur include fractures and dislocations of the proximal femur and pelvis, ligamentous disruptions of the knee, and injuries of the popliteal artery and peroneal or tibial nerves. These injuries are more likely to occur in association with high-energy trauma. Associated fractures and dislocations of the proximal femur and pelvis are most likely to occur in motor vehicle accidents as part of the "dashboard injury" complex.

The most frequently disrupted ligament is the patellar ligament. Disruption of the collaterals and cruciate ligaments also occurs. The association of multiligament knee injuries with fractures about the knee is being recognized with increasing frequency.

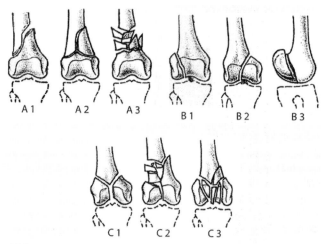

FIG. 20-1   The OTA/AO classification of distal femoral fractures.

Diagnosis and Initial Management

History and Physical Examination

Patients with a distal femoral fracture have pain and a history of a knee injury. Obvious instability and deformity are present with type A (supracondylar) and C (bicondylar) fractures but may not be present with fractures of a single condyle. The skin should be inspected for lacerations, suggesting an open fracture. Medial femoral condylar (Hoffa's) fractures frequently present with a posterior sag sign related to the femoral attachment of the posterior cruciate ligament. Accurate physical examination of the ligaments is usually not possible before fracture fixation. Radiographic signs of ligamentous injury are loss of parallelism between the articular surfaces of the femoral condyles and tibial plateaus and bony avulsion of the cruciates. After stabilization of the fracture, a thorough examination of the ligaments of the knee should be performed, with a plan for repair or reconstruction of the injured structures.

Early identification of an associated **popliteal artery** injury is crucial. The cardinal finding is decreased dorsalis pedis and posterior tibial pulses. This may be due to torsion or traction of the vessels. If aligning the fracture does not result in the return of pulses within 5 min, it should be assumed that the popliteal artery is injured and an emergent consultation with a vascular surgeon for immediate evaluation and arterial exploration is needed. Once the location of the vascular injury is determined, surgery to stabilize the fracture and restore circulation is performed emergently. If there has not been a significant delay, fracture fixation with knee-spanning external fixation or occasionally retrograde nailing provides stability prior to vascular repair. Under no circumstances, however, should revascularization of the leg be significantly delayed for fracture fixation. On rare occasions, swelling, an expanding hematoma, or an intimal tear can progress to arterial thrombosis. For this reason, vascular checks are performed every 2 h for the first 36 h after injury. Management of the normal vascular examination (arteriogram vs. clinical checks) is controversial. Vascular Doppler studies, ankle-brachial indices (ABIs), serial physical examinations, and arteriograms are all options and depend on the individual institution's protocols and surgeon preference. Recently published data support the use of serial physical examinations alone rather than arteriograms to detect significant arterial injuries.

Injuries of the **peroneal and tibial nerves** are identified by assessing sensation and the ability to plantarflex and dorsiflex the ankle. These injuries are managed with range-of-motion exercises of the ankle and foot to avoid contractures and splinting in a functional position.

Radiographic Examination

Radiographs in the anteroposterior and lateral projections are sufficient to evaluate the injury. The tunnel view of the distal femur, in which the anteroposterior radiograph is obtained with the knee flexed to 30 degrees, is helpful but painful for the patient. Radiographs must be carefully examined for minimally or nondisplaced fracture lines extending into the articular segment; these may become displaced during treatment if not recognized. Computed tomography (CT) scans can be useful for further assessment of intraarticular fracture lines or comminution. Radiographs of the pelvis, hip, femur, and tibia are obtained if clinically indicated by pain, deformity, or instability on physical examination.

Initial Management

Initial management of a distal femoral fracture begins with a gentle realigning of the leg and application of a long leg splint. If splinting does not adequately immobilize the fracture, skeletal traction can be used. A proximal tibial pin is inserted, the knee is placed on pillows, the calf is supported in a sling, and 10 to 20 lb of traction is applied. Posttraction radiographs are obtained to assess alignment and to determine whether the knee joint is being distracted because of any ligamentous disruption that may be present.

Treatment Options

Nonoperative Management

Nonoperative management has a limited role in the treatment of distal femoral fractures. In patients with minimally or nondisplaced fractures, a cast brace can be used for stabilization until the fracture heals. This approach is also used in patients with medical comorbidities precluding surgery. Typically the brace will be applied with motion at the knee limited to 30 or 40 degrees for the first few weeks. The patient is maintained at toe-touch weight bearing during this time. Once early callus is noted, the hinges of the brace can be released to allow full knee motion.

External Fixation

External fixation also plays a limited role in the treatment of these injuries. Definitive treatment with external fixation is very difficult. The large capsular reflection on the femoral side of the knee joint makes it difficult to get pins or wires distal enough to control the distal fracture segment without having the pins become intracapsular, which can lead to septic arthritis.

External fixation can play an important role in the initial management of distal femoral fractures in polytrauma patients, fractures with vascular injuries, and open fractures. External fixation in these circumstances is usually in the form of a knee-spanning external fixator. Pins should be placed in the proximal tibia and either the anterior or lateral femur. The fracture is pulled out to anatomic length and placed into slight flexion. It is advisable to avoid placing fixator pins laterally in the distal femur if plating is planned for eventual definitive fixation, as this may result in drainage in the area of the future incison. If the fixator is being placed prior to vascular exploration of a popliteal artery injury, it is beneficial to place the pins in the anterior femur, as lateral pins can interfere with externally rotating the hip to allow access to the medial approach to the popliteal fossa. In placing a spanning fixator for a distal femur fracture, it must be realized that it is impossible to prevent the articular segment from remaining in extension compared to the shaft unless a pin can be placed into this segment, which is usually not practical. Despite this extension alignment, the fracture can still be held at appropriate length and with sufficient stability to allow some patient mobilization until definitive fixation.

Intramedullary Nailing

Supracondylar femoral fractures may be stabilized with an intramedullary nail. **Antegrade nailing** of a supracondylar fracture is performed as described in Chap. 19. To decrease the incidence of nail breakage through a distal locking hole, there should be at least 5 cm of intact bone proximal to the distal screw holes; therefore this method can be used only for more proximal supracondylar fractures. Additionally, because the fracture is usually toward the end of the nail, it can be difficult to control the valgus and extension deformity that usually occurs in this fracture.

Fracture stabilization with a **retrograde nail** inserted through the intercondylar notch is a more commonly used technique (Fig. 20-2). It is easier to control the distal fragment because it is closer to the entry portal for the nail. Negatives of this approach include the intraarticular entry portal. It is unknown whether this portal will have long-term deleterious effects on the knee. Additionally, injury to the origin of the posterior cruciate ligament can occur if care is not taken during creation of the entry portal. Retrograde nails for the distal femur initially were developed as short nails. The use of these, however, was complicated by a high incidence of deformity at the fracture site and fracture of

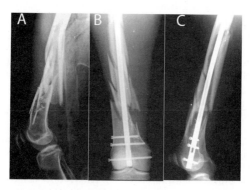

FIG. 20-2   *A.* Preoperative lateral radiograph of a type A3 distal femoral fracture. *B.* Postoperative AP and lateral radiographs in the sagittal and coronal planes showing reestablishment of proper alignment of the distal femur. (*Courtesy of Walter W. Virkus, M.D.*)

the nail. Currently, short retrograde nailing of distal femoral fractures should be limited to patients with an ipsilateral total hip arthroplasty.

Open Reduction and Internal Fixation

Open reduction and internal fixation (ORIF) was historically the primary mode of fixation in distal femoral fractures. The array of plates included blade plates, dynamic condylar screw (DCS) plates, and condylar plates. Although these are still occasionally useful in the fixation of distal femoral fractures, the introduction of locking plates has made them nearly obsolete. Locking plates provide better stability with less bone removal and easier insertion vs. these older devices. For more stable fracture patterns, nonlocking plates are available that are anatomically contoured to the distal femur, allowing easier application.

The development of locked plating represents a major advance in the surgical treatment of supracondylar femoral fractures over the past 5 years. Some locked plating systems use a minimally invasive submuscular approach, protecting the vascular structures around the fracture. While a detailed discussion of locked plating is beyond the scope of this chapter, it is critical to understand the benefits and indications for this important new technique. Locked plating involves a plate system where the head of the screw is threaded and locks into a threaded hole in the plate. This forms a fixed angle (not unlike a blade plate) at each screw-plate interface. Biomechanically, eliminating motion at the screw-plate interface significantly increases fracture stability and fixation rigidity. The result is a construct that functions much better than conventional screws and plates, especially when implanted in comminuted or osteoporotic bone. This decreases the likelihood of implant pull-out or axial collapse of the fracture. Some authors also report early and aggressive callus formation, allowing for early weight bearing and functional rehabilitation.

Definitive Management

The definitive management of supracondylar fractures in almost all circumstances is surgical. The surgical approach, stabilization device, and use of bone grafting are based on the type of fracture and surgeon experience.

Type A (Supracondylar) Fractures

These fractures are amenable to treatment either by intramedullary nailing or ORIF. They are nearly always in extension due to the pull of the gastrocnemius muscle on the distal fragment and the pull of the extensor mechanism on the proximal tibia. In the coronal plane, the fracture can be in varus or valgus, depending on whether the fracture is proximal or distal to the insertion of the adductors. Care must be taken to reduce these deformities regardless of the implant used for fracture fixation.

Retrograde nailing is performed as described in Chap. 19. In very distal fractures, it is important to make sure that the nail being used will have at least two locking screws in the distal fragment. Because supracondylar fractures by definition occur in the metaphysis, there will not be close contact between the nail and the cortex of the distal segment. As a consequence, the nail will not completely reduce the fracture, as it does in fractures at the femoral isthmus. This is particularly true in older patients with very thin cortices and decreased metaphyseal cancellous bone. Therefore care must be taken to maintain the fracture reduction in both the sagittal and coronal planes while reaming, inserting the nail, and inserting locking screws (Fig. 20-2). A slight residual translation at the fracture site often results in these cases, but this can be accepted if sagittal and coronal alignment is adequate.

Locked plating with a submuscular or standard open approach is also an acceptable technique for these fractures. This technique requires only a small incision laterally with stab holes in the skin to accommodate the locking screws proximally. Reduction is obtained by indirect means, usually by manipulating the leg over a bolster to reduce the distal segment out of extension and applying varus or valgus force to the knee to obtain the correct coronal alignment. This technique is particularly appropriate in elderly patients with poor-quality bone, thus minimizing the possibility of devascularization of the fracture fragment.

Supracondylar fractures proximal to total knee arthroplasty are increasingly common. As with other supracondylar fractures, they can be treated with either retrograde nailing or plate fixation. These fractures often have very short distal segments; therefore a nail with very distal locking screws must be utilized. Additionally, the design and manufacturer of the arthroplasty must be determined. Some older, smaller femoral components do not have an intercondylar opening large enough to allow the passage of a nail. If a short distal segment occurs in osteoporotic bone, locking-plate fixation is often more stable than a nail with two locking screws.

Type B (Unicondylar, Hoffa's) Fractures

Fractures of the medial or lateral condyles in the sagittal plane are exposed through a medial or lateral parapatellar surgical approach. The condyle is reduced and held in place with lag screws or a buttress plate. Adequacy of reduction in these fractures should be confirmed by direct visual inspection, because a malreduction in rotation can be difficult to detect with fluoroscopy. Fractures in the coronal plane usually involve the posterior portion of the condyle (Fig. 20-1, B3). These are referred to as Hoffa's fractures. They can occur in isolation or as part of a bicondylar complex fracture pattern. They are exposed through a midmedial or midlateral incision or, alternatively, through a parapatellar incision on the involved side. The fractured condyle is very posterior and must be visualized well to confirm an anatomic reduction. Lag fixation is placed from the anterior surface of the femur or trochlea into the fractured posterior condyle (Fig. 20-3). Screws placed through the cartilaginous surface of the trochlea should be headless or countersunk to avoid injuring the patellar cartilage.

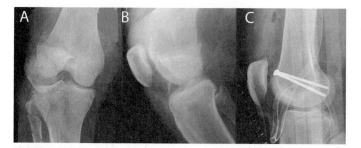

FIG. 20-3 *A* and *B*. AP and lateral radiographs showing a Hoffa's fracture of the lateral femoral condyle (OTA/AO B3) with a dislocated patella. *C*. Intraoperative lateral radiograph view showing reduction and location of countersunk 3.5-mm screws. (*Courtesy of Walter W. Virkus, M.D.*)

Type C (Bicondylar, Intercondylar) Fractures

Type C fractures vary widely from simple supracondylar/intercondylar fractures (Type C1) to very complex fractures with comminution of the articular and metaphyseal components (Type C3).

Supracondylar fractures with an intercondylar split (C1) can also be treated with either intrameduallary nail or plate fixation. If an intramedullary nail is to be used, the two condyles must be anatomically reduced to each other and held together while the nail is inserted. The nail portal is usually directed through this fracture line, so the tendency is for the nail to separate the fracture as it is reamed and inserted. The reduction should be held with lag screws (3.5 mm) placed out of the path of the nail. The articular reduction should then be reconfirmed after nail insertion. Plate fixation is performed through either a lateral or lateral parapatellar approach (Fig. 20-4).

More severely comminuted intercondylar fractures are best managed with ORIF (Fig. 20-5). Anatomically contoured plates are very useful for this location. If the metaphyseal component is very comminuted, locking plates have a clear advantage, as they can prevent the fracture from settling into varus without the need for a medial plate. Locked plating techniques on fractures with intraarticular extension require reduction and stabilization of the articular surface prior to implanting the locking plate. Although this technique can be performed through a straight lateral incision, visualization is much better with a lateral parapatellar approach if the articular fracture is comminuted (Fig. 20-5*E*). The articular surface can be stabilized either definitively with multiple 3.5-mm screws or temporarily with multiple large Kirschner wires. Anatomic reduction of comminuted metaphyseal fragments is not mandatory

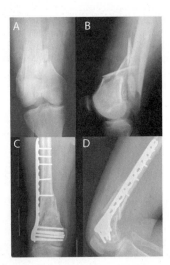

FIG. 20-4   *A* and *B.* AP and lateral radiographs showing comminuted distal femoral fracture (OTA/AO A3). *C* and *D.* AP and lateral radiographs after healing, showing how the comminuted area was spanned by a locking plate. Note that the locking plate does not have to be flush against the bone to maintain stability. (*Courtesy of Walter W. Virkus, M.D.*)

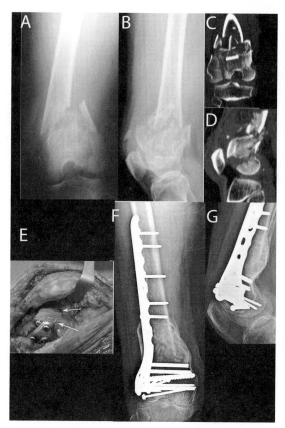

FIG. 20-5 *A* and *B*. AP and lateral radiographs of a comminuted intraarticular fracture of the distal femur (OTA/AO C3). *C* and *D*. Sagittal and coronal reconstruction CT scans showing intraarticular comminution. *E*. Intraoperative clinical photograph showing visualization of the reduced articular surface through a lateral parapatellar approach. *F* and *G*. AP and lateral radiographs showing healing of the distal femoral fracture. (*Courtesy of Walter W. Virkus, M.D.*)

as long as the relationship of the condyles to the distal diaphysis (axial alignment, length, rotation) is restored. The locking-plate systems placed submuscularly play a crucial biological and biomechanical role in the stabilization of this fracture. The advent of locked plating has reduced the number of cases that require bone grafting. One indication for grafting that still remains is the occurence of massive bone loss at the time of injury. Furthermore, the use of locking plates laterally virtually eliminates the need for a second plate medially.

One of the best indications for the use of locked plating is severe osteopenia. The stability of these plates in poor-quality bone is far superior to that of conventional implants. On very rare occasions, polymethylmethacrylate (PMMA) can be used to further augment fixation. After the fragments have been reduced, PMMA while in its doughy state is inserted into the medullary cavity across the fracture. This is done through a cortical window at the level of the fracture. This is rarely necessary if locked plates are used, but it may be needed with conventional implants.

Rehabilitation

After stabilization of supracondylar, intercondylar, and single-condyle fractures, early motion is encouraged as soon as incisional pain becomes tolerable. Continuous passive motion is rarely useful in these patients unless other injuries prevent them from participating in a therapy program. Hinged knee bracing is used only in cases where the fixation is not felt to be stable or if there is an associated ligamentous injury. The length of time during which weight bearing must be avoided depends on the stability of the fracture, the stability of fixation, and the expected rate of healing. Patients fixed with locking submuscular plates can begin partial weight bearing as soon as callus appears on radiographs. This is frequently as early as 4 to 6 weeks, which can be 6 weeks earlier than allowed with conventional implants. Full weight bearing should generally be delayed until 10 to 12 weeks in articular fractures.

Complications

Complications are commonly nonunion, malunion, arthrofibrosis, and posttraumatic arthritis. **Nonunion** is managed with autogenous bone grafting and rigid stabilization. Revision of the internal fixation device is frequently necessary, depending on the time from initial injury and surgery. A stiff knee remarkably worsens the prognosis. Great care must be taken to encourage aggressive knee motion during rehabilitation. In cases of **arthrofibrosis** that are not responsive to aggressive rehabilitation, arthroscopic or open lysis of adhesions and manipulation is indicated. If surgical intervention fails and painful arthrofibrosis persists, arthrodesis is performed. If there is no prior history of infection, an intramedullary rod is used for knee fusion fixation. If there is a history of infection, a circular external fixater with progressive compression is used to stabilize the knee fusion construct.

Varus and valgus **malunions** are invariably symptomatic and can lead to secondary arthritis and abnormalities of gait. Extension and flexion malunions are better tolerated than those occurring in the coronal plane. Symptomatic malunion is managed with corrective osteotomy of the femur.

Posttraumatic arthritis is managed with nonsteroidal anti-inflammatory drugs and local injection of steroids. Arthroscopic debridement provides only short-term relief of symptoms and recently has been shown to be of little benefit for degenerative joint disease. Surgical options for degenerative joint disease not responding to conservative means include arthroplasty or arthrodesis. While the indications are changing, arthroplasty is frequently reserved for patients who are at least 40 years old.

SELECTED READINGS

Albert MJ. Supracondylar fractures of the femur. *J Am Acad Orthop Surg* 5(3):163–171, 1997.
Ker NB, Maempel FZ, Paton DF. Bone cement as an adjunct to medullary nailing in fractures of the distal third of the femur in elderly patients. *Injury* 16(2):102–107, 1984.

Kregor PJ, Stannard JA, Zlowodzki M, Cole PA. Treatment of distal femur fractures using the less invasive stabilization system: surgical experience and early clinical results in 103 fractures. *J Orthop Trauma* 18(8):509–520, 2004.

Meyer RW, Plaxton NA, Postak PD, et al. Mechanical comparison of a distal femoral side plate and a retrograde intramedullary nail. *J Orthop Trauma* 14(6):398–404, 2000.

Zlowodzki M, Williamson S, Cole PA, et al. Biomechanical evaluation of the less invasive stabilization system, angled blade plate, and retrograde intramedullary nail for the internal fixation of distal femur fractures. *J Orthop Trauma* 18(8):494–502, 2004.

21 | Knee Dislocations

Robert C. Schenck, Jr.   James P. Stannard

This chapter reviews and describes the diagnosis and management of knee dislocations.

ANATOMY

The osseous anatomy of the knee is discussed in Chap 20. The soft tissue anatomy includes the anterior and posterior cruciate ligaments, the medial collateral ligament and associated medial structures, the lateral collateral ligament (LCL)/posterolateral corner (PLC) complex and associated lateral structures, and the medial and lateral menisci. The anterior cruciate ligament (ACL) originates posteriorly on the medial side of the lateral femoral condyle and travels anterior, medial, and distal to insert just anterior and lateral to the medial tibial spine. The posterior cruciate ligament (PCL) originates on the posterior portion of the lateral side of the medial femoral condyle and courses distal to insert on the midportion of the posterior proximal aspect of the tibia.

The medial-sided structures include the medial collateral ligament, the hamstring tendons, and the medial capsule. The medial collateral ligament (MCL) has a deep and a superficial component. Both components originate from the medial femoral epicondyle. The deep component inserts onto the peripheral rim of the medial meniscus and the proximal rim of the medial tibia. The superficial component inserts on the tibia more distally, directly posterior to the pes anserinus.

The PLC complex includes the lateral collateral ligament, the iliotibial band, the biceps femoris, and the thickened lateral capsule, which includes the arcuate ligament and fabellofibular ligament. The lateral collateral ligament originates on the lateral femoral epicondyle and inserts on the head of the fibula.

Classification

Classification of knee dislocations can be by energy of injury, position of dislocation, and the ligaments involved. Clinical experience has shown that the tibiofemoral joint can dislocate with either the ACL or PCL intact (bicruciate or cruciate intact knee dislocations). The direction of dislocation is frequently not known, as over one-third of dislocations reduce spontaneously. Furthermore, the position of the tibia on the femur does not identify what ligaments are involved. Magnitude of injury is useful in consideration of soft tissue involvement and risk of arterial injury but again does not identify which ligaments may have been torn. We classify knee dislocations according to the ligaments that are disrupted.

Four ligaments may be disrupted: the ACL, PCL, LCL/PLC, and MCL. The determination of which ligaments are disrupted is based on the physical examination, either immediately after the injury or later under anesthesia, and MRI. Common dislocation patterns include: ACL/PCL/MCL,

ACL/PCL/LCL/PLC, ACL/PCL/PLC, ACL/PCL/LCL, and ACL/PCL/MCL/LCL/PLC.

Associated Injuries

Injuries associated with knee dislocations are vascular, neurologic, or skeletal.

The incidence of **popliteal artery** injury reported in the literature varies from 5 to 40% (Fig. 21-1). The presence of pedal pulses does not rule out a minor arterial injury such as an intimal tear. Treatment should be guided by serial vascular physical examinations. If the examination is abnormal or there is any other reason to be highly suspicious of an arterial injury, emergent vascular consultation should be obtained. Ankle-brachial pressures can also be obtained. A value of 0.8 or lower suggests possible arterial injury. Disruption of the popliteal artery is a surgical emergency. Circulation must be reestablished within 8 h or the chance of salvaging the leg is minimal. Stabilization of the knee with external fixation is the most effective means of protecting the vascular repair. The external fixator can be left in place and used to manage the ligamentous injury.

The **peroneal and tibial nerves** are at risk in a knee dislocation. The peroneal nerve is injured more frequently than the tibial nerve, with an incidence of about 20%. The peroneal nerve is most commonly injured in association with the lateral ligamentous complex (e.g., adduction injury to the knee: ACL/PCL/LCL/PLC torn, MCL intact). It is usually a traction injury that cannot be repaired. The differential diagnosis of peroneal and tibial nerve deficit includes compartment syndrome.

Bony avulsions of ligamentous origins and insertions are distinct from fracture-dislocations of the knee, in which ligamentous injury is associated with a fracture of the tibial or femoral condyles. Frequently, a bony avulsion facilitates ligamentous repair. Examination by magnetic resonance imaging can make the diagnosis of an avulsion injury much clearer.

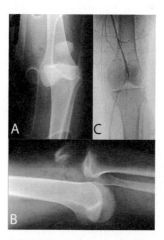

FIG. 21-1   *A* and *B*. AP and lateral radiographs of an anterior knee dislocation. *C*. Angiogram of same patient showing interruption of flow in the popliteal artery. (*Courtesy of Walter W. Virkus, M.D.*)

Diagnosis and Initial Management

History and Physical Examination

The mechanism of injury is important because the incidence of associated injuries, in particular popliteal artery disruption, is less with low-energy (e.g., sports-related) injuries. However, the clinician should be cautioned against assuming vascular integrity based on mechanism of injury.

The diagnosis of a displaced knee dislocation is often obvious because of the gross deformity. However, frequently, the dislocation has been reduced during transit to the emergency department, and swelling may be the only obvious physical finding. Lacerations are assumed to communicate with the joint unless proven otherwise. A medial skin furrow may indicate that the dislocation is complex (posterolateral dislocation) or irreducible with closed methods.

A focused vascular evaluation includes palpation of pedal pulses, examination of leg and foot compartments, and assessment of skin color and capillary refill. A focused neurologic evaluation includes examination of the peroneal nerve (i.e., sensation on the dorsum of the foot and ability to dorsiflex the ankle) and tibial nerve (i.e., sensation on the plantar aspect of the foot and ability to plantarflex the ankle, foot, and toes).

The initial ligamentous evaluation is performed in a standardized manner with reference made to the contralateral knee for comparison. The knee is stressed in varus and valgus with the knee in both full extension and 30 degrees of flexion; knee opening in full extension indicates an injury to both cruciates and the associated collateral. Instability in 30 degrees of flexion indicates a torn MCL (valgus) or LCL (varus). Hyperextension indicates a torn ACL and PLC (a positive hyperextension recurvatum test). A positive Lachman's test indicates a torn ACL. A Lachman's test is performed by flexing the knee to 25 degrees. One hand stabilizes the thigh and the other stresses the tibia to displace the knee anteriorly and posteriorly. If there is an abnormal amount of motion anteriorly, the test is positive. The resting position in knee flexion may demonstrate a posterior sag, suggesting a PCL injury (Fig. 21-2). Anterior and posterior drawer tests are performed by flexing the knee to 90 degrees and applying anterior and posterior stresses, respectively. Instability indicates a torn ACL and capsule or PCL and capsule, respectively.

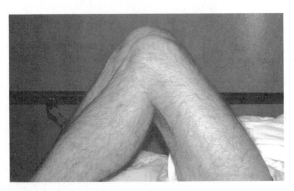

FIG. 21-2 Clinical image showing the posterior sag sign seen in injury of the PCL. (*Courtesy of Charles Bush-Joseph, M.D.*)

Radiographic Examination

The neurovascular and radiographic examinations are performed prior to reduction (Fig. 21-1*A* and *B*). Anteroposterior and lateral radiographs aid in classifying the injury by the position of the tibia on the femur and in determining whether there are associated fractures. After the initial closed reduction, the injury is further evaluated with magnetic resonance imaging (MRI). MRI identifies which ligaments are disrupted and distinguishes midsubstance tears from avulsions. This is particularly useful in planning the management of a PCL disrupted knee dislocation.

Radiographs are obtained while the patient is anesthetized. The extended knee is stressed in varus and valgus. Joint-line opening indicates complete disruption of both cruciate ligaments and of either the MCL or LCL. Anterior and posterior drawer tests are also performed. Fluoroscopy may add to the clinical exam (Fig. 21-3).

Thus, with the initial evaluation, pre- and postreduction radiographs, MRI, examination under anesthesia, and occasionally, if needed, stress radiographs, an accurate prediction of the damaged structures can be made.

Initial Management

Reduction is usually straightforward and accomplished with longitudinal traction and manipulation. Once the joint is reduced, the vascular and neurologic examinations are repeated. The knee is splinted and iced. Postsplinting radiographs are obtained to ensure a concentric reduction. Ongoing residual subluxation should be avoided, especially if definitive treatment is to be delayed. In most cases, ankle-brachial indices or serial physical examinations are performed to rule out an associated arterial injury. At a minimum, the patient is admitted for observation.

Definitive Management

Timing

Arthroscopy of the acute knee dislocation (within 14 days of injury) is contraindicated because of the risk of fluid extravasation due to capsular disruption.

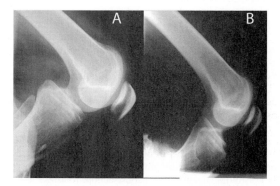

FIG. 21-3   *A* and *B*. Lateral stress radiographs demonstrating abnormal posterior (*A*) and anterior (*B*) translation due to multiligament instability. (*Courtesy of Charles Bush-Joseph, M.D.*)

With the recent advances in ligamentous reconstruction and repair, including the use of allografts, it has become preferable to delay cruciate reconstruction until after a functional range of motion is obtained. The surgeon's experience and preference go into this decision, but acute repair or reconstruction of the ACL is associated with a high incidence of arthrofibrosis. The exception to this rule is an ACL avulsion, where reattachment increases the stability of the knee without increasing the complexity or duration of surgery. Associated injuries to the PLC are also best treated early (within 1 month of injury) with either repair or reconstruction. Repair of collateral injuries adds to stability and is especially useful in treatment of the PLC.

There are no clear clinical data regarding the benefits of repair compared to reconstruction of the collaterals and corners in patients with dislocated knees. The cruciate ligaments should be reconstructed unless a bony avulsion has occurred. Occasionally, closed management of knee dislocation is required because of associated injuries (soft tissue, multiple trauma, infection).

Closed management consists of immobilization of the knee in extension, using an external fixator for 7 to 8 weeks, followed by manipulation under anesthesia, arthroscopic arthrolysis, and range-of-motion exercises. This length of time frequently allows for satisfactory healing of the PCL. Frequently, manipulation under epidural anesthesia is required to regain full motion. Bracing is an acceptable alternative to external fixation if radiographs confirm a concentric reduction while the knee is in the brace.

Surgical Management

As mentioned, it has become clear that the knee can dislocate with an intact PCL or ACL. This is a key point: a functioning PCL directs surgical management to the treatment of the torn ACL. In contrast, the dislocation in which both cruciate ligaments are torn is a much more complicated and unstable pattern, requiring treatment of both cruciate ligaments.

One or both of the collateral ligaments may be disrupted during a knee dislocation. Disruption of a collateral ligament implies disruption of underlying capsular structures and directs the surgical approach to ligamentous repair or, more commonly, reconstruction.

Fundamental techniques and principles of surgical management include the following. **Midline incisions** are used whenever possible to minimize the incidence of wound-healing problems in the event that other surgical procedures should be performed in the future. Reattachment of ligamentous avulsions can be accomplished with the **locking whip stitch**, as described by Krackow et al. (1988). **Bony avulsions are repaired with suture or screw fixation**. Direct repair of midsubstance cruciate tears is not advocated; these are reconstructed, while midsubstance collateral and corner injuries are repaired or reconstructed depending on the residual tissue available. Ligaments avulsed from their insertions or origins are **reattached with a screw and spiked washer or reconstructed**. Fixation of an autograft or allograft is accomplished by **fixing the graft in bony tunnels** in the femur and tibia (Fig. 21-4). The key to reconstruction of the dislocated knee is first **reconstructing the PCL**. Multiple ligamentous reconstructions routinely use allograft due to their availability and the desire to avoid further trauma to the knee by harvesting autografts.

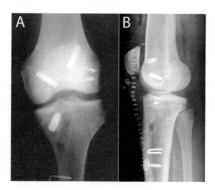

FIG. 21-4   *A* and *B*. Postoperative AP and lateral radiographs following ACL, PCL, and PLC reconstruction. (*Courtesy of Charles Bush-Joseph, M.D.*)

Specific Surgical Techniques

The following descriptions of surgical management of the dislocated knee are based on the ligaments involved.

Type I: ACL/MCL/LCL torn, PCL intact. PCL integrity directs the treatment of this type of dislocation to the ACL. Reconstruction of the ACL is delayed until range of motion is restored and collateral healing has occurred.

Type II: ACL/PCL torn, MCL/LCL intact. This injury pattern is rare, and its management is simplified by the intact collaterals. The key to successful management is reconstruction of the PCL and ACL.

Type III: ACL/PCL/MCL torn, LCL/PLC intact. The primary goal is reconstruction of the torn structures. Simultaneous bicruciate reconstruction can be performed with an arthroscopically assisted technique after functional range of motion has been obtained. Depending on healing of the PLC, reconstruction of this collateral structure may be required and is usually performed through an open approach. The use of PCL inlay vs. tibial tunnels is complex and dependent on the surgeon's experience. The inlay or onlay technique, accomplished using a trough in the back of the proximal tibia, has been associated with improved results in both clinical and cadaveric studies.

Type IV: ACL/PCL/LCL/PLC torn, MCL intact. The tearing of both the LCL and PLC complicates treatment. It is important to reestablish the PLC and associated tendinous structures (i.e., biceps femoris and/or iliotibial band) in addition to the PCL. The incision is posterolateral. The peroneal nerve is identified and protected, and the knee is inspected by subluxing the tibiofemoral joint. The locking whip stitch is used to reattach or repair the LCL and associated posterolateral structures. Alternatively, a reconstruction that recreates the LCL, the popliteal, and the popliteofibular ligament can be performed. Again, the timing of reconstruction of the ACL and PCL must be based on clinical experience. Acute PLC repair combined with simultaneous ACL/PCL reconstructions will pose a high risk of stiffness.

Type V: ACL/PCL/MCL/LCL/PLC torn. This pattern is most frequently a high-energy injury characterized by gross instability and frequently accompanied by neurovascular compromise. Repair of the PCL and posterolateral corner is the primary goal. By using a posterolateral incision, these two structures can be explored and repaired or reconstructed. A medial incision may be required to reattach the PCL to the femur or to reconstruct it with an autograft or allograft. ACL reconstruction, simultaneous or staged, allows for functional knee stability. The presence of multiple trauma complicates postoperative management.

Rehabilitation

Postoperatively, the leg is maintained in a postoperative reconstruction brace. Aggressive physical therapy concentrating on range of motion is critical. An ankle-foot orthosis is used if foot drop is present.

Complications

Complications unique to a dislocation of the knee are arthrofibrosis, residual laxity, and incompetent lateral structures.

Arthrofibrosis results in loss of motion. It is best avoided by following the surgical repair with rigorous physical therapy or by delaying reconstruction until motion has been regained and inflammation diminished. We prefer the latter approach. If 90 degrees of flexion has not been obtained by 6 weeks postsurgery, manipulation under epidural anesthesia and arthroscopic scar excision are performed. Epidural anesthesia is continued postoperatively for 2 to 3 days to maintain motion. In our experience, even in the best of situations, stiffness occurs in reconstructive bicruciate surgery and, once seen, requires careful observation and early aggressive treatment. Stiffness resulting from surgical reconstruction can be severely limiting and difficult to treat. It is best avoided by initially reestablishing range of motion after definitive reconstruction.

Residual laxity is frequently seen in dislocated knees treated nonoperatively. Although laxity is problematic for the patient, stiffness, as outlined above, is a more difficult problem functionally than is instability. Residual laxity after an attempted reconstructive effort requires careful evaluation of graft source, tunnel or inlay placement, and the functional stability of the corners.

Incompetent lateral structures result in **posterolateral rotary instability** (PLRI). Repair of the lateral structures can be difficult (midsubstance tears of the LCL are particularly difficult) but may be attempted. Alternatively, the PLC can be reconstructed. Unlike combined ACL/LCL injuries, in which the LCL is frequently treated nonoperatively, the LCL in a knee dislocation is repaired or reconstructed to promote lateral stability. Biceps tenodesis can be used to augment an LCL injury. The ACL reconstruction is necessary after initial LCL/PCL surgery (ACL functioning as an internal collateral) to provide stability in extension.

SELECTED READINGS

Dedmond BT, Almekinders LC. Operative versus nonoperative treatment of knee dislocations: a meta-analysis. *Am J Knee Surg* 14(1):33–38, 2001.

Frassica FS, Franklin HS, Staeheli JW, Pairolero PC. Dislocation of the knee. *Clin Orthop* 263:200–205, 1992.

Harner CD, Waltrip RL, Bennett CH, et al. Surgical management of knee dislocations. *J Bone Joint Surg Am* 86A(2):262–273, 2004.

Krackow KA, Thomas SC, Jones LC. Ligament–tendon fixation: analysis of a new stitch and comparison with standard techniques. *Orthopaedics* 11:909–917, 1988.

Liow RY, McNicholas MJ, Keating JF, Nutton RW. Ligament repair and reconstruction in traumatic dislocation of the knee. *J Bone Joint Surg Br* 85(6):845–851, 2003.

Mills WJ, Barei DP, McNair P. The value of the ankle-brachial index for diagnosing arterial injury after knee dislocation: a prospective study. *J Trauma* 56(6):1261–1265, 2004.

Richter M, Bosch U, Wippermann B, et al. Comparison of surgical repair or reconstruction of the cruciate ligaments versus nonsurgical treatment in patients with traumatic knee dislocations. *Am J Sports Med* 30(5):718–727, 2002.

Rihn JA, Groff YJ, Harner CD, Cha PS. The acutely dislocated knee: evaluation and management. *J Am Acad Orthop Surg* 12(5):334–346, 2004.

Stannard JP, Sheils TM, Lopez-Ben RR, et al. Vascular injuries in knee dislocations: the role of physical examination in determining the need for arteriography. *J Bone Joint Surg Am* 86A(5):910–915, 2004.

Wascher DC, Dvirnak PC, Decoster TA. Knee dislocation: initial assessment and implications for treatment. *J Orthop Trauma* 11(7):525–529, 1997.

| Fractures of the Proximal Tibia

Robert C. Schenck, Jr.   James P. Stannard

This chapter reviews fractures of the proximal tibia (the tibial spines and medial and lateral condyles). Commonly referred to as tibial plateau fractures, they involve the proximal articular surface of the tibia.

ANATOMY

The knee is a compound joint consisting of a sellar joint between the trochlea of the femur and the patella and two condylar joints between the condyles of the femur and the tibial plateaus.

The **proximal tibia** includes the medial and lateral condyles, or plateaus, and the tibial tuberosity. The articular surface of the tibia comprises the cartilage-covered medial and lateral plateaus, which articulate with the corresponding articular surfaces of the femur. The medial and lateral menisci provide congruency between the convex femoral surface and the relatively flat tibial plateaus. They also bear a portion of the load as it is transmitted from the distal femur to the proximal tibia. The two plateaus are separated by the anterior and posterior tibial spines (i.e., the intercondylar eminence). The anterior tibial spine is the insertion of the anterior cruciate ligament and the attachment of the anterior and posterior horns of the lateral meniscus and anterior horn of the medial meniscus. The posterior tibial spine is the attachment of the posterior horn of the medial meniscus. The posterior intercondylar area is the insertion of the posterior cruciate ligament. The fibular facet on the lateral tibial condyle faces laterally, distally, and posteriorly.

The **tibial tuberosity** is the anterior projection of the tibia, onto which the patellar ligament inserts. It is approximately 2 cm distal to the articular surface of the tibia.

Classification

Tibial plateau fractures have been classified by many systems. The classification of the Orthopaedic Trauma Association (OTA/AO) for the proximal tibia is similar to that for other anatomic areas. Type A is extraarticular fractures, type B is unicondylar fractures, and type C is bicondylar fractures. A subtype 1 to 3 is added to describe increasing comminution. Despite this comprehensive classification system, the system described by Schatzker et al. (1979) is currently the most commonly used by practitioners (Fig. 22-1). It is as follows: type I, split fracture of the lateral plateau; type II, split-depression fracture of the lateral plateau; type III, depression fracture of the lateral plateau; type IV, fracture of the medial plateau; type V, bicondylar fracture of the proximal tibia; and type VI, bicondylar plateau fracture and associated metaphyseal-diaphyseal fracture. Types I to III are low-energy fractures. Types IV to VI are usually high-energy injuries.

Split fractures (Schatzker I) of the lateral plateau occur in young patients with dense bone. The mechanism of injury is usually a blow to the lateral side of the knee. This fracture, which is best seen on the anteroposterior projection,

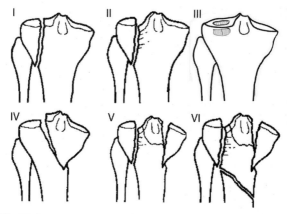

FIG. 22-1   The Schatzker classification of tibial plateau fractures.

is vertical and seldom widely displaced (Fig. 22-1, I). The lateral meniscus may be torn peripherally and dislocated into the fracture site.

Split-depression fractures (Schatzker II) are the most common type of tibial plateau fracture. These tend to occur in slightly older patients than Schatzker I fractures. The mechanism of injury is a valgus stress that impacts the lateral femoral condyle against the plateau, fracturing the lateral portion of the plateau from the proximal tibia. As the femoral condyle continues to impact the remaining medial portion of the lateral plateau, it drives a segment of articular surface into the metaphysis. This depressed segment is always on the medial side of the fracture, not on the lateral split fragment (Fig. 22-1, II). Whether the depressed segment is anterior or posterior depends on the degree of knee flexion at the time of injury (extension is associated with anterior depression, flexion with posterior depression).

Lateral-depression fractures (Schatzker III) occur in osteopenic bone. The mechanism of injury is a low-energy valgus stress: the lateral femoral condyle sinks into and depresses the lateral plateau. The lateral rim can be intact, or the entire lateral plateau may be depressed (Fig. 22-1, III).

Medial plateau fractures (Schatzker IV) range from low-energy medial-depression fractures similar to those described above on the lateral side to severe fracture-dislocations frequently associated with neurovascular injuries. Low-energy fractures are caused by a varus load to the knee. High-energy fractures are caused by axial and valgus forces across the knee, causing the lateral femoral condyle to hit the tibial spines along a vector directed medially and distally. The medial tibial condyle and the tibial spines are fractured and driven along this vector. A variety of ligamentous injuries may occur in association with this fracture; in fact, this injury may often represent a fracture-dislocation (Fig. 22-1, IV).

Bicondylar plateau fractures (Schatzker V) involve both condyles and are the result of complex high-energy trauma. Associated neurovascular (including compartment syndrome), ligamentous, and extensive soft tissue injuries are common (Fig. 22-1, V).

Plateau fractures associated with a fracture of the proximal metaphyseal diaphyseal junction (Schatzker VI) are similar to bicondylar fractures in that they are the result of high-energy trauma and frequently are associated with neurovascular, ligamentous, and soft tissue injuries. Historically, there is a high incidence of nonunion and postoperative infection in these cases due to the magnitude of the soft tissue injury and the extensive surgical exposure occasionally necessary to reduce and stabilize the fractures (Fig. 22-1, VI).

Associated Injuries

Injuries frequently associated with fractures of the tibial plateau are soft tissue injury to the ligaments or mensci, injury to the popliteal artery or trifurcation, compartment syndrome, and injury of the tibial or common peroneal nerve.

Fracture of the medial or lateral plateau **may be associated with rupture of any ligament or a tear of either meniscus**. Studies have suggested these injuries occur in 50% of tibial plateau fractures. It is important to pay specific attention to the contralateral-collateral ligament. This combination of fracture and ligamentous injury about the knee has been described by Moore as a fracture-dislocation. In low-energy injuries, while dislocation is unlikely, ligamentous injury on the side of the knee opposite the fracture may result in residual knee laxity despite anatomic reduction of the fracture.

Injuries of the **popliteal artery or trifurcation** are most likely to occur with high-energy medial tibial plateau and bicondylar fractures. If distal pulses are absent, emergency consultation with a vascular surgeon should be obtained immediately.

Compartment syndrome is indicated by the presence of the classic signs of increased intracompartmental pressure: pain at rest, pain with passive stretch of involved muscles, tense compartments, and numbness in the foot. This is a common complication following high-energy tibial plateau fractures and must be ruled out.

Injuries of the **tibial and peroneal nerves** are identified by assessing sensation on the plantar aspect of the foot and in the first web space and by assessing active contraction of the flexor and extensor hallucis longus, respectively.

Diagnosis and Initial Management

History and Physical Examination

There is pain, swelling, and a history of injury with virtually any fracture of the proximal tibia. There may be no discernible deformity, but there is usually a large knee effusion, which, when aspirated, has blood with fat in it, indicating an intraarticular fracture. Physical examination of the knee, even under anesthesia, can be quite difficult. The accuracy of the exam is limited due to the skeletal instability, pain, and swelling. Apparent ligamentous laxity may be a misinterpretation of motion occurring through the fracture site or due to the femoral condyle falling into a depression. It is equally easy to assume that motion is from the fracture and to miss a significant ligamentous injury. Accurate diagnosis requires a careful examination of the knee under anesthesia (including fluoroscopy). Failure to diagnose and treat ligamentous injuries either surgically or through rehabilitation can seriously undermine the patient's functional recovery.

Radiographic Examination

Radiographs in the anteroposterior and lateral planes are standard. Tilting the beam 10 degrees caudally, so that it profiles the articular surface, provides more accurate information regarding the amount of depression. In some instances, obtaining a traction view with either radiographs or fluoroscopy can provide valuable information for the surgeon. Computed tomography (CT) scans, and more recently magnetic resonance imaging (MRI), can be very helpful for the evaluation of associated injuries and preoperative planning for bony fixation. MRI can yield crucial information regarding the status of the ligaments and menisci while providing adequate bone detail as well. However, an MRI scan can be time-consuming to obtain and may be impossible if a spanning external fixator is in place; it is also much more expensive than CT. Although CT scanning has been the classic secondary radiographic study for preoperative planning, the information obtained through an MRI regarding bone and soft tissue may lead to MRI being the study of choice in the future.

Initial Management

Initial management of these injuries depends on their severity. For low-energy injuries without any axial shortening, a well-padded long leg splint that maintains the leg in the proper alignment is adequate. For more severe injuries, management should be directed by the status of the soft tissue. If the soft tissue envelope of the proximal tibia is only mildly swollen, a long leg splint may be adequate. If soft tissue injury is severe, heralded by blisters or severe swelling, definitive management will likely have to be delayed. In these cases, **a knee-spanning external fixator** has many benefits. A spanning fixator provides a provisional reduction and allows the fracture to be held out to anatomic length, which facilitates the recovery of the soft tissues and makes eventual surgical reduction of the fracture easier (Fig. 22-2). It also greatly increases patient comfort until definitive fixation can take place. A spanning external fixator is also often indicated in patients with an open fracture or associated vascular injury.

Definitive Management

The goals of management of tibial plateau fractures are to decrease the risk of posttraumatic osteoarthritis and provide a stable knee with a normal axis of alignment. Indications for operative management are reducible intraarticular incongruity, intraarticular displacement (i.e., a gap without a step-off) of 3 mm or more, ligamentous instability, or a deviation in the alignment of the

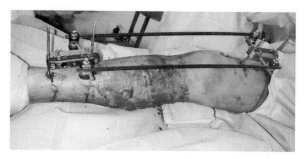

FIG. 22-2   A knee-spanning external fixator on a patient with a high-energy tibial plateau fracture and severe soft tissue injury. (*Courtesy of Walter W. Virkus, M.D.*)

knee. Residual articular incongruity of the lateral tibial plateau is better tolerated than similar incongruity of the medial plateau. Indications for nonoperative management are a fracture that cannot be satisfactorily reduced and stabilized, usually due to extensive comminution or blisters, or preexisting arthritis. Furthermore, fractures in the elderly patient where there is less than 10 degrees of valgus instability also have been shown historically to do well with nonoperative treatment.

Nonoperative Treatment

The nonoperative management of tibial plateau fractures consists of approximately 12 weeks of protected mobilization in a long leg cast-brace. Knee motion in the brace is limited to 30 or 40 degrees for the first 3 to 6 weeks and then allowed in the full arc. Minimally displaced plateau fractures are best evaluated with a careful examination (frequently under anesthesia) to look at varus and valgus stability in full knee extension. Less than 10 degrees of valgus instability is a clinical finding that indicates good potential for nonoperative management. Rasmussen (1973) described this finding initially.

The goal of **operative management** is restoration of length, alignment and rotation, anatomic alignment of the joint surface, and stabilization adequate to allow early motion. The surgical exposure and method of stabilization are based on the type of fracture and the status of the soft tissue.

Split fractures are reduced closed under fluoroscopy and stabilized with percutaneous screws. To reduce the fracture, the knee is flexed to 30 degrees and a varus stress is applied. At the same time, the lateral plateau is pushed medially toward the proximal tibia. If this maneuver does not result in reduction, the fracture is exposed through a lateral parapatellar approach. The block to reduction (frequently the lateral meniscus) is identified and removed. Non–weight bearing is maintained for 6 to 8 weeks.

Split-depression fractures are exposed through a lateral parapatellar or lateral incision. The coronary ligament of the lateral meniscus is incised and the meniscus is elevated. The fracture is "booked open" through the split component, thereby exposing the depressed segment. The depressed segment is elevated and the resulting defect bone-grafted. The split fragment is then reduced and stabilized with a buttress plate, with the screws or wires placed directly under the subchondral bone to serve as a "raft" for the elevated articular segment. A 3.5-mm plate is adequate for most unicondylar lateral fractures (Fig. 22-3).

Depression fractures are managed operatively through a parapatellar or lateral incision. The tibial attachment of the meniscus is incised and the meniscus is retracted superiorly to expose the plateau. The lateral plateau is elevated with a bone tamp inserted through a window in the lateral metaphysis. The resulting defect is packed with bone graft, bone graft substitute, or calcium phosphate cement. The articular surface is stabilized with multiple 3.5-mm screws placed immediately under the subchondral bone, using a "rafting" technique. A plate is applied laterally if the lateral rim of the plateau is depressed as well. Some cases may be amenable to arthoscopic evaluation of the reduction if screws alone are planned for fixation.

Medial plateau fractures are managed operatively through a medial parapatellar or posteromedial incision. Depending on the location of the fracture, the medial meniscus can be elevated. There may be minimal compression with high-energy fractures, in which case bone grafting is not necessary. A plate is required for stabilization because simple lag screws do not provide adequate

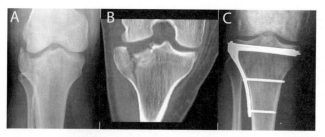

FIG. 22-3   *A.* AP radiograph of a Schatzker II split-depression tibial plateau fracture. *B.* Coronal reconstruction CT scan showing lateral split fragment and depression of the medial portion of the lateral tibial plateau. *C.* AP radiograph 3 months following ORIF. Note screw and Kirschner-wire placement directly below the subchondral bone. (*Courtesy of Walter W. Virkus, M.D.*)

stability to prevent displacement. Such fractures call for a word of caution: anatomic plate fixation placed posteromedially is often required to prevent displacement. In high-energy injuries, ligamentous repair or reconstruction may be necessary, but this may be best delayed until osseous healing has occurred and range of motion has been restored.

Bicondylar fractures with or without a metaphyseal dissociation are treated similarly. The options are open reduction and internal fixation (ORIF) with anatomic joint reduction and plate fixation of the articular segment to the tibial shaft or limited reduction and fixation of the articular fracture with external fixation to stabilize the articular segment to the tibial shaft. In choosing the best option, the surgeon must consider the amount of articular comminution and the status of the soft tissue envelope of the proximal tibia.

If the articular segment is very comminuted and the soft tissue severely injured, limited internal fixation and stabilization with a thin-wire fixator or pin monolateral fixator may be the best option. If the articular segment is reconstructable but the soft tissue injury is severe, then a knee-spanning external fixator can allow the soft tissues to recover and formal ORIF with plate fixation can be performed 7 to 14 days after injury.

Limited internal fixation and external fixation is an excellent option in cases of severe articular comminution, open fractures, fractures associated with compartment syndrome, and unresolving soft tissue injury (Fig. 22-4). This method should be performed in the first 7 to 10 days, when fracture fragments are still mobile. The articular surface is reduced by closed manipulation or manipulation of fracture fragments through small incisions. These fragments are then stabilized with multiple lag screws. The articular segment is then reduced to the tibial shaft and stabilized with a thin-wire or half-pin fixator. These pins or wires must be placed at least 14 mm distal to the joint line to prevent them from traversing the reflection of the joint capsule and potentially leading to septic arthritis. Distally, fixation in the tibial shaft is obtained with thin wires or half pins.

ORIF with anatomic proximal tibial plates is an excellent option for fixation of tibial plateau fractures either acutely or after a short duration of joint-spanning external fixation. **It is critical, however, that extensile exposures not be performed through severely swollen soft tissue**, as rates of wound dehiscense and deep infection are high. It must be determined whether the

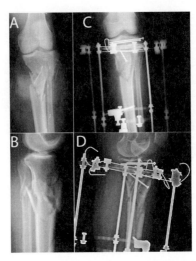

FIG. 22-4   *A* and *B*. AP and lateral radiographs of a comminuted fracture of the proximal tibia with a split into the tibial plateau. *C* and *D*. Postoperative AP and lateral radiographs showing an Ilizarov-type thin-wire external fixator and lag screws stabilizing the proximal tibia. (*Courtesy of Walter W. Virkus, M.D.*)

medial condyle will have to be reduced open and whether it will require a medial plate for stable fixation. If the medial fragment is minimally displaced, it can be reduced closed. Often, however, the medial condyle is rotated or displaced posteriorly, and in this situation the medial plateau should be reduced open, because anatomic closed reduction is very difficult. If the medial plateau fragment is large, it can be adequately stabilized by a lateral locking plate. If the fragment is small, comminuted, or osteoporotic or if a locking plate is not being used, a separate medial or posteromedial plate should be used to stabilize the medial fragment. **If a medial plate is used, it is critical that it be inserted through a separate medial incision and not placed through the same incision that is used to insert the lateral plate**. Plating both sides of the proximal tibia through one incision leads to excessive soft tissue stripping, bone devascularization, and a high incidence of nonunion or infection.

After the medial fragment is reduced, either to the lateral plateau or the metaphysis, the lateral plateau is reduced and stabilized. This may require elevation of a depressed portion of the plateau and can be performed through a lateral parapatellar or anterolateral approach. A 4.5-mm anatomic plate is then used for fixation. Locking plates provide excellent fixation and, as mentioned, can prevent axial collapse of a medial plateau fragment (Fig. 22-5).

For fractures that are minimally displaced or that can be reduced through small incisions, minimally invasive plating with locking plates is an excellent option (Fig. 22-6). A hockey-stick incision is recommended if the LISS plating system is employed. Alternatively, it can be placed using a lateral parapatellar approach. The incision should be the minimum necessary, with the plate slid into the submuscular plane and the distal screws placed percutaneously. Depending on the degree of displacement, the reduction can be accomplished with either indirect techniques, using traction and fluoroscopy,

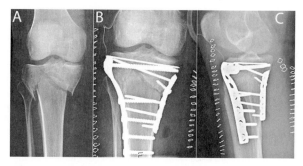

FIG. 22-5   *A.* AP radiograph of a bicondylar fracture of the tibial plateau. *B* and *C.* Postoperative AP and lateral radiographs showing a posteromedial 3.5-mm LCD plate and a lateral 4.5-mm locking plate placed through separate incisions. (*Courtesy of Walter W. Virkus, M.D.*)

arthroscopy-assisted techniques, or under direct visualization using a submeniscal arthrotomy.

Rehabilitation

Early postoperative motion is critical to attaining a good functional result. With the exception of split fractures, non–weight bearing is maintained for 12 weeks when conventional implants are used. Patients with split fractures can bear weight as tolerated at 6 weeks. If a locked plate is used, weight bearing is allowed as soon as there is any evidence of callus formation on radiographs. This frequently occurs in 6 weeks.

Complications

Complications of tibial plateau fractures include arthritis, nonunion, malunion, arthrofibrosis, infection, and late subsidence of a reduced plateau.

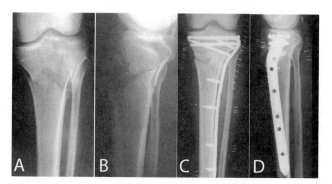

FIG. 22-6   *A* and *B.* AP and lateral radiographs of a minimally displaced bicondylar fracture of the tibial plateau. C and D. Postoperative AP and lateral radiographs following placement of lag screws and percutaneous plating using the LISS device.

Arthritis results from articular incongruity or injury to the articular cartilage that occurred at the time of fracture. Patients below 50 years of age are managed with nonsteroidal anti-inflammatory drugs and local steroid injections. If the symptoms warrant, an arthrodesis or a varus or valgus high tibial osteotomy designed to "unload" the involved condyle is performed. Patients above 50 years of age with arthritis are managed with an arthroplasty. The incidence of functionally limiting arthritis after tibial plateau fractures is not well defined but does not appear to be directly related to the quality of the articular reduction.

Nonunion of tibial plateau fractures is rare; when it occurs, it is often accompanied by infection. In evaluating the nonunion, it is important to determine whether it is infected, whether the knee joint is arthritic, and how much motion is occurring through the knee as opposed to through the nonunion. If there is no evidence of infection and there is severe arthritis, the nonunion is managed with an arthroplasty in patients above 50 years of age. In patients below age 50, the nonunion is managed with an arthrodesis by using an intramedullary nail.

Management of aseptic nonunions without arthritis consists of rigid stabilization in the form of plates and screws and autogenous cancellous bone grafting. Restricted knee motion is associated with a high incidence of failure of fixation.

The principles of management of **infected nonunions** of tibial plateau fractures are debridement of necrotic tissue, stabilization of the nonunion (with plate and screws or an external fixator), management of dead space with antibiotic-impregnated beads or muscle flaps, soft tissue coverage with local or free tissue transfer, and antibiotic coverage based on the sensitivities of the pathogenic organisms. Septic nonunion of the tibial plateau is frequently associated with destruction of the joint. In these cases, knee arthrodesis is performed with an external fixator.

Malunion usually results from inadequate reduction of one or both condyles. If malunion results in malalignment of the limb or joint, a corrective osteotomy should be performed.

Arthrofibrosis is common following tibial plateau fractures and is best treated by prevention with stable fixation and early aggressive physical therapy. In refractory cases, after fracture healing and soft tissue equilibrium has been obtained, arthroscopic or open resection of adhesions and rarely quadriceps-plasty followed by aggressive physical therapy may improve knee motion.

Late subsidence of a reduced tibial plateau occurs in osteopenic patients who have sustained a depressed fracture of the lateral plateau or a low-energy fracture of the medial plateau. At-risk patients are followed closely after weight bearing has been initiated. If subsidence is suspected, weight bearing is discontinued and aggressive physical therapy, in particular active range of motion, is instituted. After 2 to 4 weeks, partial weight bearing in a varus (lateral plateau) or valgus (medial plateau) orthosis is reinstituted and gradually increased. Radiographs are obtained weekly until the patient is bearing full weight. If subsidence has occurred and instability or alteration in the axis of the knee is symptomatic, management with osteotomy or arthroplasty can be considered.

SELECTED READINGS

Ali AM, Burton M, Hashmi M, Saleh M. Treatment of displaced bicondylar tibial plateau fractures (OTA-41C2&3) in patients older than 60 years of age. *J Orthop Trauma* 17:346–352, 2003.

Barei DP, Nork SE, Mills WJ, et al. Complications associated with internal fixation of high-energy bicondylar tibial plateau fractures utilizing a two-incision technique. *J Orthop Trauma* 18:649–657, 2004.

Cole PA, Zlowodzki M, Kregor PJ. Treatment of proximal tibia fractures using the less invasive stabilization system: surgical experience and early clinical results in 77 fractures. *J Orthop Trauma* 18:528–535, 2004.

Gosling T, Schandelmaier P, Marti A, et al. Less invasive stabilization of complex tibial plateau fractures: a biomechanical evaluation of a unilateral locked screw plate and double plating. *J Orthop Trauma* 18:546–551, 2004.

Karunakar MA, Egol KA, Peindl R, et al. Split depression tibial plateau fractures: a biomechanical study. *J Orthop Trauma* 16:172–177, 2002.

Lansinger O, Bergman B, Korner L, Andersson GB. Tibial condylar fractures. A twenty-year follow-up. *J Bone Joint Surg* 68:13–19, 1986.

Moore TM. Fracture-dislocation of the knee. *Clin Orthop* 156:128–140, 1981.

Rasmussen PS. Tibial condylar fractures. *J Bone Joint Surg* 55A:1331–1350, 1973.

Schatzker J, McBroom R, Bruce D. The tibial plateau fracture. The Toronto experience 1968–1975. *Clin Orthop* 138:94–104, 1979.

Weigel DP, Marsh JL. High-energy fractures of the tibial plateau. Knee function after longer follow-up. *J Bone Joint Surg* 84A:1541–1551, 2002.

23 | Injuries to the Knee Extensor Mechanism

Miguel A. Pirela-Cruz   Enes M. Kanlic

Anatomy

The knee extensor mechanism consists of the quadriceps muscles, quadriceps tendon, patella, patellar retinacula, and patellar ligament. Disruption of any of these components will impede active knee extension.

The extensor muscles of the thigh (rectus, vastus lateralis, vastus medialis, and intermedius) form the quadriceps and its tendon, which inserts at the base of the patella. The patella is the largest sesamoid bone in the body. Its anterior surface is convex, lying just under the subcutaneous tissue, which makes it more susceptible to injury. Its posterior surface has three facets covered by thick cartilage that articulate with the trochlea of the femoral condyles. The apex (distal third of the patella) is not covered by cartilage. The patella provides a fulcrum for knee extension, improving the knee's strength. The medial retinaculum is formed from extensions of the fascia lata and the vastus medialis aponeurotic fibers and the lateral retinaculum from the vastus lateralis and the iliotibial tract. The retinacula insert into the proximal tibia and serve as a secondary extensor mechanism. It is possible to have active extension in minimally displaced patellar fractures with preserved retinacula. The patellar ligament is a strong, 5-cm-long structure connecting the patellar apex to the tibial tuberosity.

Biomechanics

Getting from a sitting to a standing position imposes on the patella forces that are three to seven times the weight of the body. That is why the patella has the thickest cartilage (4 to 5 mm) in the body and the fixation of fractures must be sound. The height (thickness) of the patella increases the lever arm in knee extension. Terminal extension (the last 15 degrees) is up to 60% weaker in knees without a patella than in those with the patella intact.

Classification and Nomenclature

The Orthopaedic Trauma Association (OTA) classification describes three main fracture groups (Fig. 23-1). Type A (extraarticular) fractures present with an avulsion of the apex. Type B are partial articular fractures, often vertical, with a preserved extensor mechanism. Type C fractures are articular, with various degrees of complexity and a completely disrupted extensor mechanism.

Division into nondisplaced and displaced fractures is simpler and more practical. Surgery is indicated for displaced fractures distracted more than 3 mm and/or with an intraarticular step-off of more than 2 mm.

Mechanism of Injury

Patellar fractures are caused by a direct blow to the patella, as in an impact against the dashboard of a motor vehicle or a fall on the bent knee. Indirect fractures are avulsion injuries caused by the ligamentum patellae or quadriceps ten-

Group A   Group B   Group C

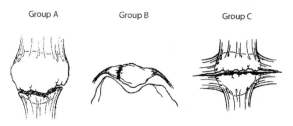

FIG. 23-1   OTA/AO classification: *A*. Extraarticular fracture. *B*. Partial articular fracture. *C*. Complete articular fracture with disrupted extensor mechanism.

don. A transverse patellar fracture may develop from the eccentric contraction of the quadriceps mechanism while a person is landing from a height.

Physical Examination

Patients present with acute pain and a history of trauma. Deformity can be significant in cases with a disrupted capsule or less marked with an intraarticular effusion and hemarthrosis where there is less displacement. The skin must be evaluated to make sure there are no wounds communicating with the fracture or joint. The gap in the knee extensor area is often easily palpable in significant displacements. The most important part of the local exam is to evaluate the integrity of the extensor mechanism (especially if there is no displaced patellar fracture on the radiographs). If the patient is not able to lift the extended leg from the exam table's surface or to hold it extended, there is probably a disruption of the extensor mechanism. Palpation can help to determine the level of rupture (above, below, or at the patella). If pain and swelling are significant, one must aspirate the blood from the joint and inject a local anesthetic. If palpation suggests a higher probability of quadriceps tendon or ligamentum patellae rupture, those areas can be infiltrated. The absence of active extension (when pain is absent or controlled by a local anesthetic) suggests disruption of the extensor mechanism and the need for a surgical repair. One must exclude femoral nerve palsy and evaluate the rest of the lower extremity (active and passive motion of the hip, ankle, and foot as well as sensation and pulses).

Initial Management

If the fracture is not displaced and there is little traumatic effusion, a knee immobilizer or cylinder cast with weight bearing as tolerated is recommended.

A displaced fracture with complete disruption of the extensor mechanism must be treated surgically. In the meantime, the patient needs a knee immobilizer, ice, elevation, and pain medication. If swelling is significant, aspiration and an intraarticular anesthetic with a compressive dressing will provide comfort and a faster recovery.

Associated Injuries

Patellar fractures caused by high-energy direct blows to the knee must be evaluated for additional injuries of the involved extremity. Some 5% of ligamentous injuries of the knee that require treatment occur with patellar fractures.

Radiographic Examination

Anteroposterior and lateral radiographs (including the distal femur and proximal tibia) (see Fig. 23-5A) are essential in evaluating patellar fractures. A skyline view is useful in cases of suspected vertical fractures and/or osteochondral fragments. This is obtained by placing the knee in 45 degrees of flexion and directing the beam from distal to proximal through the anterior aspect of the knee joint (uncomfortable and unnecessary for patients with obvious fractures).

If there is no patellar fracture, the position of the patella must be evaluated. Low position (baja) indicates possible quadriceps disruption (see Fig. 23-7A). High position (alta) suggests injury to the ligamentum patellae (avulsion or rupture) (see Fig. 23-5A).

Magnetic resonance imaging (MRI) is helpful in evaluating associated injuries (ligaments, menisci, or cartilaginous defects).

A bipartite patella, with a rounded lucency in the superior lateral corner (not sharp, as in fresh fractures), is a congenital anomaly and occasionally bilateral.

Nonsurgical Treatment

Injuries with a preserved extensor mechanism are treated with rest, immobilization, ice, and elevation. Patients can bear weight as tolerated for 6 weeks in a hinged brace locked in full extension. As the pain subsides, they can unlock the brace and start active, comfortable range-of-motion exercises (Fig. 23-2A and B).

Displaced fractures treated nonoperatively pose a high risk of significant future problems (extension weakness, posttraumatic arthritis, pain).

Surgical Treatment

Displaced patellar fractures with a fully disrupted knee extensor mechanism require surgical repair in order to regain the best possible long-term function. A midline longitudinal incision allows good access to the injury, avoids the infrapatellar branch of the saphenous nerve, and presents fewer problems for additional surgical procedures (including knee replacement) than a horizontal approach. All displaced fractures have a ruptured retinaculum, and it must be repaired.

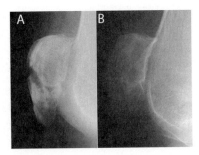

FIG. 23-2   A. Lateral radiograph of patella with less than 3 mm of distraction between fragments. B. In this 74-year-old woman, the fracture healed without surgery and with good function.

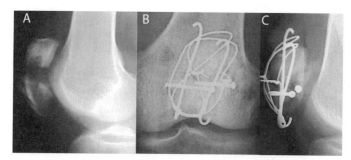

FIG. 23-3   *A.* Lateral radiograph of a complex distracted patellar fracture. *B.* Anteroposterior radiograph showing fixation with modified figure-of-eight tension band and additional screws. *C.* Lateral radiograph of the same patient showing anatomic reduction of the articular surface.

Tension-band wiring is the most commonly used technique and is very effective in transverse fractures. Two longitudinal Kirschner wires prevent intraarticular displacement and guide fragments as compression is exerted by an anterior figure-of-eight tension-band wire during knee flexion. Additional screws or cerclage wires may be necessary in more complex fractures (Fig. 23-3*A* to *C*).

The use of **cannulated screws** instead of longitudinal wires makes the construct stronger and causes less irritation to the surrounding tissues (Fig. 23-4).

Fractures of the patellar apex (distal pole) are extraarticular and repaired with a retrograde screw and washer if the distal bone fragment is large enough or with heavy, nonabsorbable sutures woven through the patellar ligament and pulled through drill holes in the proximal fragment. Distal patellar fractures must be protected by a cable around the proximal patella and through the tibial tuberosity in a figure-of-eight mode. The cable is tightened with the knee in 90 degrees of flexion (Fig. 23-5*A* and *B*).

Patellectomy

In some cases it is impossible to reconstruct badly comminuted fractures. In order to preserve quadriceps strength, the bone debris is removed (**partial**

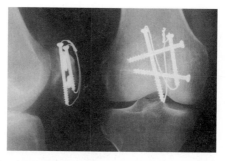

FIG. 23-4   Cannulated screws with figure-of-eight wire pulled through them, providing stable fixation and less irritation of surrounding tissues than would have been possible with prominent K wires.

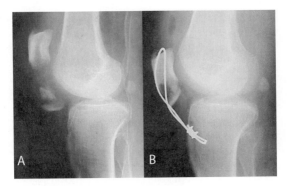

FIG. 23-5　Extraarticular avulsion of the patellar apex with small bone fragments. *B*. Reconstructed ligamentous avulsion with sutures and supporting patellotibial cable.

patellectomy) and the ligamentum patellae or quadriceps tendon reattached to the major bone fragment through drill holes close to the joint surface of the patellar remnants (for better gliding biomechanics). These repairs usually require the additional protection of a cable passed above the patella and through the tibial tuberosity.

In a situation where there are no major bone fragments left, the removal of all bone fragments (**total patellectomy**) and reconstruction of the preserved soft tissue elements of the extensor mechanism is the only solution. These patients can still regain full but weak active extension (Fig. 23-6*A* and *B*).

Postoperative Treatment

After the surgical repair, the knee should be put through a range of motion and the repair tested. C-arm images must be obtained to make sure no displacement has occurred. The amount of flexion possible without displacing the repair will determine the allowed range of motion in the first 4 to 6 weeks of the rehabilitation program. A hinged brace locked in extension allows for full weight bearing; as active flexion improves, it can be adjusted accordingly.

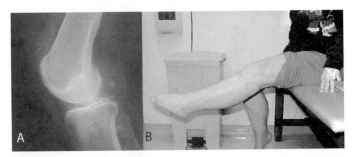

FIG. 23-6　Lateral radiograph of the knee after patellectomy. *B*. Elderly patient 20 years after surgery, with full extension.

Maximum recovery can take up to 1 year. Some 70% of patients achieve good to excellent results.

Complications

Patellofemoral posttraumatic arthritis is a common complication, particularly if there is incongruity or a significant step-off involving the articular surface. Partial patellectomies often result in patellofemoral arthrosis. A significant number of patients complain of discomfort or pain secondary to the hardware, which may require removal. If loss of fixation occurs prematurely, revision of the repair must be done to prevent further displacement and malunion. Nonunions are rare and should be treated surgically only if symptomatic. Stress fractures occur in athletes, starting in the anterior cortex. When diagnosed, they may require fixation. Pain after a patellar fracture is common, and patients should be so advised.

Patellar Dislocations

Lateral dislocation of the patella occurs in adolescents and children with predisposing conditions such as a malaligned extensor mechanism or generalized ligamentous laxity. Such injuries are easily reduced in extension with a distal and medial force on the lateral side of the patella and the patient under sedation. The knee is kept in extension for 4 to 6 weeks, with physical therapy to strengthen the quadriceps. Two-thirds of patients will have cartilage damage (on tangential radiographs, computed tomography, or MRI) and may require surgery for internal fixation of large osteochondral fragments or removal of loose bodies. Half will dislocate again, and in those situations lateral retinacular release and repair of the medial patellofemoral ligament and vastus medialis at the adductor tuberosity or medial capsular reefing is indicated. In special circumstances (e.g., athletic considerations) repair of the patellofemoral ligament and vastus medialis should be considered for an initial injury. In these instances, early protected joint mobilization is crucial to a good result.

Quadriceps Rupture

This injury is rare and occurs in persons above 40 years of age and with predisposing factors such as steroid use, kidney failure, or diabetes mellitus. Tendon ruptures occur during a violent, eccentric contraction of the quadriceps muscles (stumbling on the stairs).

Clinically, these patients present with pain and swelling above the patella. They have difficulty extending the knee, but extension is possible with complete rupture when the patellar retinacula are preserved. Radiographs will reveal patella baja, or an inferiorly positioned patella (Fig. 23-7A). If the diagnosis is uncertain, as in partial ruptures, MRI is helpful; when there is doubt, surgical exploration is prudent.

Treatment

In an acute setting (Fig. 23-7B), surgical reapproximation and direct repair of the quadriceps tendon is feasible. Nonabsorbable materials (e.g., #5 Ethabond) are used to reattach the tendon to the patella with transosseous sutures. In chronic situations or with tenuous tissues, the repair can be augmented with a

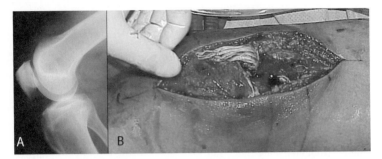

FIG. 23-7   *A.* Patella baja, ruptured quadriceps tendon. *B.* Clinical photo of ruptured quadriceps tendon.

tendon transfer (semitendinosus). The goal is to obtain a stable repair that allows for early, passive motion of the knee and quadriceps rehabilitation.

Rupture of the Patellar Ligament

This injury occurs in persons below 40 years of age, usually after an eccentric contraction of the knee musculature. It can be associated with chronic tendinitis ("jumper's knee") and local steroid injections. On physical examination, the patient is unable actively to extend the knee or to hold it extended, and pain and palpable gap are present at the apex of the patella. Radiographically, a high-riding patella (patella alta) may be observed due to the unopposed pull of the quadriceps tendon. A small avulsion fracture at the patellar apex may occur (Fig. 23-5*A*).

Treatment

Partial tears (complete extension possible) are rare and can be treated nonoperatively by immobilization; however, surgical exploration often shows the injury to be more extensive than anticipated and avoids the problem of dealing with a more complex situation of reconstruction at a later time. Complete disruption requires early surgical intervention. If the piece of bone is still present, a retrograde screw may provide fixation. If there is no substantial bone fragment, then multiple nonabsorbable sutures should capture the patellar ligament (whipstitch technique) and fasten it to the patella through longitudinal transosseous holes (close to the articular surface) for a secure fixation (Fig. 23-5*B*). The medial and lateral retinaculum also require repair.

Delayed recognition occurs with scarred and retracted tissues; in such instances the repair must be augmented with semitendinosus and/or gracilis tendon, released proximally, and pulled through the patella.

All repairs of the patellar ligament should be secured by a cable passed in a figure-of-eight tension-band mode above the patella and through the tibial tuberosity. To avoid shortening of the ligament and a flexion contracture, the cable must be tightened with the knee in 90 degrees of flexion.

The rehabilitation program is similar to that already discussed for injuries of the extensor mechanism: a hinged brace with weight bearing as tolerated in extension and early range-of-motion exercises (passive extension only in the first 6 weeks).

SELECTED READINGS

Carpenter JE, Kasman RA, Patel N, et al. Biomechanical evaluation of current patella fracture fixation techniques. *J Orthop Trauma* 11:351–356, 1997.

Hung LK, Lee SY, Leung KS, et al. Partial patellectomy for patellar fracture: tension band wiring and early mobilization *J Orthop Trauma* 7:252–260, 1993.

Kosanovic M, Komadina R, Batista M. Patella fractures associated with injuries of the knee ligament. *Arch Orthop Trauma Surg* 117:108–109, 1998.

Lieb FJ, Perry J. Quadriceps function. *J Bone Joint Surg Am* 50:1535–1548, 1968.

24 | Diaphyseal Fractures of the Tibia and Fibula

Paul Appleton Charles M. Court-Brown

This chapter reviews fractures of the tibial and fibular diaphysis.

Fractures of the tibial diaphysis are the most common long bone fractures treated by orthopedic surgeons. They have always been regarded as difficult to treat, as—until comparatively recently—cast management was the treatment of choice and the soft tissue defects associated with open fractures could be treated only by basic plastic surgery techniques. Nonunion was common and complications such as compartment syndrome and infection were frequently devastating. However, recent advances such as intramedullary nailing, the detection of compartment syndrome, the management of nonunion and infection, and improved plastic surgery techniques have resulted in improved management and results.

ANATOMY

The proximal and distal 5 cm of the tibia are metaphyseal. The diaphysis of the tibia is triangular in cross section, having medial, lateral, and posterior surfaces separated by anterior, medial, and lateral borders. The anterior border is sharp proximally, but distally it becomes blunt and runs into the medial malleolus. The medial border is blunt proximally but sharpens distally as it runs into the posterior border of the medial malleolus. The lateral border of the tibia is also blunt proximally, but it sharpens as it runs distally into the lateral side of the inferior tibial metaphysis. The medial surface of the tibial diaphysis is subcutaneous, accounting for the high incidence of open tibial fractures. The lateral surface is hollowed proximally for the tibialis anterior muscle. The posterior surface is bounded by the medial and lateral borders and is crossed proximally by the soleal line. This ridge gives rise to the soleus muscle.

The shaft of the fibula is long and slender and has anterior, posterior, and lateral surfaces separated by anterior, posterior, and medial borders. It has a slight spiral twist. A major function of the tibia is to anchor the musculature that controls the movement of the ankle and foot. There are four myofascial compartments in the leg (Fig. 24-1). These compartments are of considerable importance in tibial diaphyseal fractures.

The anterior compartment is bounded by the lateral border of the tibia, the interosseous membrane, the anterior fibula, and the deep fascia. It contains four muscles: the tibialis anterior, extensor hallucis longus, extensor digitorum longus, and peroneus tertius. The muscles are supplied by the deep peroneal nerve and the anterior tibial artery, which runs through the anterior compartment and continues below the ankle joint as the dorsalis pedis artery.

The lateral compartment is contained by the lateral border of the fibula, the deep fascia, and fascial connections between the fibula and deep fascia. It contains the peroneus longus and brevis muscles, which are supplied by the superficial peroneal nerve. The superficial peroneal nerve is at risk during application of external fixators, fibular plating, and proximal cross-locking screws of a tibial nail fracture.

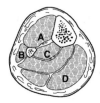

FIG. 24-1   Diagrammatic representation of the compartments of the leg. *A.* Anterior compartment. *B.* Lateral compartment. *C.* Deep posterior compartment. *D.* Superficial posterior compartment.

There are two posterior compartments: deep and superficial. The deep posterior compartment, in addition to the anterior compartment, is most often involved in compartment syndrome. It is bounded by the posterior surface of the tibia, the medial and posterior borders of the fibula, the interosseous membrane, and the fascia, which separates it from the superficial posterior compartment. It contains four muscles: the popliteus, flexor hallucis longus, tibialis posterior, and flexor digitorum longus. All these muscles are supplied by the tibial nerve and the main neurovascular bundle, containing the tibial nerve, and the posterior tibial artery, which runs through the compartment. The superficial posterior compartment is bounded by fascia and contains the gastrocnemius and soleus muscles in addition to the plantaris muscle. These are supplied by branches of the tibial nerve. The sural and saphenous nerves run between the skin and deep fascia and are not associated with specific compartments.

CLASSIFICATION

The OTA classification is widely used for fractures of the tibia and fibular diaphyses (Fig. 24-2). Type A fractures are unifocal and are distinguished by their morphology (A1 fractures are spiral, A2 fractures are short and oblique, and A3 fractures are transverse) and the presence and location of a fibular fracture. The suffix .1 indicates an intact fibula, .2 a fibular fracture distant from the tibial fracture, and .3 a fibular fracture at the same level as the tibial fracture.

Type B fractures are bifocal wedge fractures, with B1 containing intact spiral wedge fractures. B2 are intact bending wedge fractures and B3 are comminuted wedge fractures. The suffixes .1 to .3 are the same as for type A fractures.

Type C fractures are complex multifragmentary segmental or comminuted fractures. C1 fractures are spiral wedge fractures with the suffixes .1 to .3 indicating the number of intermediate fragments. C2 fractures are segmental, with the suffixes .1 to .3 indicating the number of segments and degree of comminution. C3 fractures are comminuted, with .1 to .3 indicating the extent and severity of the comminution.

EPIDEMIOLOGY

Fractures of the tibia and fibula account for 2% of all fractures. About 65% occur in males and the overall average age is about 37 years. The distribution is bimodal, with young males and older females having the highest incidences. About 23% of tibial diaphyseal fractures are open and about 22% are associated with an intact fibula. About 54% are type A unifocal fractures, 28% are type B wedge fractures, and 18% are type C comminuted or segmental fractures.

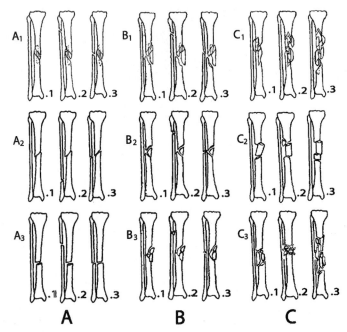

FIG. 24-2   The OTA classification of tibial diaphyseal fractures. [*Orthopaedic Trauma Association Committee for Coding and Classification. Fracture and dislocation compendium.* J Orthop Trauma *10(suppl):51–55, 1996.*]

The most common causes are motor vehicle accidents and sports in young males and falls in older females. There is evidence that the epidemiology of tibial diaphyseal fractures is changing in many countries. Improved road safety and a growing incidence of osteopenic fractures has resulted in an increasing incidence of fractures in the elderly.

CLINICAL HISTORY AND EXAMINATION

Fractures of the tibial diaphysis are usually obvious, the patient presenting with local pain, swelling, and deformity. The possibility of a tibial fracture should be considered in all unconscious or severely injured patients and a thorough physical examination undertaken. A complete history should be obtained from the patient, relative, or caregiver. The cause of the fracture will indicate the extent of the injury and the possibility of coexisting injuries. In the elderly, the history should include details about any comorbid conditions, the patient's prefracture ambulatory status, and his or her domicile, as these factors may alter the treatment and play a role in outcome. Physical examination should include a complete examination of the limb while looking for other injuries. The knee, ankle, and hindfoot must be carefully examined and the vascular and neurologic status of the leg checked. The soft tissues should be checked for evidence of an open fracture. In the multiply injured patient, a complete examination must be undertaken, according to Advanced Trauma Life Support (ATLS) principles.

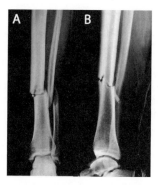

FIG. 24-3   Anteroposterior (*A*) and lateral (*B*) radiographs of an A3.3 fracture of the tibia and fibula. This was a sports injury and a Gustilo type I open fracture.

The possibility of compartment syndrome must be considered in all patients with fractures of the tibial diaphysis. This syndrome may occur within a few hours of the accident, and a thorough examination of the level of pain, sensory loss, muscle function, and pulses is mandatory. Ideally, compartment monitoring should be undertaken at this stage. If there are signs of skin crushing, the possibility of underlying myonecrosis should be considered. This may occur in motor vehicle accidents and may also be seen in drug addicts, alcoholics, and the elderly, all of whom may lie on the ground or a floor for a prolonged period after fracture.

Radiologic Studies

Anteroposterior and lateral radiographs should be sufficient to diagnose a tibial diaphyseal fracture (Fig. 24-3). The knee and ankle must be included to see whether the fracture extends proximally or distally and to check for other musculoskeletal injuries.

A number of features should be looked for on the anteroposterior and lateral radiographs; these are listed in Table 24-1. Computed tomography (CT) and magnetic resonance imaging (MRI) scans are not usually required, although MRI may be useful in diagnosing a stress fracture or an associated ligamentous injury of the knee. Arteriography or Doppler studies may be required if there is suspicion of vascular injury.

TABLE 24-1   Important Features in Anteroposterior and Lateral Radiographs of the Tibia and Fibula

The location and morphology of the fracture
The presence of secondary fractures that might displace intraoperatively
Comminution, which signifies a high-energy injury or osteopenic bone
Widely displaced bone fragments, which may suggest significant soft tissue damage
Bone defects
Damage to knee or ankle joints
The state of the bone—osteopenia, metastases, or previous fracture
Periprosthetic fracture
Gas in the tissues—open fracture or anaerobic infection

Associated Injuries

About 15% of patients with tibial fractures have other musculoskeletal injuries. Approximately 70% of associated injuries are in the lower limbs, and surgeons should be aware of the possibility of an ipsilateral femoral fracture ("floating knee") as well as other fractures of the femur, tibia, and foot. There may be damage to the ipsilateral knee ligaments or a knee dislocation. About 4% of tibial diaphyseal fractures are bifocal, there being other fractures of the tibial plateau, plafond, or ankle in association with the diaphyseal fracture.

TREATMENT

There are four major treatment methods for tibial diaphyseal fractures: intramedullary nailing, external fixation, plating, and nonoperative management. In the last 10 to 15 years, surgeons have focused on intramedullary nailing, although the other methods are used as well. Plating is now less popular, and although nonoperative management is still used for some closed tibial diaphyseal fractures, it is now deemed inappropriate for use in the management of open fractures and it is less commonly used for unstable closed fractures. Traction should not be used, as it confines patients to bed, increases joint stiffness, and may cause compartment syndrome by raising the intracompartmental pressure.

Intramedullary Nailing

In recent years there has been debate about the advantages of reaming the intramedullary canal prior to tibial nailing. Reaming permits the insertion of wider nails, and animal and clinical studies have suggested that it stimulates the periosteal vasculature and is therefore osteogenic. Both reamed and unreamed nails are used to treat tibial diaphyseal fractures; an analysis of the results of both methods in the management of closed and open fractures is given in Table 24-2. The results are taken from the major papers in the literature.

This analysis shows that reamed nails give better results in closed fractures (Fig. 24-4) with a lower incidence of infection, nonunion, and malunion. In open fractures, the benefit of reaming disappears, presumably because the prognosis is governed by the effects of the soft tissue damage, which negates any beneficial effect of reaming.

Fractures of the proximal third of the tibia are difficult to nail. They are usually high-energy comminuted fractures and nailing often results in excessive varus or an anterior bow. Techniques have been described to compensate for this, but external fixation or locked plating is usually easier in proximal tibial fractures, particularly if they are OTA type B or C. Distal tibial fractures can usually be nailed if they are more than 4 cm from the ankle joint. However, if

TABLE 24-2 The Results of Reamed and Unreamed Intramedullary Nailing in Closed and Open Tibial Fractures

	Reamed nails		Unreamed nails	
	Closed	Open	Closed	Open
Union (weeks)	17.1	32.3	25.2	29.3
Infection (%)	1.4	6.5	1.7	6.2
Nonunion (%)	2.1	14.0	15.6	21.4
Malunion (%)	2.1	5.5	5.3	9.2

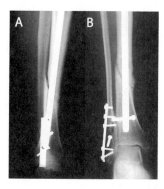

FIG. 24-4   Lateral (*A*) and anteroposterior (*B*) radiographs of a bifocal fracture of the tibia and fibula treated by intramedullary nailing. The ankle fracture was treated conventionally using an interfragmentary screw and a plate.

they are oblique or spiral fractures within 4 cm of the ankle joint, plating or external fixation may be easier.

Complications of Intramedullary Nailing

The complications associated with intramedullary nailing of the tibia are listed in Table 24-3.

The main complication of tibial nailing is knee pain. This is probably multifactorial, being caused by local soft tissue damage, prominent nails, and prominent proximal cross screws. Although about 60% of patients complain of knee pain, about 80% have no pain or only minimal discomfort. It correlates with age, with younger, more active patients complaining of more symptoms. It is usually but not invariably relieved by nail removal. Surgeons have considered that it might be caused by damage to the patellar tendon during nail insertion, but there is no evidence that this is the case. Nail breakage is uncommon and is usually associated with an untreated nonunion. Screw breakage is higher with unreamed nails (25%) vs. reamed nails (3%). Thermal necrosis is caused by excessive reaming with blunt reamers. It may present as osteomyelitis and is usually treated with bone resection and reconstruction.

External Fixation

There has been considerable debate about the ideal type or configuration of external fixator and the ideal stiffness with which tibial diaphyseal fractures should be held by a fixator. There are three basic designs of external fixator:

TABLE 24-3 The Average Results from the Literature of the Main Complications of Tibial Intramedullary Nailing

Knee pain	60%
Neurologic damage	5%
Nail breakage	1%
Screw breakage	3–25%
Thermal necrosis	<1%

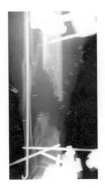

FIG. 24-5   Anteroposterior radiograph of a Gustilo IIIb open fracture of the tibia and fibula treated with a multiplanar external fixator. Note the bone loss and the distal tibial malposition. Malunion is a complication of external fixation.

the uniplanar fixator applied to the subcutaneous border of the tibia; the multiplanar device (Fig. 24-5), which can be constructed in many different configurations; and the ring fixator, which is usually applied with fine wires rather than half pins. There is, however, no evidence that one design or configuration is better than another.

The results of the use of uniplanar and multiplanar external fixators in mixed series of both open and closed tibial diaphyseal fractures are given in Table 24-4.

Precise comparison of papers dealing with external fixation and intramedullary nailing is difficult. However, comparison of the results shown in Tables 24-2 and 24-4 suggests that external fixation is associated with a higher degree of nonunion and malunion vs. intramedullary nailing, although there is a similar incidence of infection. The main complications are pin-tract sepsis, which averages about 32%, and patient compliance. Studies directly comparing intramedullary nailing and external fixation show that intramedullary nailing is associated with faster union, fewer secondary operative procedures, better hindfoot function, and improved walking distance.

Primary external fixation and secondary intramedullary nailing are increasingly used in "damage-control surgery" for the management of tibial diaphyseal fractures in severely injured patients. The primary external fixator can be applied quickly; then the patient can be returned to the operating room from the intensive care unit for definitive nailing when his or her condition has sta-

TABLE 24-4 Results of the Use of Uniplanar and Multiplanar External Fixation in the Treatment of Tibial Fractures[a]

	Uniplanar	Multiplanar
Union (weeks)	25.1	30.7
Nonunion (%)	9.4	18.6
Infection (%)	5.4	9.7
Malunion (%)	24.5	27.9

[a] The quoted series contained 90 to 95% open fractures.

TABLE 24-5 Results of Plating of Tibial Fractures

Union (weeks)	32.1
Infection (%)	4.8
Nonunion (%)	9.5
Malunion (%)	7.4

[a]The results are mostly from mixed series of closed and open fractures (average about 35% open fractures).

bilized. Studies suggest that, provided the nailing is not undertaken in the presence of discharging pin sites, good results can be achieved.

Plating

Primary plating of tibial diaphyseal fractures is now less common than it was 10 years ago. The results from the literature are given in Table 24-5. Plating can give good results, but it is technically more demanding than intramedullary nailing or external fixation.

The results of plating tibial fractures are not as good as those of intramedullary nailing and external fixation; this technique is usually reserved for proximal tibial diaphyseal fractures, where locked plates have been particularly successful. Complications of plating include refracture and fixation failure.

In the last few years the development of locked plates (Fig. 24-6) has elicited renewed interest in the plating of tibial fractures. In locked plates, the screws screw into the plate as well as into the bone. This provides a very strong construct that is particularly useful for osteopenic bone. When used around the tibial metaphyses, these plates can be inserted with minimally invasive techniques under fluoroscopic control. They are particularly useful for those proximal tibial diaphyseal fractures that often occur in older patients; it is likely that their use will increase, although it is unlikely that they will replace intramedullary nailing as the optimal treatment for most diaphyseal fractures.

Nonoperative Management

There are three basic methods of treating tibial diaphyseal fractures nonoperatively: the long leg cast; the patellar tendon–bearing cast, designed to permit knee movement; and the functional brace, designed to allow movement of both knee and hindfoot. The results of all three methods are given in Table 24-6.

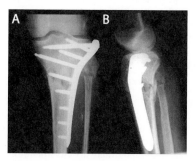

FIG. 24-6   Anteroposterior (A) and lateral (B) radiographs of a LISS locked plate used to treat a proximal tibial fracture.

TABLE 24-6 Results of the Use of Different Casts and Braces in the
Treatment of Mixed Series of Closed and Open Tibial Fractures[a]

	Long leg casts	Patellar-tendon–bearing casts	Functional braces
Union (weeks)	16.5	17.3	18
Nonunion (%)	20.4	12.3	19.5
Malunion (%)	15.7	26.4	16.3
Joint stiffness (%)	26.3	36.1	34.6

[a] Nonunion includes both "delayed" union and nonunion.

Table 24-6 shows that the three different types of casts and braces give similar results. The complications of nonoperative management are not insignificant. The incidence of nonunion is higher with nonoperative than with operative treatment. The incidence of malunion is relatively high, as is the incidence of hindfoot stiffness. The problems associated with such stiffness are often underestimated, but studies have indicated that only 47% of patients managed nonoperatively report a good or excellent result and only 27% report no problems with running.

More recent studies of nonoperative management have tended to concentrate on less severe fractures, as surgeons have adopted operative treatment for the more severe fractures. The technique still has a place in the treatment of low-energy stable fractures in young patients, in whom union is rapid and the incidence of hindfoot stiffness low. A number of studies have directly compared intramedullary nailing and nonoperative treatment; these have highlighted the improved rates of union and better functional outcome associated with intramedullary nailing.

OPEN FRACTURES

The successful treatment of open tibial fractures involves two key components: adequate debridement and rapid, expert soft tissue reconstruction. Debridement should be performed as an emergency procedure and consists of the surgical excision of all contaminated and devitalized tissue. All devitalized bone fragments should be removed. Bone stabilization will usually be with an intramedullary nail or an external fixator. A "second-look" procedure after 36 to 48 h should be undertaken, as adequate assessment of the soft tissues is not always possible initially. If flap cover is required, this should be performed as soon as possible once the wound is "clean." Bone reconstruction may involve grafting or bone transport. The soft tissue defect associated with open tibial fractures may be of a considerable size (Fig. 24-7).

COMPLICATIONS

Nonunion

The incidences of nonunion associated with the different treatment techniques are given in Tables 24-2 and 24-4 to 24-6. Nonunions are either aseptic or infected. The management of infected nonunions is described in the section on infection, below. Aseptic nonunions are best classified as hypertrophic and atrophic. In hypertrophic nonunions, there are clear radiologic signs of incipient fracture healing, and it is likely that the nonunion has occurred for mechanical reasons. Conversely, atrophic nonunions show no evidence of fracture

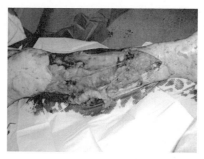

FIG. 24-7   A Gustilo IIIb open tibial fracture in a 52-year-old woman. Note the large area of soft tissue loss and the skin degloving.

union radiographically and occur because of impaired vascularity at the fracture site. This type of nonunion is common after severe open fractures.

The management of hypertrophic nonunion calls for altering the biomechanical environment of the fracture. If the nonunion has followed treatment with a cast or brace, the application of a plate, external fixator, or intramedullary nail will stimulate union. If the hypertrophic nonunion has followed the use of a plate or external fixation device and the nonunion is well aligned, closed intramedullary nailing is the treatment of choice. Atrophic nonunions are managed with autogenous cancellous bone grafting. Should the nonunion persist, the surgeon will have to consider vascularized bone grafts or bone transport.

Exchange intramedullary nailing is useful in the treatment of both hypertrophic and atrophic nonunions that occur after intramedullary nailing. The technique consists of nail removal, reaming of the intramedullary canal by a further 1 to 2 mm, and then the introduction of a wider-diameter nail. In hypertrophic nonunions, the technique is about 90% successful in stimulating union in an average of 10 weeks. It is also useful in atrophic nonunions, although two exchange nailing procedures may be required. It is usually unsuccessful if there is a bone defect greater than 2 cm in size or more than 50% of the bone circumference or if the nonunion is infected.

Malunion

There is no clear definition of malunion; however, 5 degrees of angulation or rotational abnormality and 1 cm of shortening provide a reasonable working definition. There is some evidence that tibial malunion may be associated with an increased incidence of knee and ankle osteoarthritis. If a patient presents with a malunion, care must be taken to determine whether further surgery is worthwhile. Management is corrective osteotomy and stabilization with any of the previously described methods.

Compartment Syndrome

The clinical features of compartment syndrome are discussed in Chap. 1. It is often diagnosed by assessing the patient's clinical signs but is best diagnosed by the use of a pressure monitoring system with a catheter placed in the anterior compartment. The diastolic blood pressure and the intracompartmental pressures are thus assessed on a continuous basis; when the pressure difference (DP) is greater than 30 mmHg, a compartment syndrome has developed.

Studies have highlighted the superiority of this technique over the use of clinical signs. The condition is rare in patients above 35 years of age and mainly affects young males. It occurs in about 7% of closed tibial fractures and in 3 to 6% of open fractures, depending on the extent of the soft tissue damage. Treatment is by four-compartment fasciotomy, which must be implemented emergently. The operation is done through medial and lateral incisions, with the anterior and lateral compartments being decompressed through the lateral incision and the deep and superficial compartments through the medial incision.

Infection

The incidence of infection varies with the treatment method, but the main factor is the degree of soft tissue injury associated with the fracture. In most series, the infection rate for closed fractures is about 2%, rising to about 15% for severe type III open fractures. Treatment depends on the speed of diagnosis. If infection is diagnosed early, before an abscess has formed, high-dose antibiotics will usually be adequate. If a pyogenic collection is present, it should be drained, with reaming of the intramedullary canal to remove any pyogenic membrane. If there is devitalized bone and soft tissue, it should be removed with flap cover and bone reconstruction using bone graft or lengthening. Infected nonunions usually fall into this category.

SPECIAL CONSIDERATIONS

Isolated Tibial Fractures

Until comparatively recently there was considerable debate as to whether an intact fibula conferred a better or worse prognosis than a fracture of the tibial diaphysis. Isolated tibial fractures are common, accounting for about 22% of tibial fractures. They occur in younger patients and are usually low-energy injuries with a predominantly OTA type A morphology. Table 24-7 gives the results of nonoperative management, reamed intramedullary nailing, and external fixation.

There are very few studies of the operative management of these fractures, but Table 24-7 shows that while the nonunion rate is low, the use of nonoperative management is associated with a very high rate of varus malalignment and a high incidence of refracture. It has been shown that the only isolated tibial fracture that maintains its position in a cast is the A3.1 transverse fracture. All other fracture types tend to displace and should be managed operatively using a reamed intramedullary nail.

Isolated Fibular Fractures

Most "isolated fibular fractures" are either type C ankle fractures or avulsion fractures of the proximal fibula associated with a ligamentous knee injury. True isolated fibular fractures are very rare. They are usually caused by a fall or a direct blow. Treatment is symptomatic, with supportive strapping or use

TABLE 24-7 Results of Treating Isolated Tibial Fractures

	Nonoperative	Reamed IM nailing	External fixation
Nonunion	3.1	0	0
Varus deformity	32	0	17.6
Refracture	13.7	0	11.8

of a below-knee walking cast or brace. Nonunions are extremely rare and are best treated by plating and grafting if symptomatic. Proximal fibular fractures may cause damage to the superficial peroneal nerve.

Stress Fractures

Stress fractures are either fatigue fractures occurring in young patients as a result of excessive repetitive loading on normal bone or insufficiency fractures, which result from normal loading on abnormal bone (Fig. 24-8). These generally occur in older patients as a result of age-related osteopenia, osteoporosis, inflammatory joint disease, Paget's disease, and other associated conditions. Tibial stress fractures are usually transverse, although longitudinal fractures have been described. Fatigue fractures are usually seen in the proximal and middle thirds of the tibia, whereas insufficiency fractures are often seen in the distal third of the tibia, frequently close to the ankle joint. With increasing numbers of knee arthroplasties in this population, however, insufficiency fractures of the proximal tibia are becoming more common. Most tibial fatigue fractures occur in military recruits, long-distance runners, and ballet dancers. They usually follow an increase in training or activity. Most insufficiency fractures are associated with osteoporosis or age-related bone loss. Stress fractures of the fibula usually occur just above the lateral malleolus in runners.

The treatment of tibial fatigue fractures is usually nonoperative, with the use of a below-knee cast or patellar tendon–bearing cast. When such fractures fail to unite, they are best treated by reamed intramedullary nailing. Insufficiency fractures of the proximal tibia related to the presence of the cemented or uncemented arthroplasty can be treated nonoperatively if there is no evidence of loosening of the implant. However, if the implant is loose, revision arthroplasty is required. Distal tibial insufficiency fractures are managed nonoperatively.

Metastatic Fractures

Metastatic deposits in the tibia are very uncommon and usually associated with a poor prognosis. Treatment depends on the patient's prognosis, but unless the condition is terminal, stabilization of the tibia should be undertaken. It is best to stabilize the bone before a pathologic fracture occurs; this is usually done with an intramedullary nail. Surgeons should be aware that a mortality rate of up to 10% has been reported in the nailing of pathologic femora.

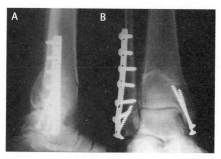

FIG. 24-8 Lateral (*A*) and anteroposterior (*B*) radiographs of an insufficiency fracture in a 78-year-old woman. It occurred shortly after an ankle fracture.

TABLE 24-8 Suggested Protocol for the Treatment of Tibial Fractures

Proximal diaphyseal fractures	
Good alignment	Reamed intramedullary nailing
Poor alignment (comminuted)	Locked plating or periarticular external fixation
Middiaphyseal fractures	Reamed intramedullary nailing
Distal diaphyseal fractures	
Beyond 4 cm of ankle joint	Reamed intramedullary nailing
Within 4 cm of ankle joint	
Transverse fracture	Reamed intramedullary nailing
Other fractures	Plating or periarticular external fixation
Metastatic fractures	Reamed intramedullary nailing
Stress fractures	Nonoperative
Open fractures	Reamed or unreamed intramedullary nailing
	External fixation if comminution is close to joints
Multiple injuries	Consider primary external fixation and later nailing

SUGGESTED TREATMENT

A suggested protocol for the treatment of tibial fractures is presented in Table 24-8. Clearly a number of factors—such as the age, health, and function of the patient—must be taken into consideration in deciding treatment.

SELECTED READINGS

Court-Brown CM. Fractures of the tibial and fibula. In Bucholz RW, Heckman JD (eds). *Rockwood and Green's Fractures in Adults*, 5th ed. Philadelphia: Lippincott Williams & Wilkins, 2001:1939–2000.

Court-Brown CM, Christie J, McQueen MM. Closed intramedullary tibial nailing. Its use in closed and type 1 open fractures. *J Bone Joint Surg* 72B:605–611, 1990.

Court-Brown CM, McQueen MM, Quaba AA, Christie J. Locked intramedullary nailing of open tibial fractures. *J Bone Joint Surg* 73B:959–964, 1991.

Court-Brown CM, Will E, Christie J, McQueen MM. Reamed or unreamed nailing for closed tibial fractures. *J Bone Joint Surg* 78B:580–583, 1996.

Gaebler C, Berger U, Schandelmaier P, et al. Rates and odds ratios for complications in closed and open tibial fractures treated with unreamed, small diameter nails: a multicenter analysis of 467 cases. *J Orthop Trauma* 15:415–423, 2001.

Keating JF, O'Brien PJ, Blachut PA. Interlocking intramedullary nailing of open fractures of the tibia. A prospective, randomised comparison of reamed and unreamed nails. *J Bone Joint Surg* 79A:334–341, 1997.

OTA fracture and dislocation compendium. *J Orthop Trauma* 10(suppl 11):51–55, 1996.

Riemer BL, DiChristina DG, Cooper A, et al. Nonreamed nailing of tibial diaphyseal fractures in blunt polytrauma patients. *J Orthop Trauma* 9:66–75, 1995.

Sarmiento AA, Gersten LM, Sobol PA, et al. Tibial shaft fractures treated with functional braces. Experience with 780 fractures. *J Bone Joint Surg* 71B:602–609, 1989.

Schandelmaier P, Krettek C, Rudolf J, et al. Superior results of tibial rodding versus external fixation in grade 3b fractures. *Clin Orthop* 342:164–172, 1997.

Tornetta P, Bergman M, Watnik N, et al. Treatment of grade-IIIb open tibial fractures. A prospective randomised comparison of external fixation and non-reamed locked nailing. *J Bone Joint Surg* 75B:13–19, 1994.

Trafton PG. Tibial shaft fractures. In Browner BD, Jupiter JB, Levine AM, Trafton PG (eds). *Skeletal Trauma*, 3d ed. Philadelphia: Saunders, 2003:2131–2255.

| Indirect Fractures and
Dislocations of the Ankle

Arsen M. Pankovich   *John A. Elstrom*
Chris John Dangles

Indirect ankle fractures are among the most common fractures in the body. They fascinated surgeons in the nineteenth century, who, as a result, (1) described the gross and functional anatomy of the ankle; (2) discovered various mechanisms of injury by extensive studies in cadavers; (3) classified various fracture types and described their clinical appearance; and (4) established the basic principles of conservative treatment, which influenced generations of surgeons well into the middle of the twentieth century. Initially, at a time when invasive surgery was at its very beginnings, these surgeons had no radiography with which to visualize a fracture in all its complexity (Fig. 25-1). A number of surgeons from many different countries have described ankle injuries (Potts, Dupuytren, Maisonneuve, Lauge-Hansen). Some eponyms still linger, although they are fading steadily away with the universal acceptance of classification systems based on the mechanism of injury or anatomic description. The fascination with ankle fractures has shifted to other subjects, as successful surgical treatment has become commonplace owing to the wide influence of the Association for Osteosynthesis (AO) materials and methods.

The topics covered in this chapter are ankle anatomy, mechanisms of ankle injuries, classification of various lesions, diagnosis, initial and definitive management, and complications and their management.

ANATOMY

Three bones form the ankle: the body of the talus with its trochlea (superior articular surface) and the medial and lateral articular surfaces, the distal tibia with articular surfaces of the plafond and medial malleolus, and the articular surface of the lateral malleolus of the fibula (Fig. 25-2).

The distal tibia consists of the plafond, the weight-bearing articular surface, the medial malleolus, the anterior and posterior processes, and the lateral surface. The **plafond** is concave from front to back (sagittal plane) and flat or more often slightly convex from side to side (coronal plane). **The medial malleolus** is formed by the slender, distally protruding anterior colliculus and a broader posterior colliculus, which are separated by the intercollicular groove. The **lateral surface**, lying between the anterior (Tillaux-Chaput) and posterior (Volkmann) tibial tubercles, is concave and triangular; it forms the tibiofibular syndesmosis with the corresponding surface on the fibula and contains the interosseous ligament. The plafond and the medial and lateral malleoli form the **ankle mortise**, and the body of the talus fit perfectly into it.

The **talus** consists of a head, neck, and body. The head articulates with the navicular bone. The body of the talus viewed from above shows various degrees of wedging of its trochlea, being wider anteriorly at an average of 2.4 mm (up to 6 mm). When viewed from the front, the trochlea looks concave; when viewed from the side, it looks convex. The medial and lateral articular surfaces are slightly concave and convex, respectively, to various degrees, which gives the trochlea a conical shape.

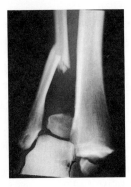

FIG. 25-1   Dupuytren's fracture, described c. 1810.

The mortise closely approximates the shape of the talus, and these elements have a close, congruent fit throughout the arc of motion. Only slight rotatory or lateral motion of the lateral malleolus (from zero to not more than 2 mm) has been observed in cadaver testing when the talus was dorsiflexed, and this depended on the amount of the anterior wedging of the trochlea. Thus, the mortise only rarely becomes too narrow after a tight syndesmotic screw fixation. Dorsiflexion of the ankle prior to insertion of a screw is prudent, as it cannot be predicted which ankle mortise will become too tight to permit full dorsiflexion.

It was determined that ankle motion occurs around a single axis in 80% of cases. Practically, the axis extends, with some variation in its plane, between the tips of the medial and lateral malleoli.

Nine ligaments and the capsule provide stability to the ankle during weight bearing and at rest (Fig. 25-3). On the lateral side of the ankle, the **tibiofibular syndesmosis** is held together by the anterior tibiofibular ligament, the interosseous ligament, the interosseous membrane, the posterior tibiofibular ligament, and the inferior transverse ligament (Fig. 25-3; 1a, 1b, 1c, and 1d).

The **deltoid ligament** provides a strong medial support. It consists of two portions (layers). The superficial deltoid ligament originates mostly from the

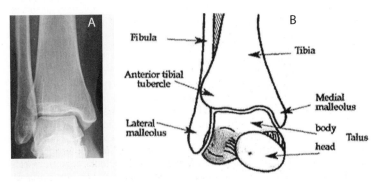

FIG. 25-2   Normal ankle. *A.* Anteroposterior radiograph. *B.* Drawing of osseous anatomy of the anterior ankle.

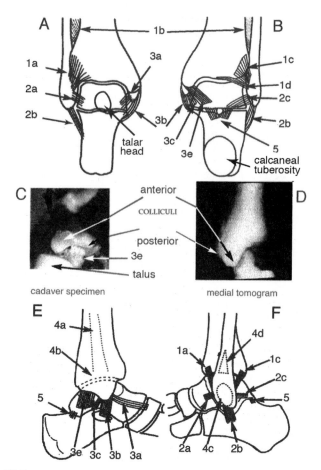

FIG. 25-3 Ligaments of the ankle, 1 (a, b, c, and d). Ligaments of the syndesmosis, 2 (a, b, and c). Lateral collateral ligaments, 3 (a, b c, and d). Deltoid ligament, 4. Landmarks: a. Outline of the fibula on the medial ankle view. b. Outline of the ankle joint in a lateral projection. c. Outline of the syndesmosis, the site of the interosseous ligaments. 5. Posterior talocalcaneal ligaments.

anterior colliculus and has three distinct parts that attach to the navicular bone (naviculotibial ligament), the sustentaculum tali on the os calcis (calcaneotibial ligament), and the anterior part of the medial tubercle of the talus (superficial talotibial ligament) (Fig. 25-3; 3a, 3b, and 3c). The deep deltoid ligament originates from the posterior colliculus and the intercollicular groove and consists of two parts: a small band between the posterior colliculus and the medial talar tubercle (deep anterior talotibial ligament) lying under the superficial deltoid and the strong and wide ligamentous band (deep posterior talotibial ligament), which is the main stabilizing structure that holds the talus reduced in the ankle mortise (Fig. 25-3; 3d and 3e).

Lateral collateral ligaments on the lateral side, the anterior and posterior talofibular and calcaneofibular ligaments, bridge both the ankle and subtalar joints and provide their lateral stability (Fig. 25-3; 2a, 2b, and 2c).

The **crural fascia** envelops the tendons, which pass over the ankle. Four fibrous bands, which serve as pulleys for tendons, reinforce the crural fascia: anteriorly the transverse and cruciate crural ligaments, medially the laciniate ligament, and laterally the peroneal retinacula. In addition, they provide stability to the ankle by holding tendons, when contracted, in proximity to bones.

Tendons that pass over the ankle are anteriorly, from medial to lateral, the tibialis anterior, extensor hallucis longus, extensor digitorum longus, and peroneus tertius; laterally, the peroneus longus and peroneus brevis; and, posteriorly, the flexor hallucis longus, flexor digitorum longus, posterior tibialis, and Achilles tendon.

The **blood supply** to the ankle and foot is derived from the dorsalis pedis and the posterior tibial and peroneal arteries, accompanied with their veins. The saphenous vein is situated anteromedially.

Nerves that cross the ankle are, anteriorly, the deep and superficial branches of the peroneal nerve; posteromedially, the tibial nerve; and posterolaterally, the sural nerve.

PATHOMECHANICS OF ANKLE INJURIES

It is obvious and accepted by most authorities that indirect ankle fractures and dislocations occur because of the action of various forces or combinations of forces on the normal ankle structures, in particular on the talus.

In order for such forces to cause pathologic motions of the talus, the subtalar joint must be locked from positioning of the foot. The force that locks the subtalar joint further forces the talus in a particular direction. These talar motions, responsible for injuries of the ligaments and of the adjacent parts of the tibia and fibula, are all pathologic and do not occur during normal ankle motion with weight bearing. Obviously, body weight is transmitted to the ankle and foot and increases the amount of force delivered to the talus.

In order to lock the talus, the foot moves to either supination or pronation; thus these motions are included in the descriptions of particular injuries.

The following **pathologic motions** have been observed:

Abduction. Essentially no medial tilting of the talus occurs in the ankle, as the deltoid ligament holds it firmly in place.

Adduction. Lateral talar tilt even up to 20 or 30 degrees is known to exist in some normal ankles; the collateral ligaments must be relatively taut for the talus to cause injuries to the collateral ligaments, although slack ligaments would allow the tilting talus to engage the medial malleolus and produce a typical vertical fracture.

External rotation. Only 1 to 2 degrees of external rotation is known to occur in some ankles when full dorsiflexion is reached; any further rotation is considered pathologic.

Internal rotation. This does not occur during normal ankle motions.

These facts constitute the basis of the functional classification of ankle injuries as described by Lauge-Hansen.

CLASSIFICATION OF INDIRECT ANKLE FRACTURES

A great deal has been written and much more argued about the usefulness of any of the available classifications of the indirect fractures and the dislocations. Most commonly cited are the AO anatomic classification as accepted by the Orthopaedic Trauma Association (OTA) and the Lauge-Hansen functional classification and its extension. It seems that both classifications are useful, though both have been considered too complex and impractical for general use in clinical practice.

OTA/AO Classification

The classification, originally developed by Danis and Weber, was accepted and refined by the AO group and was adopted by OTA and the *Journal of Orthopaedic Trauma*. It remains the most popular for its simple grouping of the three main fracture types (A, B, C), which are based on the state and the level of the lateral bone–ligament complexes and the level of the fibula where they occur. Three subtypes and further three sub-subtypes of each main type have been described; they reflect the significant anatomic variety of the indirect fractures. Although an extensive group of fractures is presented in this classification, the lesions are catalogued in a systematic and logical order that is easy to understand and use.

The Lauge-Hansen Classification and Its Extended Modification

This classification is based on the mechanism of the injury and presents four main types. Each fracture type has incremental and sequential stages of injuries, specific and typical to each type. The four common types are the supination–external rotation (SE) type (Fig. 25-4), the pronation–external rotation (PE) type, the supination–adduction (SA) type (Fig. 25-5), and the pronation–abduction (PA) type (Fig. 25-6). There are some other specific fracture types, which are encountered less often in the practice.

Typical Lesions

In using either classification, one must understand the typical lesions that occur in any given type. The basic ligamentous structure is the **ligamentous complex**, which consists of a particular ligament and of the insertion sites at both ends. When the ligamentous complex is injured, the lesion can occur at five points: the ligament can be partially or completely ruptured in its substance, it can be avulsed at each end, and it can avulse the bone at the insertion site. The specific sites of bone avulsion have been described:

1. **Tillaux-Chaput's fracture**, an avulsion of the anterior tibial tubercle of the same name by the anterior tibiofibular ligament
2. **Wagstaffe's or Le Fort's fracture**, an avulsion of the anterior fibular tubercle by the anterior tibiofibular ligament
3. **Volkmann's fracture**, an avulsion of the posterior tibial tubercle by the posterior tibiofibular ligament

One further typical lesion should be recognized: **fracture of the posterior process of the tibia**. The fragment is large and often takes the posterior third of the tibial plafond. The lesion is caused by a vertical shearing force of the talus driven proximally while the ankle is plantarflexed. The lesion causes ankle instability and a tendency for posterior subluxation or dislocation of

AO CLASSIFICATION SYSTEM

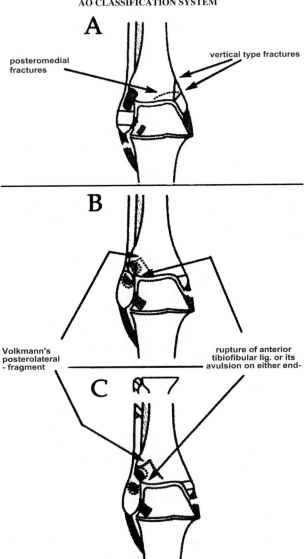

A

posteromedial fractures

vertical type fractures

B

C

Volkmann's posterolateral - fragment

rupture of anterior tibiofibular lig. or its avulsion on either end-

A

In all A type: intact syndesmosis
                    never a deltoid rupture

A1:_1_2_3 -rupture of lateral collateral ligaments
or
-fracture of lateral malleolus below syndesmosis

A2:_1_2_3 -one of the A1 lesions
plus
-a fracture of the medial malleolus

A3:_1_2_3 -one of the A1 lesions
plus
-a posteromedial fracture of the
medial malleolus

B

B1:_1_2_3 -simple oblique or comminuted
fracture of the lateral malleolus at syndesmosis
-rupture of the anterior tibiofibular ligament
-intact medial side

B2:_1_2_3 -one of B1 lesions
plus
-fracture of medial malleolus, or
rupture of deltoid ligament

B3:_1_2_3 -lesions as in B2
plus
-Volkmann's fragment posterolaterally

C

In all C types:
-medially--malleolar fracture or deltoid rupture
-complete rupture of syndesmosis

C1:_1_2_3 short oblique ⎫
                              ⎬ | fractures of fibula
                              ⎭ | above syndesmosis |
C2:_1_2_3 comminuted

C3:_1_2_3 injuries at ——————— upper fibula
plus
Volkmann's fragment posterolaterally

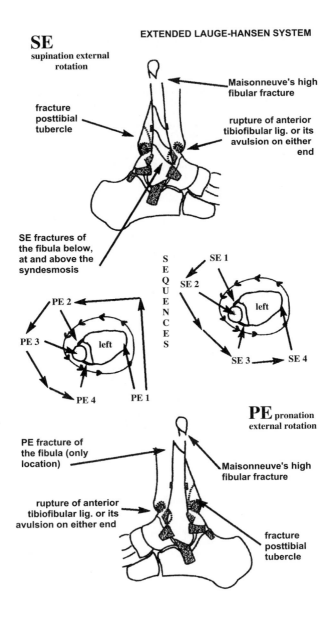

SE supination external rotation

EXTENDED LAUGE-HANSEN SYSTEM

Maisonneuve's high fibular fracture

fracture posttibial tubercle

rupture of anterior tibiofibular lig. or its avulsion on either end

SE fractures of the fibula below, at and above the syndesmosis

SEQUENCES

SE 1
SE 2
left
SE 3 ⟶ SE 4

PE 2
PE 3
left
PE 4   PE 1

PE pronation external rotation

PE fracture of the fibula (only location)

Maisonneuve's high fibular fracture

rupture of anterior tibiofibular lig. or its avulsion on either end

fracture posttibial tubercle

EXTENDED LAUGE-HANSEN SYSTEM

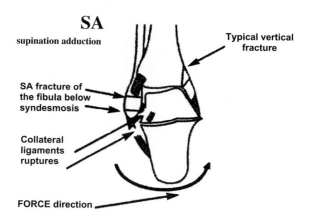

SA
supination adduction

Typical vertical fracture

SA fracture of the fibula below syndesmosis

Collateral ligaments ruptures

FORCE direction

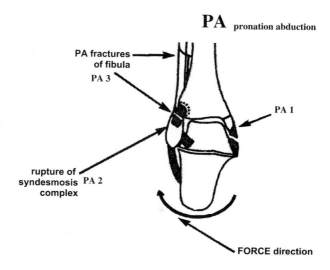

PA
pronation abduction

PA fractures of fibula

PA 3

PA 1

rupture of syndesmosis complex   PA 2

FORCE direction

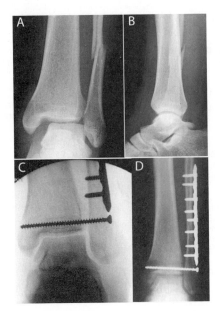

FIG. 25-4   SE-4 (above the syndesmosis) Lauge-Hansen ankle fracture. *A.* Initial anteroposterior view. *B.* Lateral view. *C.* Intraoperative spot image. *D.* Treated with plate fixation and a syndesmotic screw. (*Courtesy of Robert F. Hall, Jr., M.D.*)

the ankle. Surgical fixation of this fragment in an anatomic position is mandatory (Fig. 25-7).

DIAGNOSIS AND INITIAL MANAGEMENT

History and Physical Examination

The history of injury is rarely helpful because the patient can seldom describe the direction of the injuring force. On physical examination, areas of ecchy-

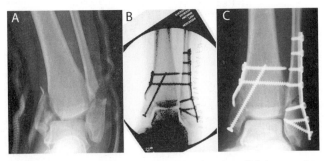

FIG. 25-5   SA fracture. *A.* Initial anteroposterior view. *B.* Intraoperative spot image. *C.* Treated with plate-and-screw fixation and an antiglide spring plate to stabilize the vertical medial fracture. (*Courtesy of Robert F. Hall, Jr., M.D.*)

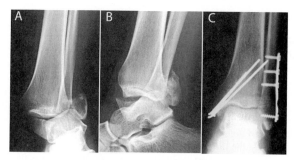

FIG. 25-6   PA fracture (low at the syndesmosis). *A.* Initial anteroposterior view. *B.* Intraoperative spot film. *C.* Treated with ORIF.

mosis, swelling, and tenderness are assessed over the anteromedial and posteromedial joint line and laterally over the entire length of the fibula. The condition of the skin is noted. Frequently, the skin will be contused or even damaged. Gentle manipulation of the ankle may show gross instability.

Ottawa Rules

A great number of ankle injuries are seen in emergency departments; only about 15 to 20% of these are found to involve a fracture. Obviously the number

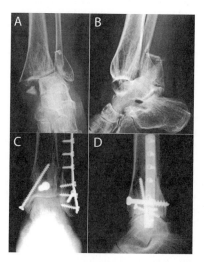

FIG. 25-7   SE-4 fracture with a large posterior tibial fragment that requires AP compression screw fixation. Initial anteroposterior view shows the fracture of a fibula, lateral displacement of the talus, and a fracture of the anterior colliculus of the medial malleolus (*A*). The lateral view shows a large, proximally displaced fragment of the tibia (*B*). Postoperative anteroposterior (C) and lateral (*D*) views show fracture fixation. The cortical screw used in the medial malleolus was inserted as a lag screw by overdrilling the distal fragment. (*Courtesy of Robert F. Hall, Jr., M.D.*)

of negative radiographs is substantial. The Ottawa group has proposed a specific protocol to exclude the presence of a fracture by clinical examination, thus eliminating unnecessary radiographs from the workup in some instances (30 to 40%). However, although significantly reduced, the number of negative radiographs is still high (40 to 50%). This protocol, known as **Ottawa rules**, states that a patient requires ankle radiography if there is subjective pain in the malleolar areas and at least one of the following: (1) tenderness over the posterior edge and surface of the lateral malleolus (which should include palpation along the entire length of the fibula to look for a more proximal fracture), (2) tenderness of the posterior edge of the medial malleolus, and (3) inability to bear weight at the time of injury upon examination.

Almost 100% accuracy in excluding ankles without a fracture has been experienced; thus there can be a significant reduction, with a high degree of confidence, in the number of negative radiographs taken in the emergency department. In spite of convincing reports, the Ottawa rules are not yet in wide use, perhaps related to a degree of uncertainty and the need for radiographic reassurance on the part of the examiner as well as potential legal implications.

Radiographic Examination

The standard radiographic examination consists of anteroposterior, lateral, and mortise views. The mortise view or true anteroposterior view of the ankle is obtained with the foot in 20 degrees of internal rotation. The radiographs are examined with the following six points in mind:

1. Presence and type of a fracture of the medial malleolus or its colliculi.
2. Presence, type, and location of a fracture of the fibula. The direction of the fracture usually mirrors the mechanism of injury. In addition, the level of the fibular fracture indicates the extent of the injury, as fractures above the syndesmosis indicate a more severe injury and an unstable syndesmosis.
3. The state of the deltoid ligament and its deep portion, particularly when the initial radiographs show no widening of the medial clear space. When a pronation fracture of the fibula is present, the deltoid ligament is ruptured. When a supination fracture of the fibula is present and the medial malleolus is intact, the deltoid ligament may or may not be ruptured. Stress radiographs are required.
4. When there is an injury of the medial ligamentous complex without a fracture of the fibula at the ankle, the entire length of the fibula is radiographed to determine whether there is a high fibular fracture.
5. Other associated fractures should be recognized, such as those involving the posterior tibial process, the anterior and posterior tibial tubercles, and the anterior fibular tubercle.
6. The dome of the talus is examined for osteochondral fractures.

Stress Radiographs

External rotation stress radiographs are obtained when there is an indication that the deltoid ligament may be ruptured despite the fact that the mortise appears intact. The foot is gently rotated externally and a mortise view of the ankle obtained. The width of the clear space between the lateral tibial plafond and the lateral talus is determined. Likewise, the width of the clear space at the corner where the tibial plafond joins the medial malleolus and the medial corner of the talus is determined. A difference greater than 3 mm between these two measurements indicates a ruptured deltoid ligament (Fig. 25-8).

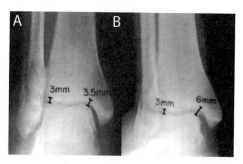

FIG. 25-8 Stress radiograph in assessment of medial instability. *A.* A normal ankle where the joint space is equal medially and laterally. *B.* A rupture of the deep deltoid ligament, as shown by widening of the medial clear space.

Other Imaging Techniques

Tomography, computed tomography (CT), magnetic resonance imaging (MRI), and arthrography are rarely necessary in evaluating indirect fractures of the ankle. These studies can be useful in evaluating a soft tissue injury, the presence of bone comminution, or the location of an occult fracture.

Initial Management

Subluxations or frank dislocations are reduced by pulling in line with the deformity. The ankle is splinted, elevated, and iced. Excessive swelling, ecchymosis, and blisters usually improve sufficiently with this regimen that surgery can take place within 4 to 7 days.

While stable and undisplaced fractures can be treated conservatively by splinting and discharge from the emergency department, more advanced lesions are splinted and the patients admitted for surgical treatment.

Associated Injuries

Associated injuries of neurovascular structures are rare, but they should be ruled out with a careful focused examination of the extremity. Compartment syndrome is occasionally associated with indirect fractures of the ankle; if it is suspected on the basis of the clinical examination, compartment pressures are measured.

Definitive Management

The decision on the definitive method of management depends on the evaluation of the particular injury. The following factors must be considered.

Is the fracture stable? Even an undisplaced fracture can be inherently unstable. Probably the most deceiving lesion is a PE fracture of the fibula located above syndesmosis that is usually undisplaced; it is accompanied by a rupture of the deltoid ligament and the unstable syndesmosis, yet may look on the radiographs like a simple fracture of the fibula. Casting, even a stress radiograph, would be a waste, since the talus would inevitably displace in a cast. On the other hand, an SE fracture of the fibula above syndesmosis can be stable, as the medial side and the posterior tibiofibular complex might be intact. Stress radiographs usually resolve the question of instability. Cast immobilization is indicated if the medial side proves to be stable. Generally most lesions with a fracture of both malleoli or a deltoid rupture are unstable and require surgical reduction and stabilization.

Most displaced fractures of the fibula, particularly if there is any shortening, require open surgical reduction and internal fixation, even when the medial complex is intact. Shortening of the fibula at the fracture site has been shown to reflect incongruity at the distal articulation, probably because there is also anterior or posterior displacement of the lateral malleolus, which also contributes to the incongruity.

Displaced and even many nondisplaced fractures of the medial malleolus require internal fixation, as most such complete fractures tend to displace in a cast. If the fibular fracture is treated by internal fixation, any undisplaced fracture of the medial malleolus should also be internally fixed to avoid subsequent procedures that might be necessitated by displacement, which can occur even weeks later. Closed reduction of a displaced fracture of the medial malleolus is not an acceptable treatment, as redisplacement and nonunion occur too often. The high incidence of nonunion in conservatively treated fractures is attributed to interposition of the periosteum between the fracture fragments and to inhibition of healing by synovial fluid from the ankle joint. Undisplaced fractures of the anterior colliculus can sometimes be left unfixed, when isolated and undisplaced, although any subsequent displacement would require internal fixation, considering that the fragment is a part of the medial articular surface. Vertical fractures of the medial malleolus are extremely unstable and invariably are better treated by internal fixation. Fractures of the posterior colliculus are rare and most often remain undisplaced as a single large fragment, as they are held in place by the the flexor tendons situated in the fibrous canal over the posterior malleolar groove. Unless displaced, fractures of the posterior colliculus require no internal fixation.

Smaller fracture fragments of the Tilluax-Chaput or Volkmann tubercles rarely need internal fixation. A larger posteromedial or posterolateral fragment requires anatomic reduction and internal fixation.

A Wagstaffe–Le Fort's fragment is often a part of comminution of the lateral malleolus; as such, it is routinely fixed with the main fracture.

The tibiofibular syndesmosis is generally destabilized in all complete lesions of fractures at or above the syndesmosis and in some SE fractures below the syndesmosis (mixed oblique fracture of the lateral malleolus, Destot). In some of these fractures, the anterior tibiofibular complex is intact, even in a complete lesion, where there is also a fracture of the medial malleolus and injury of the posterior tibiofibular complex. Isolated displaced fractures of this type are rare. Unstable syndesmosis has also been noted in a lesion often referred to as a complete ligamentous diastasis of the ankle, where the deltoid ligament is ruptured as well as all ligaments of the syndesmosis, including the interosseous membrane. The lesion is the second stage of a posteroanterior lesion. An unstable syndesmosis requires recognition at surgery, as it is usually part of a complete lesion. It is thought that persisting fibular instability is the result of a complete rupture of the interosseous ligament and of multiple smaller anterior and posterior interosseous fibers as well as a rupture of the interosseous membrane to and often above the site of the fibular fracture. Although all ligaments of the syndesmosis might appear disrupted, the decision to stabilize it should be made only after the fixation of all fractures. Although instability of the fibula at the syndesmosis can be diagnosed by grasping it with an instrument and pulling it anteroposteriorly and laterally, many surgeons prefer to do an intraoperative stress radiograph, which seems more objective. If unstable, the fibula is transfixed with a 3.5-mm (4.5 mm in a large or heavy individual) cortical screw, which transfixes the fibula and engages the medial cortex of the tibia (Fig. 25-5). In doing this, it is recommended to dorsiflex the ankle maximally before inserting the screw across the tibial cortex in order to prevent the overapproximation of the fibula to the tibia. In situations where the anterior width of the talar trochlea is increased, a reduction of ankle dorsiflexion can result from a tight ankle mortise. In situations where the fibular fracture is proximal (e.g., Maisonneuve injury) and not stabilized by internal fixation, it may be prudent to use two 4.5-mm cortical screws.

The deltoid ligament is rarely if ever repaired. It constantly heals without significant residual instability. When repair is indicated, it requires attachment to the talus, where it is commonly detached, or to the medial malleolus, by passage of the sutures through the drill holes in the bone and by partially decorticating the bone at the site of the attachment.

Surgical Techniques

Open Reduction

The procedure is usually done under tourniquet hemostasis.

Incisions and exposure. An incision is made laterally over the fibula. When practical it is extended distally and anteriorly directly over the distal syndesmosis. In a high fibular fracture, a second smaller incision can be made at the syndesmosis. Exposure of the medial side is through a curved incision centered over the anterior medial corner of the mortise, or a straight incision is sometimes made and centered over the medial malleolus. The skin is handled carefully to avoid injuring it further. The crural fascia is detached from its attachment to the lateral fibula and allowed to retract. This sometimes releases the swollen tendons and muscles and allows easier reduction of the fibula, which is often displaced anteriorly by the taut crural fascia. The dome of the talus is examined, as are the anterior tibiofibular and talofibular ligament complexes. The joint is inspected for the presence of loose (osteo)chondral fragments, which should be removed or washed out. The articular defects, particularly on the talar dome, are common and must not be overlooked; they should be debrided and drilled to facilitate their repair and possible regeneration of cartilage.

Fixation of the fibular fracture. A standard **interfragmentary screw fixation** is done or, when necessary, in a case of comminution, temporary or permanent cerclage **wire** or **pin fixation** in order to reduce and hold together the reduced fragments of the fibula. Then a one-third **semitubular neutralization plate** is attached posterolaterally to the fibula. Alternatively, **antiglide fixation** with a more posteriorly placed one-third semitubular plate can provide a good stabilization.

Fixation of medial malleolar fractures. The medial malleolus is reduced and held with a clamp while a 4.0-mm cancellous screw is inserted over a guidewire. Two screws are rarely needed in fixation of a noncomminuted malleolar fragment. A fracture of the anterior colliculus should not be overlooked on preoperative radiographs. It must be handled very carefully to avoid splitting it. A single 4.0-mm cancelous screw, inserted over a guidewire, provides good fixation. The temptation of inserting two screws should be resisted, since irreparable comminution of the small fragment can lead to unsatisfactory reduction and fixation. Instead, it is advisable to fix smaller fragments with a wire tension band.

Deltoid ligament repair. When repair is indicated, it requires attachment to the talus, where it is commonly detached, or to the medial malleolus, by passage of the sutures through the drill holes in the bone and by partially decorticating the bone at the site of the attachment.

Fixation of the posterior fragments. Larger posteromedial or posterolateral fragments require anatomic reduction and internal fixation. Depending on their size, they can be fixed with a front-to-back lag screw after the fragment is reduced by forced dorsiflexion (Fig. 25-9). Direct exposure and reduction and internal fixation are also utilized in many cases. The stability of the distal fibula at the syndesmosis is examined in the last step and handled as described above.

Bone grafting. If bone grafting of an impacted medial or lateral plafond is required, cancellous bone is obtained from the ipsilateral distal femur or the tibia or an allograft or commercial bone substitute can be used. Careful assessment of the reduction is paramount for avoiding articular incongruity and preventing the development of posttraumatic osteoarthritis.

Postoperative management. A short leg splint is applied at the end of the procedure and a short leg cast prior to discharge. At 2 weeks, the cast is taken

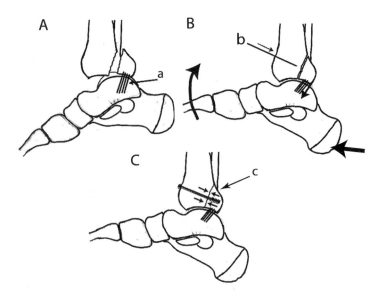

FIG. 25-9   Fixation of a large posterior fragment by a front-to-back lag screw. *A.* The fragment is displaced posteriorly and superiorly and the talus subluxed. *B.* Forward translation and dorsiflexion of the foot reduces the talus by pull of the posterior capsule and remaining intact ligaments. *C.* A lag screw is inserted over the guidewire and it compresses fracture fragments (*C*).

off, the sutures are removed, and a commercial removable cast is applied. Range-of-motion exercises are undertaken at that time. In simple noncomminuted fractures, cast immobilization is discontinued at this time if the deltoid ligament is intact. The patient is allowed full weight bearing at 6 weeks.

Closed Reduction

Closed reduction of displaced fractures is rarely indicated because redisplacement is common and the outcome uncertain. It is indicated when local conditions at the ankle, such as infected cellulitis and deep abrasions, make open reduction undesirable. Closed reduction, preferably under general or regional anesthesia, is performed by applying traction on the foot and supinating it after obtaining the length to reduce the medial malleolus or to reduce the talus in the mortise, which also reduces the fibula into the syndesmosis by a pull of the collateral ligaments. Residual mild displacement of the fibula at the fracture site is commonly unavoidable. During the procedure, radiographic imaging is mandatory. Postoperatively and after casting, conventional radiographs are obtained. When reduction is lost, the procedure is repeated during the same session. If reduction is lost on subsequent radiographs, another operative reduction is justified in a few days and after a further reduction in swelling. A long leg cast is commonly applied after closed reduction; it is changed or adjusted as required. The cast is usually worn for 8 to 10 weeks. Weight bearing is allowed only after the fracture has healed.

Cast Immobilization without Reduction

An isolated, usually undisplaced or minimally displaced fibular fracture at any level is treated by cast immobilization after the stability of the syndesmosis and the deltoid complex has been determined. Sometimes immediately and very often after a few weeks of immobilization in a cast, a commercially available removable cast is prescribed for further immobilization. After 2 to 3 weeks and once the local pain has subsided, range-of-motion exercises are started. Weight bearing is begun at about the same time. Immobilization is continued for 4 to 6 weeks, when periosteal callus bridging the fracture site is usually observed.

Complications

Complications of indirect ankle fractures include posttraumatic osteoarthritis, infection, and nonunion. **Posttraumatic osteoarthritis** is rather rare after an indirect ankle fracture. The cause can be attributed to the unrecognized and untreated impaction fractures of the plafond, to scuffing or compression of the articular cartilage surface at the time of injury, and from comminution of the articular surface even after an anatomic reduction. Healing of inadequately reduced fractures is seen less often nowadays, with an understanding of the benefits of an anatomic reduction achieved by open reduction and internal fixation.

Postoperative infection is rare though more common on the lateral side. Breakdown of skin over the plate has been observed. Treatment with antibiotics and local wound care will often suffice. Any infection can be controlled, and although the wound will be open, the fibular fracture will still heal. The plate can then be removed to allow wound healing, which is usually rather rapid. Chronic osteomyelitis is indeed rare.

Nonunion of the fibula is very infrequent and responds well to local bone grafting. Nonunion of the medial malleolus is essentially nonexistent after open reduction and internal fixation.

The dictum in the treatment of ankle fractures, as in fractures of other joints, is achieving a healed fracture in an anatomic position as well as a stable joint. The patient should know that despite an excellent anatomic surgical result, the absence of complications, early joint mobilization, and physical rehabilitation, residual pain and stiffness can spoil the final result.

INJURIES OF THE LATERAL COLLATERAL LIGAMENT COMPLEX

Facts concerning ankle sprains include the following: (1) Rupture of the anterior talofibular ligament is usually an isolated injury. (2) Simultaneous rupture of all three collateral ligaments is rare, the posterior talofibular ligament being the least vulnerable. (3) Rupture of the anterior talofibular ligament is usually a complete, or grade III, injury. This is not the case with injury of the calcaneofibular ligament, which is frequently partial. (4) Sprains (syndesmotic) of the anterior tibiofibular ligament are separate injuries with a different mechanism of injury and prognosis.

Classification

Injuries of the lateral collateral ligament complex of the ankle are classified into three groups:

First degree: Complete rupture of the anterior talofibular ligament only, the mechanism of injury being internal rotation of the pronated ankle.

Second degree: Complete rupture of the anterior talofibular and calcaneofibular ligaments but with an intact posterior talofibular ligament; the mechanism of injury is internal rotation of the supinated foot.

Third degree: All three lateral collateral ligaments of the ankle are ruptured; the mechanism of injury is adduction of the supinated ankle.

Two patterns of medial malleolar fracture are associated with injuries to the lateral collateral ligament: a vertical fracture (SA pattern) and a supination–internal (SI) rotation fracture. The latter is a transverse or slightly oblique fracture of the medial malleolus and indicates a second-degree lateral sprain.

Diagnosis and Initial Management

History and Physical Examination

The clinical evaluation is most important because radiographs are frequently of little help. Specifically, there is a history of injury (usually inversion of the foot from stepping on an irregular surface, with the sensation of a pop), the immediate onset of pain, swelling, and difficulty in bearing or inability to bear weight.

There is swelling over the site of injury and tenderness directly over the involved ligament (most often the anterior talofibular ligament). Manual motor testing determines the integrity of the major musculotendinous units important to gait and stability of the foot and ankle. Not all painful swollen ankles are the result of a sprain and some sprains result from underlying problems. The pulses and sensation (both deep and superficial pain) are evaluated. A bad sprain in a young athlete is not the same problem as it is in an overweight diabetic with peripheral neuritis or vascular insufficiency.

Stability of the talus in the coronal plane (adduction) and sagittal plane (anterior drawer) is assessed.

Tenderness over the anterior tibiofibular ligament and/or the deltoid ligament suggests injuries to these ligaments and a syndesmotic and/or deltoid ligament sprain. In this situation, pain is present with external rotation, and stability of the ankle mortise with external rotation must be determined. A Maisonneuve's fracture of the proximal fibula is ruled out by physical and/or radiographic examination. The squeeze test of the proximal fibula to the tibia will cause pain in the distal syndesmosis if its ligaments have been injured.

Radiographic Examination

Plain films are usually of little value and indicate only soft tissue swelling. An SA or SI medial malleolar fracture may be present on the mortise view. The Ottawa rules, outlined in the discussion of ankle fractures, are a valuable guide in determining which patients require radiographs.

Stress films are valuable but require substantial analgesia and are difficult to obtain with validity in unanesthetized patients. Stability in the coronal plane is assessed by adducting the midfoot while a mortise view is obtained. This view is compared with a stress film of the uninjured side. Varus tilt of the talus, which is 10 degrees greater than that of the uninjured side, indicates a third-degree sprain. Stability in the sagittal plane is assessed with a lateral film of the ankle taken while an anterior drawer test is performed. To perform the anterior drawer test, the heel is held in one hand while the other pushes the tibia posteriorly. Anterior displacement of greater than 3 mm when compared with the normal side indicates at least a first-degree sprain. In most instances (except when there is obvious instability on the clinical examination), these stress views underestimate severity and do not determine management.

In special situations (e.g., when primary repair is a consideration), examination under anesthesia or MRI can be undertaken. In severe injuries, MRI will also show the extent of bone bruising (edema), which may be of prognostic interest.

Differential Diagnosis

Other important considerations are those of the differential diagnosis and confounding problems. Not all painful swollen ankles are ankle sprains! The following is only a partial list of injuries or other diagnoses that may be associated with or mistaken for an ankle sprain: peroneal tendon subluxation, osteochondral fracture of the talar dome, lateral fracture of the talar wall, fracture of the calcaneal process, Maisonneuve's fracture, stress fracture (especially in diabetics with neuropathy or the osteopenic patient), peroneal nerve palsy, tendon rupture (Achilles or tibialis), and superficial injury of the peroneal nerve.

Initial Management

There is no dislocation or deformity to reduce; therefore splinting, crutches, ice, analgesic medication, and elevation are customary and are used in proportion to the severity of injury. Significant injuries with substantial pain and swelling and an inability to bear weight require adequate splinting in the plantigrade position of weight bearing. There is no sadder sight than the patient who comes from the emergency department with an inexpertly applied, poorly padded posterior splint, the foot in equinus, who cannot get it off soon enough because the pain and swelling have in fact been made worse. Splinting is not a job for the inexperienced.

Definitive Management

Functional treatment is desirable and is done in a manner proportionate to the severity of injury and with proper consideration of the kind of patient who has the injury. A grade I sprain in a young athlete will be treated differently than a grade II sprain in an overweight middle-aged diabetic.

Functional treatment means the use of support (elastic anklet, air-filled clamshell splint, prefabricated removable walking cast, or, rarely, a wrapped-on fiberglass cast) that will allow the patient to bear weight as soon as possible with reasonable comfort. As the symptoms resolve, the encumbrance of support diminishes and self-rehabilitation begins. Weight bearing is the sine qua non of rehabilitation and is followed by active range-of-motion exercises, double toe rises, light resistance exercises, and formal physical therapy with proprioceptive reeducation, which always includes balancing-board exercises. Long-term protection with an ankle lacer or pneumatic splint will be advisable in certain situations, again depending on the activity level, stage and quality of recovery, and body habitus and proprioceptive skills of the patient in question. The author has yet to see a skateboarder or roller-park habitué who has required long-term support to return to his or her venue.

Primary ligamentous repair is rarely carried out even in patients whose activities require strong lateral support at the ankle. Well-controlled investigations have brought to our attention two points: (1) acute surgical repair will prolong the initial recovery and confer no advantage with regard to stability at follow-up when compared with functional treatment and (2) posttraumatic arthrosis does not usually occur in patients with chronic lateral instability.

When operative repair is elected, the exposure is through an incision that parallels the peroneal tendons. The peroneal sheath is opened and the tendons are retracted anteriorly to reach the posterior talofibular and calcaneofibular ligaments. The anterior talofibular ligament is the easiest to expose and repair. Suture anchors or drill holes through bone are useful when the ligament has been avulsed at its insertion. Postoperatively, the ankle is protected with a short leg cast for 4 weeks and a removable cast for 2 weeks.

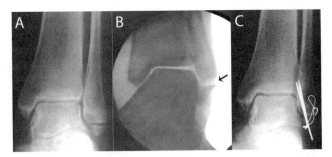

FIG. 25-10   Patient with recurrent inversion ankle sprains. *A.* Radiograph of the ankle showing an ununited fracture of the lateral malleolus. *B.* Inversion stress radiograph showing movement of the ununited fracture fragment and a talar tilt (*arrows*). *C.* Radiograph following surgical repair of the nonunion and attached calcaneofibular ligament as well as modified Ahlgren-Larsson advancement of the anterior talofibular ligament and anterior capsule.

Complications

The complication unique to this injury is laxity of the lateral collateral ligament complex, resulting in "giving out" when a varus force is applied to the foot (e.g., when the patient walks on uneven ground). Management is conservative, with a broad heel on the shoe (occasionally a lateral shoe wedge), peroneal strengthening, proprioceptive exercises, and an ankle support.

Numerous operative repairs for lateral instability have been described. Currently, anatomic reconstruction by advancement or plication of the lax tissue (as described by Karlsson or Brostrom) is preferred (Fig. 25-10). Procedures using the peroneus brevis as a tenodesis frequently do not hold up well.

Before any reconstruction is undertaken, the diagnosis of instability must be confirmed by a careful history and hopefully objective physical evidence; rehabilitation must have been attempted and other causes of instability eliminated. Undiagnosed pain is not an indication for ligamentous reconstruction.

SELECTED READINGS

Kaikkonen A, Kannus P, Järvinen M. Surgery versus functional treatment in ankle ligament tears. *Clin Orthop* 326:194–202, 1996.

Krips R, Brandsson S, Swensson C, et al. Anatomical reconstruction and Evans tenodesis of the lateral ligaments of the ankle: clinical and radiological findings after follow-up for 15–30 years. *J Bone Joint Surg* 84B:232–236, 2002.

Lauge-Hansen N. Fractures of the ankle. Combined experimental–surgical and experimental–roentgenologic investigations. *Arch Surg* 60:957–985, 1950.

Löfvenberg R, Kärrholm J, Lund B. The outcome of nonoperated patients with chronic lateral instability of the ankle. *Foot Ankle Int* 15:165–169, 1994.

Muller ME, Nazarian S, Koch P, Schatzker J. *Classification of Fractures.* Berlin-Heidelberg: Springer-Verlag, 1990.

Orthopaedic Trauma Association Committee for Coding and Classification. Fracture and dislocation compendium. *J Orthop Trauma* 10(suppl 1):559–581, 1996.

Pankovich AM. Acute indirect ankle injuries in the adult. *J Orthop Trauma* 16:58–69, 2002.

Pijnenburg A, Bogaard K, Krips R, et al. Operative and functional treatment of rupture of the lateral ligament of the ankle: a randomized prospective trial. *J Bone Joint Surg* 85B:525–530, 2003.

Ruedi TP, Murphy WM. *AO Principles of Fracture Management.* Stuttgart and New York: Thieme, 2000.

26 | Fractures of the Tibial Pilon

Walter W. Virkus   *John L. Lin*

Fractures of the articular surface of the distal tibia are common and often occur in association with other injuries. These injuries have a severe impact on the patient's quality of life. Patients typically have ankle stiffness and some degree of chronic discomfort. Many require a change in occupation due to limitations imposed by their injuries. The physician's role is to minimize early complications, maximize return to activities of daily living and work, and educate the patient as to the poor prognosis of these injuries. If operative treatment is selected, careful attention to both the soft tissue and osseous injury is required to prevent iatrogenic complications and subsequently poor or even disastrous results.

MECHANISM AND PATHOANATOMY

Pilon fractures occur from either an axial load or, less commonly, a severe torsional injury. With an axial load, the talus is driven up into the tibial plafond, causing segmentation and impaction. The position of the foot plays a role in the fracture pattern. Dorsiflexion or plantarflexion directs the force anteriorly or posteriorly, respectively. This typically leads to more comminution of the affected portion of the articular surface.

Increasingly higher amounts of energy are dissipated into the surrounding soft tissues, producing a soft tissue injury with a severity that parallels the severity of the osseous injury. Higher levels of energy can lead to increasing comminution in either the articular segment, metaphyseal segment, or both or even extension into the diaphysis. The typical primary fracture lines of an intraarticular pilon fracture form a triradiate pattern separating the articular surface into anterolateral, posterolateral, and medial segments. The two lateral fragments are typically attached to the fibula by the syndesmotic ligaments, which facilitates the use of the fibula in restoring anatomic length of the tibia. Increasing energy adds additional fracture lines to this pattern, increasing the number of fragments. Often a "die punch" fragment exists in the middle of the articular surface that has no soft tissue attachment and therefore is not reduced with longitudinal traction.

HISTORY

The history of a patient with a pilon fracture is usually straightforward. Most commonly such injuries are due to motor vehicle accidents and falls from a height. Less commonly they can occur through a rotational injury, as in skiing. The patient will complain of pain in the ankle and typically will be unable to bear weight. Patients with a history of a fall should be questioned about back pain. Concomitant injuries also often occur, such as other lower extremity fractures, head injuries, and upper extremity fractures. Medical history—including diabetes, peripheral vascular disease, hypertension, coronary artery disease, history of smoking, occupation, and other musculoskeletal complaints—is important in guiding treatment and assessing prognosis.

PHYSICAL EXAMINATION

Careful assessment of the whole patient is vital in all cases of severe trauma to an extremity. Particular attention should be paid to the thoracic and lumbar spine, pelvis, and hips to make sure that there is no concomitant proximal injury. The diagnosis of a plafond fracture is usually obvious on physical examination. The examination reveals swelling, ecchymosis, and often deformity of the ankle. Open injuries are found in 12 to 56% of high-energy fractures and 3 to 6% of low-energy fractures. It is important not to miss a small puncture wound marking an open injury. Careful assessment of the condition of the soft tissues (i.e., presence of fracture blisters) and neurovascular status must be carried out. Examination of the skin for normal wrinkles, known as the "wrinkle test," will often serve to determine the level of swelling; the condition of the skin in this regard should be noted for future comparison (Fig. 26-1). Compartment syndrome is found in 0 to 5% of cases and must be ruled out, especially in higher-energy injuries. Firm compartments, decreased sensation, pain out of proportion, and pain with passive stretch are suggestive of compartment syndrome.

DIAGNOSTIC IMAGING

Initial imaging should consist of plain radiographs. Orthogonal images of the ankle (anteroposterior and lateral) and entire tibia/fibula should be obtained. A mortise view of the ankle is also useful. If operative intervention is anticipated, further imaging with computed tomography utilizing 2-mm sections through the articular surface is highly recommended. These images can be obtained either during the initial workup or preferably after placement of a spanning external fixator. Axial images are most helpful in defining the number and size of fracture fragments and can help in preoperative planning (Fig. 26-2). Sagittal, coronal, and three-dimensional reconstructions may also yield additional information about the fracture pattern.

CLASSIFICATION

Two classification systems are commonly used in describing fractures of the tibial plafond. The Ruedi and Allgower classification was the first in common use. A type I fracture is a nondisplaced intraarticular fracture, a type II fracture is a displaced intraarticular fracture with minimal or no comminution, and a type III fracture is a comminuted fracture of the articular surface and

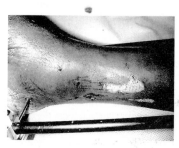

FIG. 26-1   The "wrinkle" test showing wrinkles and epithelialized blisters indicating a recovered soft tissue envelope.

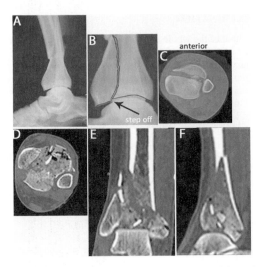

FIG. 26-2 Radiologic evaluation of pilon fractures. *A.* A lateral radiograph shows a simple pilon fracture with extension into the diaphysis. *B.* A closer view shows a step-off at the fracture site. *C.* An axial CT of a more severe injury at the plafond shows an anterior articular fracture, slightly comminuted. *D.* An axial CT view shows extensive comminution of the plafond. Coronal (*E*) and sagittal (*F*) CT reconstruction of the distal tibia clearly defines the morphology of the fracture.

metaphysis. Its use has recently diminished, and now the most commonly used classification system is the one proposed by the Orthopedic Trauma Association (OTA/AO) (Fig. 26-3). This system consists of three fracture **categories**:

Type A—extraarticular fracture
Type B—partial intraarticular fracture in which part of the articular surface maintains attachment to the metaphysis and diaphysis of the tibia
Type C—complete articular fracture in which the entire articular surface is separated from the metaphysis and/or diaphysis of the tibia

Each category is then further divided into three fracture **groups**:

Type 1—minimal or no comminution
Type 2—minimal articular comminution with severe metaphyseal comminution
Type 3—severe comminution of the articular surface and metaphysis

The above groups in each category are then further divided into three **subtypes**.
Overall there are 27 fracture types of the distal tibia. The purpose of so many subtypes is to allow accurate classification of the fractures and to facilitate meaningful research on these difficult injuries. For general practice, it is useful to simplify the classification to a fracture involving the entire articular surface (type C), part of the articular surface (type B), or not involving the articular surface (type A). Adding a digit (1 to 3) to this letter indicates an increasing degree of fracture comminution. For example, an A3 fracture is a severely comminuted fracture of the metaphysis with no articular fracture. A C1 fracture is a simple fracture dividing the entire articular surface into two or three fragments.

Classification of Pilon Fractures

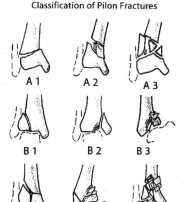

FIG. 26-3   OTA/AO classification of pilon fractures.

The additional subtypes do not have a role in the day-to-day use of this classification system.

INITIAL MANAGEMENT

After the history and physical examination, radiographs should be obtained promptly. After radiographic confirmation of the injury, the extremity should be placed in a well-padded splint, iced, and elevated to reduce pain and prevent further soft tissue injury. Open injuries should be assessed, large debris removed, and a sterile saline or povidone-iodine dressing applied. Appropriate antibiotics and tetanus prophylaxis should be administered. If an open injury is present, formal operative debridement should also be accomplished during this initial procedure and should be undertaken in a timely manner (within less than 6 h). Provisional reduction of articular fragments can be accomplished through the open wound if contamination is not severe. Fracture fragments visible through the wound or its extension are manipulated with Kirschner wires or sharp picks and then held in place with lag screws or wires. Hardware should not be placed if a clean wound bed is not achieved. If traumatic wounds cannot be closed, placement of an antibiotic bead pouch can decrease the rate of infection and prevent desiccation of exposed tendons and neurovascular structures. This is performed by placing polymethylmethacrylate beads that are mixed with antibiotics over the wound and covering them with an adhesive dressing, such as Ioban. The fluid that collects under the dressing then has a very high antibiotic concentration. If definitive treatment is to be deferred until swelling diminishes, provisional length should be obtained as described in the section on staged open reduction and internal fixation (ORIF), below.

DEFINITIVE TREATMENT OPTIONS

After the initial management described above, a definitive management plan should be determined. The treatment plan should include timing, provisional restoration of length, method of articular reduction, and fixation. Regardless of the method, the basics of pilon fracture fixation include anatomic reconstruction of the articular surface and reestablishment of the length, alignment, and rotation of the tibia and fibula with some form of neutralization construct in the form of a plate or external fixator.

Nonoperative Treatment

Nonoperative treatment has a diminishing role as an improved understanding of the importance of the soft tissues and better surgical techniques develop. Casting can be used in minimally or nondisplaced extraarticular fractures without comminution (OTA A1) or in nondisplaced articular fractures in patients with multiple risk factors.

External Fixation/Limited ORIF

An external fixator can be used for definitive fixation with or without internal fixation. Factors making this treatment option preferable include severe osseous comminution of either the articular surface or metaphysis (OTA C3), proximal extension into the diaphysis, severe soft tissue injury, and patient risk factors including smoking, diabetes, and peripheral vascular disease. This method works best when done in the acute period, so it should be chosen early. It is, however, possible to revert to this treatment approach if a staged protocol is complicated by failure of limb swelling to decrease or by other adverse events.

While many variables are involved in this treatment approach, it has three basic components:

1. Articular reduction
2. Limited internal fixation
3. Application of an external fixation device

Limited internal fixation can range from a few lag screws to multiple Kirschner wires or small plates. *Limited* refers not only to the amount of implanted hardware but also to the amount of exposure used to achieve reduction and fixation. The external fixator can range from a simple monolateral frame to a complicated ring fixator. These decisions are based on the specifics of the bone and soft tissue injury as well as surgeon preference. The decision to plate the fibula is also controversial, as described below.

The basic technique of external fixation/limited ORIF is first to obtain articular reduction, usually by indirect reduction methods. Small incisions can then be made to place reduction clamps, fine-tune the reduction, and place screws, wires, or small plates. Most commonly, lag screws are placed anterior to posterior to stabilize the coronal split that is typical of this injury. Additionally, screws are placed to stabilize a large medial malleolar fragment if necessary. Short plates can be used to buttress small areas of comminution. Axial CT scans can help in determining the ideal placement and direction of these implants based on the fracture lines present. The external fixator in this technique acts to neutralize forces and to maintain alignment of the reduced articular surface. The external fixator serves the same function as the plate used in formal ORIF.

A wide range of fixators can be used in the treatment of pilon fractures. These include fixators that span the ankle joint or attach to the distal tibia and those that are on only one side of the leg (monolateral), both sides of the leg (delta frame), or circumferential with rings. Monolateral fixators and delta frames are typically bridging external fixators used to protect the articular surface and stabilize the metaphysis until healing occurs, at which time they are removed so that ankle motion can begin. Monolateral fixators are usually placed medially, with pins in the calcaneus and talus connected to pins in the tibia. Delta frames have pins that traverse the calcaneus, protruding medially and laterally, that connect to pins in the tibia to make a triangle. These may be more stable than monolateral fixators in preventing varus and valgus angulation of the distal tibia (Fig. 26-4). The potential disadvantage of both of these fixator constructs is that the ankle is immobilized until they are removed. The advantage is that they get good purchase away from the fracture site. An Ilizarov-type fixator is a multiple-ring device attached to the tibia with a combination of wires and half pins. A hybrid fixator typically has one ring with tensioned thin wires attached to more standard pin clamps and half pins. The main difference between these two fixators is that the hybrid can be slightly easier to apply, while in some cases a properly constructed Ilizarov frame can permit full weight bearing. In most pilon fractures, the use of thin-wire ring fixators is usually necessary to avoid spanning the ankle joint. Reduction of the articular surface must be obtained prior to insertion of the wires to be attached to the fixator. When wires are placed, the first wire is driven medial to lateral, parallel to the joint line. The wire should be a minimum of 2 cm from the joint line to avoid being intracapsular. A second wire with a bead or olive is driven from posterolateral to anteromedial through or anterior to the fibula. The bead prevents sliding of the distal tibial segment along the wires. The third wire is inserted just anterior to the posterior tibial tendon in the medial malleolus. Additional wires or anterior half pins can be added for stability. The wires are then tensioned after being attached to a ring. An additional ring or half pins are then placed into the proximal tibia; the proximal and distal rings are connected; proper length, alignment, and rotation are obtained; and the connecting bars are tightened.

The advantage of this approach is limited stripping of open wounds and soft tissue without sacrificing reduction of the articular surface. Disadvantages include pin-tract infections (about 20%); malalignment, requiring adjustment of the fixator (10 to 15%); and delayed motion in cases where the ankle joint is spanned. Final range of motion has been shown in several series not to differ statistically from ORIF or nonspanning external fixation.

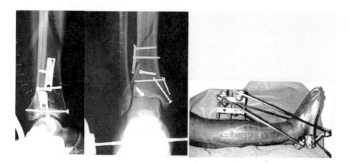

FIG. 26-4   Postoperative radiographs and clinical photo following limited internal fixation and external fixation with a delta-type frame.

Plating the Fibula

Plating of the fibula as part of the treatment of pilon fractures is controversial. Some authors advocate this procedure in the acute period to help maintain length and provisionally reduce the fracture fragments through the soft tissue attachments to the tibia. A trend toward a better final reduction has been reported with this approach when followed by formal or limited ORIF. Critics of this approach cite the increased rates of wound complications, and studies have shown equivalent clinical and radiographic results regardless of whether or not the fibula is plated acutely. Additionally, plating of the fibula can lead to varus alignment of the ankle joint if anatomic length of the tibia is not maintained until healing. Occasionally, the decision to plate the fibula will depend on whether a plate or external fixator will be used to stabilize the metaphyseal fracture. If external fixation is anticipated, it is often advantageous to allow mild shortening through the fibula, because it can be very difficult to maintain anatomic tibial length with an external fixator. If plating is performed, all incisions for definitive fixation should be anticipated and the incision for fibular plating kept a minimum of 7 cm from the anticipated site of future incisions. This often means shifting the lateral incision more posterior if a standard anteromedial approach is anticipated for ORIF. Additionally, an anatomic reduction is essential if plating of the fibula is performed. Nonanatomic reduction of the fibula will hamper anatomic reduction of the distal tibia when definitive fixation is undertaken.

Staged (Formal) ORIF

Formal ORIF is an excellent treatment method in cases where the soft tissue envelope permits. It can be used in nearly all fracture types (OTA A, B, and C). It allows early ankle motion and avoids the problems of pin-tract infections and bulky fixators. Definitive open reduction and fixation should be avoided in the immediate injury period due to a high incidence of complications when carried out in the acute setting. Complications occur in up to 50% of cases when ORIF is carried out before 5 days postinjury. A delay of 7 to 21 days has been shown to significantly decrease complications. However, to delay formal ORIF without reestablishing anatomic length acutely can make reduction of the anatomic joint and metaphysis very difficult. Therefore most staged protocols involve some method of early reestablishment of length, making use of ligamentotaxis for provisional reduction. This serves to make fracture fixation easier and speeds the recovery of the soft tissues by decreasing the outward pressure from underlying fracture fragments.

Reestablishment of the length of the tibia and fibula should be accomplished with the use of calcaneal traction (10 lb), placement of a spanning external fixator (Fig. 26-5), plating of the fibula, or a combination of these methods.

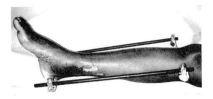

FIG. 26-5   Simple spanning external fixator.

When placing either traction or external fixation pins, care should be taken to stay clear of anticipated incisions that will be needed during the final reconstruction. Subsequently, the condition of the soft tissue is monitored while the extremity is elevated. The appearance of a wrinkle sign signals a decrease in swelling and is a prerequisite before attempting definitive fixation. Incisions through blisters should be avoided unless they are fully epithelialized.

Once soft tissue swelling has resolved, formal open reduction and internal fixation of the pilon fracture is undertaken. Classically, this follows these standard steps:

1. ORIF of the fibula
2. Anatomic reduction and stable fixation of the articular surface
3. Reduction and fixation of the articular segment to the metaphyseal/diaphyseal segment
4. Bone grafting the metaphyseal defect

Reduction of the fibula should reestablish the proper fibular length, and the ligaments from the fibula to the lateral tibia pull the anterolateral fragment (Chaput's) and the posterolateral fragment (Volkmann's) distal to their anatomic position. The anatomically reduced Chaput's fragment serves as the stable keystone on which to reduce the subsequent articular fragments.

Surgical Approaches

The approach to formal ORIF is dictated by the fracture lines. In most cases, the fracture line exiting the tibia anteriorly is entered, allowing separation of the adjacent fragments and reduction of the depressed joint fragments. Care must be taken, however, to ensure an adequate skin bridge of at least 7 cm if two incisions are used, and soft tissue stripping should be minimized. CT scans are very helpful in determining where these fracture lines exist, and which approach will offer the best exposure for joint reduction. The traditional exposure is via the anteromedial approach, which is medial to the tendon of the tibialis anterior, just lateral to the tibial crest (Fig. 26-6). However, when the fracture line exiting anteriorly is more lateral, an anterolateral incision between the extensor digitorum and the peroneus tertius is utilized. A posteromedial approach posterior to the flexor digitorum longus may be useful when there is a large posteromedial

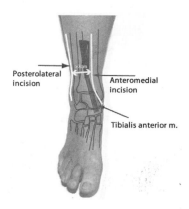

Posterolateral incision

Anteromedial incision

Tibialis anterior m.

FIG. 26-6   Anteromedial pilon incision and posterolateral fibular incision.

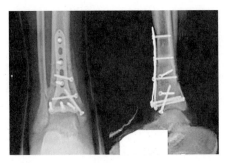

FIG. 26-7   Postoperative radiographs following staged formal ORIF. The fibula was not plated in this case owing to the condition of the local skin.

fragment. Last, a posterolateral approach that exposes both the tibia and fibula by anterior retraction of the peroneal tendons, allowing plating of the fibula and reduction of the posterolateral tibia through the same incision, can be helpful.

Once the ideal approach is determined, the operation is best begun with plating of the fibula if this has not yet been done. Then the articular surface is reconstructed through the chosen approach. Provisional reduction is maintained with Kirschner wires and lag screws. The articular surface is then secured to the metaphyseal segment with a plate applied either anteriorly or medially, depending on the fracture pattern (Fig. 26-7). Implants of small-fragment caliber are preferable to large-fragment implants. It is critical that mechanical alignment and rotation be established. If a metaphyseal defect results, it is grafted with cancellous bone or bone-graft substitute.

Percutaneous Plating

Percutaneous plating is a relatively new technique for treating pilon fractures. It is particularly useful in extraarticular fractures (OTA A1 to A3) and simple complete articular fractures (OTA C1). In this method, the articular reduction is obtained via closed or percutaneous reduction and fixation. The articular segment is then placed in the correct orientation in relation to the proximal tibia and secured by an anteromedial plate that is passed subcutaneously under the skin, just superficial to the periosteum of the tibia (Fig. 26-8). Screws are placed proximal and distal to the fracture, which is being held in proper alignment as confirmed by fluoroscopy. In most cases, the accompanying fibular fracture is also plated. Soft tissue swelling must still be sufficiently diminished prior to proceeding. This technique has the advantage of allowing early ankle motion and avoiding large incisions that may break down. The disadvantages are that reduction must be obtained indirectly, without visualizing the metaphyseal portion of the fracture. Therefore the surgeon must be comfortable with indirect reduction techniques and assessing the reduction radiographically.

TREATMENT DECISIONS

Treatment decisions in pilon fractures depend on many variables, including the osseous injury, soft tissue swelling, the patient's general medical and social status, and the surgeon's experience in treating these fractures. The method of treatment should be decided on a case-by-case basis. Early results of ORIF

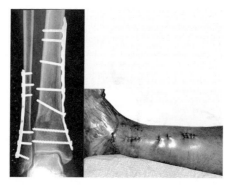

FIG. 26-8   Postoperative radiograph and surgical incisions following percutaneous plating.

were good in the low-energy injuries for which they were first described. When these methods were applied to higher-energy injuries, the complication rate increased and the good results decreased. This has led to an evolution of treatment that now includes the range of methods described above. Regardless of the method chosen, careful evaluation of the soft tissue envelope and thoughtful preoperative planning are important. If the fracture is three or four large fragments, the soft tissue swelling is minimal, and the patient has no medical risk, formal ORIF is an excellent option. If the fracture is in many small fragments, the soft tissue injury is severe, or the patient has significant risk factors, a more conservative approach of external fixation with limited ORIF is often a better choice. External fixation with limited internal fixation has a much lower rate of the severe complications that can lead to significant morbidity or even amputation. Cases in which an acceptable reduction can be obtained with closed or limited open methods may be amenable to a percutaneous plating technique, which can avoid some of the disadvantages of external fixation.

Postoperative Management

Regardless of the treatment method chosen, postoperative management must focus on edema control, wound healing, and early motion when possible. The patient should be immobilized in a bulky postoperative splint and avoid weight bearing. Protection should continue with a cam walker boot, splint, or short leg cast once the wound has healed. Patients with external fixators should be instructed on proper pin care and methods to avoid equinus contracture of the ankle. Patients are maintained without weight bearing on the involved extremity until early fracture healing in the form of bridging callus is apparent on radiographs. Most surgeons will not allow full weight bearing on articular fractures for 12 weeks.

Complications

Wound Breakdown/Infection

Although quite common in earlier reported series, the incidence of this complication has significantly decreased with staged protocols. Rates of deep infection range from 0 to 5%. Slightly higher rates of infection are seen with

ORIF than with external fixation and limited internal fixation. Skin slough or superficial infections are somewhat more common but can be treated with oral antibiotics in almost all cases, with subsequent resolution. These infections should be treated aggressively to avoid a deeper osseous infection. Pin-tract infections occur in 10 to 20% of cases in recently reported series, usually resolving with oral antibiotics. Loss of soft tissue coverage may result in the need for skin grafts or free muscle flaps. Amputation is a last resort in severe infections.

Malunion and Nonunion

Nonunion rates of 5 to 8% have been reported regardless of treatment method. Higher-energy injuries show relatively higher rates. Malunion of the articular surface is dependent on the mode of fixation. Anatomic reduction has been reported in 58 to 86% of ORIF cases in contrast to external fixation, where anatomic reduction was found in 25 to 57%. Malalignment of the distal tibia is found in 4 to 25% of cases, with a higher percentage seen when plating of the fibula was not done.

Arthrosis

Rates of arthrosis, which usually occurs in the first 2 years after injury, range from 12 to 100%. The quality of reduction influences development of degenerative changes. However, even with anatomic reduction, arthritis develops in 12% of cases. These results may be due to irreversible articular damage that occurs during the initial injury, which cannot be restored even with anatomic reduction. Although arthrosis of the tibiotalar joint is common after pilon fracture, clinical results show only a weak correlation with radiographic arthrosis. These results suggest that even if arthrosis is present radiographically, the patient may not require further intervention. Therefore there is little if any role for immediate or early arthrodesis.

Joint Ankylosis

Decreased motion of the ankle and subtalar joint is common and, in long-term follow-up, appears to be unaffected by the type of treatment. Nearly all cases result in some loss of motion in both the tibiotalar and subtalar joints.

SELECTED READINGS

Anglen J. Early outcome of hybrid external fixation for fracture of the distal tibia. *J Orthop Trauma* 13(2):92–97, 1999.

Bartlett CS, Weiner LS. Fractures of the tibial pilon. In Browner BD, Jupiter JB, Levine AM, Trafton PG (eds). *Skeletal Trauma: Basic Science, Management, and Reconstruction.* Vol II, 3d ed. Philadelphia: Elsevier Science, 2003.

Bonar S, Marsh JL. Tibial plafond fractures: changing principles of treatment. *J Am Acad Orthop Surg* 2:297–305, 1994.

Goulet JA. Tibial-pilon fractures: open reduction internal fixation. In Wiss DA (ed). *Master Techniques in Orthopaedic Surgery: Fractures.* Philadelphia: Lippincott, Williams & Wilkins, 1998:459–472.

Marsh JL, Saltzman CL. Ankle fractures. In Bucholz RW, Heckman JD (eds). *Rockwood and Green's Fractures in the Adult,* 5th ed. Philadephia: Lippincott, Williams & Wilkins, 2002:2001–2090.

Marsh JL, Weigel DP, Dirschl DR. Tibial plafond fractures: how do these ankles function over time? *J Bone Joint Surg* 85A:287–295, 2003.

Patterson MJ, Cole JD. Two-staged delayed open reduction and internal fixation of severe pilon fractures. *J Orthop Trauma* 13(2):85–91, 1999.

Pollak AN, McCarthy ML, Bess RS, et al. Outcomes after treatment of high-energy tibial plafond fractures. *J Bone Joint Surg* 85A:1893–1900, 2003.

Sands AK, Grujic L, Byck D, et al. Clinical and functional outcomes of internal fixation of displaced pilon fractures. *Clin Orthop* 347:131–137, 1998.

Sirkin M, Sanders R, DiPasquale T, Herscovici D. A Staged protocol for soft tissue management in the treatment of complex pilon fractures. *J Orthop Trauma* 13(2):78–84, 1999.

Teeny SM, Wiss DA. Open reduction and internal fixation of tibial plafond fractures: variables contributing to poor results and complications. *Clin Orthop* 292:108–117, 1993.

Thordarson D. Complications after treatment of tibial pilon fractures: prevention and management strategies. *J Am Acad Orthop Surg* 8:253–265, 2000.

Tornetta P, Gorup J. Axial computed tomography of pilon fractures. *Clin Orthop* 323:273–276, 1996.

Williams TM, Marsh JL, Nepola JV, et al. External fixation of tibial plafond fractures: is routine plating of the fibula necessary? *J Orthop Trauma* 12:16–20, 1998.

| Fractures and Injuries of the Foot

Enes M. Kanlic   Miguel A. Pirela-Cruz

This chapter reviews injuries of the foot (i.e., distal to the ankle joint). Injuries of the foot are classified according to the mechanism of injury (indirect, direct, or due to repetitive stress) and to the involved anatomic zone and specific bone.

The foot is divided into the hindfoot, consisting of the Achilles tendon, talus, and calcaneus; the midfoot, consisting of the tarsal navicular, three cuneiforms, and cuboid; and the forefoot, consisting of the five metatarsals and corresponding phalanges.

HINDFOOT INJURIES

The hindfoot converts rotatory tibial forces into foot pronation. The calcaneus is an important lever arm and vertical support during the gait and an important horizontal support of the lateral column during the stance phase.

TALUS

Anatomy and Biomechanics

The **talus** is unique in that no muscles insert on it, 60% of its surface is covered with articular cartilage, and its vascular supply is tenuous. The posterior tibial artery gives off branches going through the posterior capsule, deltoid, and sinus tarsi roof. The tibialis anterior gives off arterial branches that enter the superior neck and branch to the sinus tarsi. The peroneal artery provides branches to the posterior and lateral aspects of the body. They anastomose in the tarsal canal inferior to the talar neck. The major blood supply enters the talus posterior to the neck, and isolated neck fractures do not necessarily lead to avascular necrosis of the talar body.

Fractures of the **neck of the talus** are the most common talar fracture and are classified into four types (Fig. 27-1). Type I is undisplaced. Type II is displaced with subluxation or dislocation of the talocalcaneal articulation. Type III is displaced with a talocalcaneal and a talotibial dislocation. Type IV is a type III fracture with a dislocation of the head of the talus from the talonavicular joint (rare). The incidence of avascular necrosis and nonunion increases from approximately 0 to 13% in type I fractures to 100% in type III and IV fractures, even with early accurate reduction and stable fixation.

Some 15 to 20% of talar fractures involve only the **talar body**. Without an associated subtalar dislocation, the incidence of avascular necrosis is 25%. With an associated subtalar dislocation, the incidence of avascular necrosis is approximately 50%.

Fractures of the **head of the talus** comprise 5 to 10% of all talar fractures and frequently represent an injury of Chopart's joint.

Fractures of the **lateral process** are the second most common type of talar fracture. They are caused by hyperextension of the supinated foot and are nondisplaced.

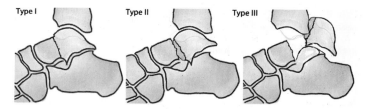

FIG. 27-1 Hawkins classification of talar neck fractures.

Osteochondral fractures involve the lateral side of the talar dome and are usually traumatic in origin. They are associated with 0.9 to 6.5% of acute ankle sprains. Similar lesions on the medial side may be degenerative in origin.

Diagnosis and Initial Management

History and Physical Examination

There is pain distal to the ankle in the hindfoot. There is obvious deformity in cases of talocalcaneal dislocation. Open wounds and skin tented over bone, which put the patient at risk for pressure necrosis, are noted. The neurovascular status distal to the injury is assessed.

Diagnostic Measures

Anteroposterior, lateral, and modified anteroposterior x-rays (described by Canale and Kelly, with 15 degrees of foot inversion and the x-ray beam aiming cranial at an angle of 75 degrees) are adequate to evaluate fractures of the talar neck and body and talocalcaneal dislocation. Lateral process fractures are best seen on a mortise view with foot in plantarflexion. Computed tomography (CT) should be obtained whenever possible in order to evaluate better the presence of comminution and lateral and posterior process fractures. The presence of osteochondral fragments in the talocalcaneal articulation and cartilage quality are best determined by magnetic resonance imaging (MRI).

The earliest signs of avascular necrosis are radiographic. The Hawkins sign is the appearance of a radiolucent line below the subchondral bone of the talar dome. This sign is best seen on a mortise view and appears between 6 and 8 weeks after injury. The Hawkins sign is due to resorption of subchondral bone, and its presence indicates the preservation of the main blood supply; its absence, however, does not necessarily mean that avascular necrosis will occur. Diffuse sclerosis of the talar body after 3 to 6 months is a more positive predictor of avascular necrosis. MRI is helpful where there is no hardware or if titanium implants have been used.

Initial Management

Fractures without significant displacement and without an associated dislocation are splinted and iced. If there is displacement or a dislocation, early reduction will lessen the risk of soft tissue necrosis and possibly prevent further vascular damage.

Closed reduction is attempted in the emergency department. If unsuccessful, open reduction is indicated. Closed reduction of talar neck fractures with subtalar subluxation (type II) is accomplished with the knee in flexion, relaxing the gastrocnemius, gentle plantarflexion of the foot, and traction to the heel. Supination or pronation of the heel to increase the deformity and then to reverse it often helps reduction. When reduction has been accomplished, it is usually stable. The foot and ankle are then splinted with the ankle in a neutral position and iced.

Open fractures are treated in the operating room as soon as possible with irrigation and debridement, reduction, and fixation tailored to the amount of soft tissue injury. Minimally damaged soft tissues allow for treatment as in closed injuries (including plate fixation and primary bone grafting). When there are soft tissue defects, the wound must be left open ("vacuum" dressings), with external fixation and additional plastic reconstructive procedures.

Associated Injuries

Fracture of the head of the talus indicates injury to the Chopart joint; therefore the calcaneocuboid joint must also be examined.

Neurovascular injuries are rare even in cases where the talar body was expulsed posteromedially and are ruled out with a careful examination.

Definitive Management

Nondisplaced fractures (type I, confirmed by CT) are managed nonoperatively with a non-weight-bearing short leg cast until the fracture heals, usually 6 to 10 weeks. Radiographs obtained weekly for the first 3 weeks determine whether displacement of the fragments has occurred.

Displaced fractures (types II to IV) are managed with open reduction and internal fixation (Fig. 27-2). Varus malunion due to shortening on the medial side because of comminution will lead to shortening of the medial arch and varus deformity of the hindfoot; this will cause weight bearing mostly on the lateral side of the foot, with consequent foot pain and local callosities. That is why it

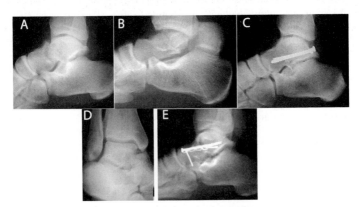

FIG. 27-2   Talar fractures and their treatment. *A.* Hawkins type II fracture with a displaced fracture of the talar neck and subtalar subluxation. *B.* Hawkins type III fracture with comminution and a large extruded fragment. *C.* Posterolateral-anteromedial parallel screws provide the best compression and excellent fixation. *D.* Medial displacement of the talar head and neck fragment. *E.* A lag screw provides interfragmentary compression and a medial buttress plate serves to prevent medial displacement.

is important to recognize varus deformity by preoperative CT scan and to obtain anatomic reduction at surgery and reliable fixation (plate) (Fig. 27-2*D* and *E*).

The lateral side of the neck has harder bone and usually less comminution; therefore an anterolateral approach will allow for easier reduction and screw placement. Also, it is possible to remove bone debris from the subtalar joint through this approach.

An anteromedial incision is used for screw placement, or, if comminution is severe, for placement of a miniplate and bone grafting.

A posterolateral incision will allow for the best biomechanical screw placement, particularly if 4.0-mm cannulated screws are inserted perpendicular to the fracture plane and parallel to the long talar axis after the reduction is first obtained through the anterior approach (Fig. 27-2*C*). The screws are countersunk to minimize impingement. Postoperatively, no weight bearing is allowed until the fracture has healed, or for at least 10 weeks. If the soft tissues are in good condition and fixation is stable, early motion will improve function and cartilage nutrition.

Displaced fractures of the talar body are managed with open reduction and internal fixation. Exposure is through the fracture site or osteotomy of the medial malleolus; vessels entering the talus through the deltoid ligament must be spared. The fracture is reduced and stabilized with Kirschner wires and headless or conventional screws. The fixation device should not penetrate the subchondral bone and project into the ankle joint; if this is recognized postoperatively, the device should be withdrawn sufficiently to prevent damage of the articular cartilage and the development of degenerative arthritis. If fixation is tenuous, an external fixator with pins in the tibia and calcaneus should be used in order to neutralize stresses across the fracture site.

Postoperatively, there is no weight bearing until healing occurs, or for at least 10 weeks. In most cases, immobilization should not be necessary beyond postoperative splinting, as fixation must be stable.

Undisplaced **talar head fractures** are managed in a non-weight-bearing short leg cast for 6 weeks and with an arch support for an additional 3 to 6 months. Unstable, large fragments are managed with open reduction and fixation with screws or Kirschner wires and absorbable pins. An external fixator with pins in the calcaneus and the first metatarsal should protect fixation. Fragments of the talar head smaller than 30% of its diameter are excised. If the joint is unstable, primary talonavicular arthrodesis should be considered.

Fractures of the **lateral process** of the talus are often unrecognized. The diagnosis should be considered in patients with a chronic lateral ankle sprain and is made by CT scan. Fractures extending into the subtalar joint will cause posttraumatic arthritis if left untreated. Larger fragments are fixed with screws, and smaller fragments, if symptomatic, are excised.

Fractures of the **posterior process** should be distinguished from a symptomatic os trigonum, usually confirmed by CT. Forced plantarflexion causes posterior pain; if splinting and the avoidance of weight bearing does not help, excision often does.

Undisplaced **osteochondral fractures** of the talar dome diagnosed by MRI are managed with a non-weight-bearing short leg cast for 6 weeks. When conservative management fails or if the fragments are displaced, surgery is indicated. Lateral osteochondral fractures are located anteriorly on the talar dome and are exposed through an anterolateral approach. Osteotomy of the medial malleolus is required to expose medial osteochondral fractures. Small fragments are excised (Fig. 27-3). Large fragments are internally fixed after curettage

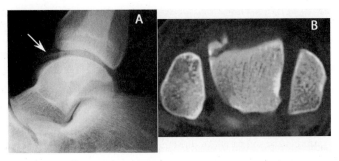

FIG 27-3.   Talar osteochondral fragment. *A.* Lateral radiograph showing the fragment (*arrow*). *B.* CT scan shows a small fragment, which can be excised.

and drilling of their bed. Postoperatively, avoidance of weight bearing is maintained until healing has been demonstrated radiographically. Alternatively, these injuries can be approached arthroscopically.

Complications

Complications of fractures of the talus are avascular necrosis, nonunion, and posttraumatic arthritis.

Avascular necrosis of the body of the talus is the complication that occurs following fractures and dislocations of the talus. It is most likely to occur following a displaced fracture of the talar neck or body. If subchondral resorption in the talar dome does not appear on radiographs (negative Hawkins sign) after 6 weeks, avascular necrosis is suspected. Diffuse sclerosis of talar body on radiographs 3 to 6 months after the injury confirms the diagnosis. Patients are allowed to bear weight after the fracture heals at 10 to 16 weeks. The revascularization process can take up to 3 years, and prolonged avoidance of weight bearing has not proven to make a significant difference in outcome. Slow collapse of the talar body and development of the posttrauamic arthritis are accompanied by significant pain with weight bearing. Talocrural arthrodesis is a definitive procedure that will give significant relief of pain and improve ambulation, although 1 to 2 in. of shortening usually occurs due to resection of the necrotic talar bone.

Posttraumatic arthritis of the subtalar joint is yet another complication of talar fractures. Patients complain of pain with walking on uneven ground. Pain on supination-inversion and pronation-eversion of the subtalar joint and a decreased range of motion are usually diagnostic. The diagnosis is confirmed by CT. It is important to identify accurately the symptomatic joints by selective injections of local anesthetic, as the talonavicular and calcaneocuboid joints can also be involved. Initial management is conservative, with anti-inflammatory medications and local injections of steroids. If this fails, **subtalar arthrodesis** is indicated. **Triple arthrodesis** is recommended if the calcaneal cuboid and talonavicular joints are involved. If the ankle and subtalar joints are involved, **pantalar arthrodesis** may be necessary. Retrograde nailing of both joints by inserting an intramedullary nail from the calcaneus through the talus and into the tibia is a surgical option.

Varus malunion is reported as a frequent complication due to an inadequate reduction and stabilization in malposition.

The rate of **delayed union and nonunion** after talar neck fractures is about 10%. Management is by a revision of the internal fixation and grafting with autogenous cancellous bone.

SUBTALAR DISLOCATION

The term *subtalar dislocation* denotes dislocation of both the talocalcaneal and talonavicular articulations.

Anatomy

The **subtalar joint** has four articulations: three between the anterior middle and posterior facets of the calcaneus and talus and one between the head of the talus and navicular. These articulations function as one multiaxial joint. Forty degrees of supination and pronation occur through the subtalar joint. The ankle and subtalar joints function together as a universal joint, with 45 degrees of dorsi- and plantarflexion.

Classification

Subtalar dislocations are classified according to the position of the forefoot in relation to the talus and whether there is an associated dislocation of the tibiotalar joint. The types of subtalar dislocation commonly encountered are medial, lateral, and pantalar. Medial dislocation is by far the most common type of dislocation (85%) and is caused by forefoot supination. Lateral subtalar dislocation is less (15%) frequent and is the result of forefoot pronation. Lateral dislocations are the result of greater force and have a worse prognosis than medial dislocations. Pantalar dislocations are most frequently a medial subtalar dislocation associated with a tibiotalar dislocation. They have a poor prognosis because of the high incidence of avascular necrosis and associated soft tissue injury.

Diagnosis and Initial Management

History and Physical Examination

The patient has pain localized to the foot. Deformity of the foot is obvious. The foot appears shortened and is in equinus, and the talar head is prominent. Medial dislocations have the calcaneus lying medial to the talus and the talar head is prominent dorsolaterally. In lateral dislocations, the calcaneus is lateral and the talar head is prominent medially. Some 10 to 40% of subtalar dislocations are open; injuries of posterior tibial nerve and artery are possible.

Radiographic Examination

The diagnosis of subtalar dislocation is obvious radiographically. Anteroposterior (most important), lateral, and oblique radiographs of the foot are obtained (Fig. 27-4). Other radiographic views and studies are not necessary to make the diagnosis. After closed reduction, coronal CT of the talocalcaneal joint determines the presence of osteochondral fragments in the joint and the congruity of reduction.

Initial Management

Once a subtalar dislocation has been diagnosed, reduction is performed as quickly as possible to minimize the incidence of skin necrosis. The reduction

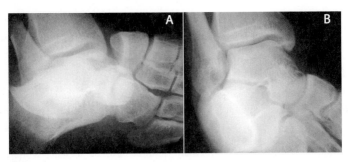

FIG. 27-4   Medial subtalar dislocation. *A.* Initial radiograph. *B.* Anatomic reduction following closed reduction.

maneuver is axial traction and deformity accentuation followed by reversal. In addition, the head of the talus is relocated with digital pressure. Some subtalar dislocations cannot be reduced by closed means. Repeated forceful attempts at closed reduction are not indicated and may jeopardize the viability of the skin over the head of the talus. If reduction is accomplished, a well-padded splint is applied with the ankle in a neutral position.

Associated Injuries

Fracture of the neck of the talus and intraarticular osteochondral fractures of the talus and calcaneus are frequently associated with subtalar dislocations. Talar neck fractures are ruled out by assessment of the lateral radiograph of the foot. The presence of intraarticular osteochondral fragments is determined with coronal CT through the talocalcaneal articulation.

Definitive Management

The goal of management is a congruous reduction. If this is obtained with closed reduction and the skin is viable, a short leg cast is applied. The patient is maintained without weight bearing for 4 weeks. Skin necrosis precludes casting.

In cases where a closed reduction cannot be accomplished, open reduction is performed. The most common obstacle to reduction of medial dislocations is "buttonholing" of the talar head through soft tissue anteriorly (the extensor retinaculum, extensor digitorum brevis, talonavicular ligament, and joint capsule). The most common cause of irreducible lateral dislocation is displacement of the posterior tibial tendon inferior to the neck of the talus. Occasionally, fractures of the head of the talus or interposed osteochondral fragments may block reduction. The surgical exposure for open reduction is through a longitudinal skin incision over the head of the talus. Interposed soft tissue is identified and incised or retracted, and osteochondral fragments are removed. If the posterior tibial tendon is disrupted, it is repaired after reduction. The joint is then inherently stable. The foot is immobilized in a short leg cast, and weight bearing is avoided for 4 weeks. If the injury is open, an external fixator is used in place of a cast.

In cases of open pantalar dislocation, if the wound is not highly contaminated, the talus should be put back and fixed to the tibia and navicular. Another option is to do a primary tibiocalcaneal fusion using an intramedullary nail.

Complications

Lateral and open dislocations (high-energy injuries) have poor outcomes. The complications of subtalar dislocations are infection secondary to skin necrosis or an open injury, subtalar arthritis, and avascular necrosis (total dislocations of talus).

ACHILLES TENDON INJURIES

The Achilles tendon (tendo calcaneus) is the largest tendon in the body. It is formed by union of the gastrocnemius aponeurosis and the tendon of the soleus muscle in the middle of the calf and extends about 15 cm distally to its insertion into the middle of the calcaneal tuberosity. The calcaneal bursa is located between the tendon and the upper surface of the tuberosity. It does not have a true synovial sheath; instead, there is a paratenon that permits about 1.5 cm of tendon glide. The blood supply to the tendon is provided by many branches; these penetrate the paratenon, particularly anteriorly. Decrease in the number of these branches with age and repeated microtrauma can lead to degenerative and inflammatory changes in the tendon, most pronounced at about 4 to 6 cm above the insertion, where the tendon is most vulnerable to rupture.

Classification

Disruption of the Achilles tendon can be caused by a laceration (direct injury). Direct injuries can affect adjacent tendons, the tibial or sural nerve, or the posterior tibial artery. Indirect injuries occur from activities requiring a vigorous push-off of the foot and are not associated with other injuries.

Diagnosis and Initial Management

History and Physical Examination

The diagnosis of an injury of the Achilles tendon usually includes a history of a sudden snap in the back of the leg, commonly associated with forceful plantarflexion of the foot and ankle. In addition to local tenderness, there is often a palpable gap in the tendon and a positive Thompson-Doherty calf squeeze test. In the Thompson-Doherty calf squeeze test, the patient is prone with the knee flexed and the examiner squeezes the calf muscle above the area of injury and tenderness. Plantarflexion of the foot occurs if the tendon is in continuity. If the tendon is ruptured, there is no response.

Radiographic Examination

Radiographic examination has little to offer, though an MRI can be diagnostic in situations where the physical findings are difficult to interpret.

Definitive Management

The treatment of acute Achilles tendon rupture is controversial, because excellent results have been reported using only cast immobilization and also by those who favor surgical repair. Since surgical repair is not difficult and provides for more exact approximation of the tendon ends, it is the treatment of choice. Percutaneous repair as described by Mann et al. and cast treatment in equinus are other options. There is a 20% risk of rerupture with cast treatment, and in those patients in whom permanent tendon healing occurs, the recovery of plantarflexion strength may be incomplete.

Operative Procedure

The patient is operated on in the prone position with general anesthesia and a thigh tourniquet. The Achilles tendon is exposed by a longitudinal curvilinear incision placed on the posteromedial aspect of the leg over the site of injury. The skin and subcutaneous tissues are opened, the peritenoneum incised, and the site of tendon rupture exposed. The tendon disruption is mop-ended and the repair carried out with a heavy 5-mm polyester suture passed transversely through the tendon approximately 3 cm proximal to the disruption. The suture is then looped proximal to the transverse limb and distally out the torn tendon end. A similar suture is placed in the distal portion of the tendon. A whip stitch can also be used. The torn surfaces are then pulled together and the suture ends tied. The ragged edges of the tendon are then brought into approximation with a few interrupted 2-0 chromic sutures. The peritenoneum is closed using 4-0 chromic sutures and the subcutaneous tissue with subcuticular stitches. Careful handling of the soft tissues is important so as to prevent complications. When the tendon rupture is near the insertion, the suture material may be passed through the proximal portion of the tendon and then through a transverse drill hole in the calcaneus. A short leg cast is applied with the foot in 20 degrees of plantarflexion for 3 weeks; then the leg is casted with the ankle at a right angle for an additional 4 to 6 weeks. On removal of the cast, the patient is placed in a double upright ankle-foot orthosis (AFO) with 90 degrees of dorsiflexion stop to prevent any accidental reinjury.

Complications

Complications of Achilles tendon rupture are rerupture, infection, and calf weakness. The risk of rerupture and calf weakness are greater with nonoperative treatment. The risk of skin necrosis and infection is greater with surgical treatment. Surgical complications are more frequent after the use of pull-out suture techniques and when avascular grafts are used to supplement the surgical repair. Should sinus formation and infection occur, nonabsorbable suture material will have to be removed in order to achieve wound healing. Patients with a history of local steroid injection, systemic steroid use, diabetes, peripheral vascular disease, and unsatisfactory local skin conditions have an increased incidence of complications after surgical repair.

Rerupture of the tendon usually occurs 1 to 2 weeks after cast immobilization is discontinued and is treated by another surgical repair.

Should skin necrosis occur, early debridement of necrotic tissue is important to prevent a deep infection of the tendon repair itself. Following debridement, the wound is left open; a wound VAC (Kinetic Concepts, San Antonio, TX) may be used to achieve closure. Adhesions of the tendon repair to the skin may be related to inadequate repair of the peritenoneum and subcutaneous tissues.

CALCANEUS

The superior aspect of the calcaneus has three facets that articulate with the talus. The posterior facet is the largest, and preservation of congruity and interrelationship of all three facets is crucial for long-lasting function. The talocalcaneal ligament runs from the superior surface of the calcaneus to the inferior surface of the talus. It lies in the sinus tarsi and is the primary stabilizer of the talocalcaneal articulation. The sustentaculum tali is on the medial side of the calcaneus. On its superior aspect is the middle facet, and on its inferior surface is the groove for the tendon of the flexor hallucis longus. Anterolaterally, the calcaneus articulates with the cuboid.

The posterior portion of the body of the calcaneus is the tuberosity that serves for insertion of the Achilles tendon. The plantar fascia and the small muscles of the foot originate from the plantar surface of the calcaneus. The anterior process is the origin of the bifurcate ligament, which runs to the cuboid and navicular, stabilizing the midfoot.

Classification

Fractures of the calcaneus are broadly classified as intraarticular (75%) or extraarticular (25%). Intraarticular fractures involve the posterior facet. Extraarticular fractures involve the tuberosity, sustentaculum tali, and anterior process. In addition to being fractured, the calcaneus is occasionally dislocated.

Intraarticular fractures of the calcaneus are caused by axial loading of the talus, which is driven into the calcaneus. The talus acts as a wedge, producing the primary fracture. This fracture is in the sagittal plane, starting at the anterolateral wall and continuing posteriorly and medially through the posterior facet to the medial wall of the calcaneus. The primary fracture divides the calcaneus into an anterior medial half and a posterior lateral half. If the force of the axial load is not dissipated, the impact of the talus produces a compression fracture of the lateral portion of the posterior facet. There are variations of this basic fracture pattern due to the position of the foot (e.g., supination of the foot medializes the primary fracture, pronation lateralizes it, plantarflexion results in a tongue-type fracture, and dorsiflexion results in a joint depression fracture (Fig. 27-5).

The therapeutically and prognostically most useful classification is based on CT evaluation of **posterior facet involvement**, as described by Sanders and coauthors (Fig 27-6). Fractures are grouped into nondisplaced, type I (nonoperative treatment); displaced (types II and III, two and three fragments, reconstruction possible); and comminuted (type IV, four or more fragments). Excellent and good results after surgical repair occurred in 73 and 70% for types II and III, and only in 9% for type IV fractures.

Extraarticular fractures of the calcaneus are caused by axial loading or by the avulsion of bony insertions and origins of ligaments and tendons. Isolated fractures of the tuberosity of the calcaneus are caused by direct impact or avulsion of the tendo-Achilles insertion. Fractures due to direct impact are minimally displaced; the plane of the fracture is sagittal. Avulsion fractures of the

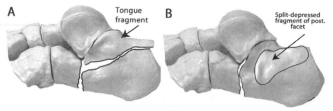

FIG. 27-5 Calcaneal fractures. *A.* Tongue type. *B.* Depression type.

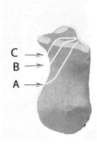

FIG. 27-6   Primary fracture lines across the posterior facet of the calcaneus (Sanders).

Achilles tendon are displaced; the plane of the fracture is horizontal, and this injury occurs mainly in osteoporotic bone.

Fractures of the sustentaculum tali are caused by the medial slide of the talus impacting the sustentaculum during axial loading of a supinated foot. Anterior process fractures are an avulsion of the origin of the bifurcate ligament caused by forefoot adduction and inversion. Dislocations of the calcaneus are extremely rare. There is usually a fracture of the calcaneus or cuboid at the calcaneocuboid articulation.

Diagnosis and Initial Management

History and Physical Examination

There is a history of an impact often caused by a fall or a twisting injury. Pain is localized to the hindfoot. When the foot is seen shortly after injury, prior to diffuse swelling, the exact location of the fracture can be determined by gentle palpation. Fracture of the sustentaculum tali is indicated by painful passive motion of the great toe (the flexor hallucis longus runs beneath the sustentaculum). An avulsion fracture of the tendo-Achilles is indicated by weakness of plantarflexion of the ankle. Loss of plantarflexion is not complete because the peroneal and posterior tibial muscles are intact.

Radiographic Examination

The radiographic projections helpful in the evaluation of calcaneal fractures are the lateral, oblique, axial, and Broden views. The **lateral projection** is the most helpful and is diagnostic of posterior facet depression and tuberosity avulsion. The Böhler tuber angle (Fig. 27-7), and the crucial angle of Gissane, which indicate the extent of displacement and angulation, are determined on the lateral view. The loss of parallelism of the articular surface of the posterior facet of the calcaneus and of the talus is also determined on the lateral view.

The **oblique view** is useful to assess the presence of a fracture of the anterior process of the calcaneus and to determine whether there is involvement of the calcaneal cuboid articulation.

The **axial view**, or Harris, or jumper's view, is obtained by placing the foot on the cassette with the ankle dorsiflexed and the tube directed 30 degrees

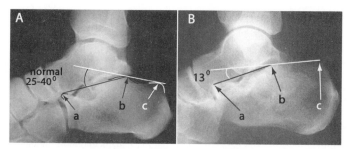

FIG. 27-7   Böhler tuber angle. A. In a normal calcaneus, the angle varies between 25 and 40 degrees. B. In a calcaneus with a depressed posterior facet, the angle is less than 25 degrees. The lines are drawn from the top of the anterior process to the highest point on the posterior facet, then to the top of the calcaneal tuberosity.

proximally. The axial view is useful in evaluating the tuberosity, the sustentaculum tali, and axial shortening.

The **Broden views** are used to assess the posterior and middle facets. For these views, lateral radiographs are obtained, with the foot passively dorsiflexed, supinated, and internally rotated, while the beam is centered on the sinus tarsi from different angles.

If the patient is active and healthy, in order to assess fully the injury and indication for surgery, it is necessary to obtain a CT scan. Semicoronal CT at 30 degrees (gantry perpendicular to inferior talar articulation) will allow for evaluation of the posterior calcaneal facet (position and number of fracture lines) and integrity of the tuberosity (Fig. 27-8A).

Axial scans in the plane of the foot will present the position of the tuberosity, a fracture location on medial wall, comminution and shortening, as well as the sustentaculum tali, anterior calcaneus, and calcaneocuboid joint (Fig 27-8B).

This information is necessary for preoperative surgical planning.

Initial Management

Initially a splint is applied. Ice and elevation will help to reduce the swelling.

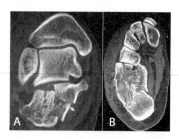

FIG. 27-8   CT scans of calcaneal fractures. A. Semicoronal view shows a comminuted three-fragment fracture of the posterior facet (Sanders III). B. Axial calcaneal view shows involvement of the calcaneocuboid joint, comminution of the body, and a longitudinal misalignment.

Associated Injuries

Some 40% of calcaneal fractures incurred in a fall are associated with a fracture of the lumbar spine, usually a stable compression fracture. Injuries of the medial and lateral plantar nerves result in decreased sensation on the plantar aspect of the foot. Compartment syndrome is suspected if there is massive swelling and severe pain not relieved by ice, elevation, and customary amounts of analgesics.

Definitive Management

Definitive management depends on the patient's medical condition and level of activity, the quality of soft tissue envelope, the type of calcaneus fracture (nondisplaced, displaced, or comminuted), and compliance.

Patients with low activity levels and medical problems (neuropathy, insulin-dependent diabetes, peripheral vascular disease, venous stasis or congestion, lymphedema, immune compromise, heavy smoking) have a high risk of wound healing problems and should not be treated operatively. Patients who develop surgery-related complications do much worse than those with the same type of injury without surgery.

Intraarticular fractures of the calcaneus that are not significantly displaced (2-mm step-off, 3-mm diastases) are managed nonoperatively with no weight-bearing for 4 weeks. Casting is counterproductive because it leads to stiffness of the subtalar joint.

Absolute surgical indications are biologically young, compliant patient with fracture subluxation of the posterior facet, beak fractures (avulsion of calcaneal tuberosity), and open injuries.

In selected patients, the management of **displaced intraarticular fractures** (Sanders types II and III) is operative. On the regular radiographs, displacement is defined as loss of articular congruity of the posterior facet or at the calcaneal cuboid joint, loss of parallelism between the posterior facets of the calcaneus and talus, more than 4 mm of shortening of the tuberosity as seen on the axial projection, and a Böhler angle of 10 degrees or less.

The surgical approach is through an extensile lateral incision. Surgery is delayed until swelling has decreased to the point that the skin on the dorsum of the foot wrinkles with ankle eversion (usually 10 to 14 days). The incision is in front of the Achilles tendon. It extends distally to the plantar skin where it turns 90 degrees and runs parallel with the plantar aspect of the foot. The incision is carried down to the calcaneus. A flap that includes the sural nerve and peroneal tendons is raised, exposing the entire lateral calcaneus, including the calcaneocuboid articulation and the posterior facet. It is necessary to re-create the lost space by reducing the tuberosity first (pulling it distally to obtain the height, taking it out of varus and pushing it medially). The posterior facet is reduced and fixed to the usually intact sustentaculum tali with lag screws under direct visualization. Anterior fragments with calcaneocuboid joint surface are reduced if needed and attached to the posterior segments. The whole construct is held together with anatomic low-profile plates (Fig. 27-9A and B) and preferably locking screws. Bone-void fillers can improve stability in areas of major defects. Intraoperative x-ray control is necessary to assure accurate reductions and hardware position (Fig. 27-9C). Open subtalar arthroscopy can provide better and faster verification of the quality of the reduction.

Comminuted fractures, Sanders type IV (four or more pieces of posterior facet), in healthy individuals should be managed by primary subtalar arthrode-

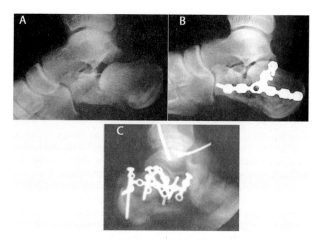

FIG. 27-9   Surgical treatment. *A.* Depression-type calcaneal fracture with a Böhler angle of 4 degrees. *B.* Reduced fracture that was fixed with an anatomic reconstruction-type Y plate. *C.* An intraoperative lateral radiograph shows a very comminuted fracture (Fig. 27-8), reduced and in good alignment, and fractures fixed with locking plates and screws.

sis, which is more effective and technically easier to perform than later reconstruction of malunited bone and scar tissues.

Occasionally, tongue-type fractures can be reduced and stabilized with the Essex–Lopresti percutaneous method (Fig. 27-10) by driving a large pin into the tongue fragment from posterior to anterior. The tongue fragment is then

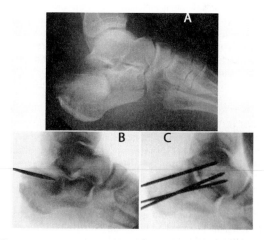

FIG. 27-10   Essex-Lopresti method of reduction and fixation of a tongue-type calcaneal fracture. *A.* Initial radiograph. *B.* Kirschner wire is introduced in the tongue fragment and used as reduction tool. *C.* Fixation of subtalar joint and percutaneous pinning.

reduced under fluoroscopy by manipulating the pin, and the pin is advanced into the talus (or anterior/inferior fragments of calcaneus if possible), thereby stabilizing the fracture. This technique seldom results in anatomic reduction but is of use when the patient has risk factors for wound healing.

Isolated fractures of the **tuberosity caused by direct impact** are almost always minimally displaced and are managed with avoidance of weight bearing for 3 to 6 weeks. In the rare case of a displaced tuberosity fracture, the displaced fragment is on the medial side. The fracture is reduced and held in place with screws.

Isolated fractures of the **tuberosity caused by avulsion** of the Achilles tendon are usually displaced. They are exposed through a medial approach, reduced, and stabilized with a large cancellous screw and a washer. If reduction is difficult, proximal recession of the gastrocnemius muscle at the muscle-tendon junction will make the reconstruction easier and more stable.

Postoperatively, if the fixation is adequate, immobilization is not required; however, no weight bearing is maintained for 4 to 6 weeks. In the rare case in which there is minimal displacement, an acceptable alternative form of management is a short leg cast in slight equinus. Immobilization is continued for 6 weeks. Throughout this period, the fracture is followed radiographically. Displacement is an indication for open reduction and stabilization.

Minimally displaced fractures of the **sustentaculum tali** are managed in a short leg weight-bearing cast for 4 to 6 weeks. Displaced fractures require a medial approach and fixation.

Undisplaced fractures of the **anterior process** are managed in a short leg weight-bearing cast for 4 to 6 weeks. Displaced large fragments are managed with open reduction and fixation. Excision of the fragment is not indicated, as it is the origin of the bifurcate ligament. The fragment is usually small and fixation may not be stable; therefore the foot is cast in a neutral position. In chronic situations, persistent pain, soft tissue reaction, and a small fragment are indications for excision.

Dislocations of the calcaneus are managed in the same fashion as subtalar dislocations. An immediate closed reduction is performed. If this cannot be achieved, open reduction is indicated. After closed reduction, it is important to assess the talocalcaneal articulation for loose bodies; if present, these are removed. The reduction is usually stable and fixation is not necessary. A short leg cast can be used for a few weeks.

Complications

Complications of fractures of the calcaneus are malunion, resulting in a widened heel and plantar fasciitis; subtalar arthritis; calcaneocuboid arthritis; and peroneal tendinitis.

A **widened heel and plantar fasciitis** are managed conservatively. Footwear is altered, and a heel cup may be necessary. Injections of local anesthetic and steroids may relieve symptoms. Rarely, excision of a spike of bone is indicated.

Subtalar and calcaneocuboid arthritis is managed conservatively with anti-inflammatory medication and local corticosteroid injections. Arthrodesis is a last resort; the preferable method is subtalar arthrodesis with distraction and a wedge-block bone graft.

Peroneal tendinitis is caused by impingement on the peroneal tendon sheath. Local injections of anesthetic and steroids may help; if not, the peroneal sheath can be decompressed by removing a portion of the displaced lateral wall of the calcaneus.

INJURIES OF THE MIDFOOT

Injuries of the midfoot include fractures and dislocations of the navicular, cuneiform, and cuboid bones and dislocations of the Chopart joint.

The talonavicular and calcaneocuboid joints form a functional transverse tarsal joint **(Chopart joint)** (Fig. 27-11) that is mobile during the foot's flat gait phase and locked (inverted heel) during the toe-off phase, allowing for effective transfer of propulsive forces. Talonavicular and cuboidometatarsal joints are more mobile than the rest of the midfoot and their fusion is to be avoided. If subtalar fusion is indicated, it should be done with the calcaneus slightly pronated, providing for more flexibility.

The **navicular** articulates with the head of the talus and the three cuneiform bones. The posterior tibial tendon inserts on the tubercle of the navicular, supporting the medial longitudinal arch.

The bones of the foot form **longitudinal and transverse arches**. The longitudinal arch is higher medially than laterally. The medial segment (talus, navicular, cuneiforms, and first, second, and third metatarsals) is the dynamic portion of the foot and flattens during weight bearing. The lateral segment (calcaneus, cuboid, and fourth and fifth metatarsals) is flatter, more rigid, and contacts the ground first during weight bearing. The transverse arch is formed by the shape of the tarsals and bases of the metatarsals, which are broader on the dorsal than the plantar aspect, forming a stable "Roman arch." The bones of the foot are connected by fibrous structures (e.g., the plantar fascia), intrinsic muscles, and extrinsic muscles. The muscles and the tensioned plantar fascia act as a "tie" at the base of the longitudinal arch, which prevents it from flattening during weight bearing.

Classification

There are three types of fractures of the tarsal **navicular:** dorsal chip fractures, fractures of the tuberosity, and fractures of the body of the navicular. The dorsal chip fracture, the most common type of navicular fracture, is a capsular

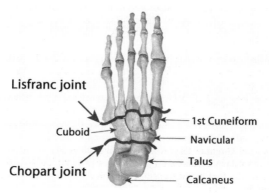

FIG. 27-11   Chopart and Lisfranc joints.

avulsion caused by plantarflexion and pronation of the foot. Fracture of the tuberosity is an avulsion of the posterior tibial tendon and occurs during eversion of the foot. Fractures of the body of the navicular are the least common type and are caused by forceful hyperextension and inversion. Stress fractures occur in athletes and cause chronic midfoot pain.

Fractures of the **cuneiforms** are often overlooked and are usually caused by direct trauma.

Fractures of the **cuboid** are due to direct trauma, capsular avulsion during inversion or eversion of the forefoot, or compression during abduction of the forefoot.

Chopart dislocation is a rare injury. There are three types: medial, lateral, and plantar. The mechanism of injury is inversion, eversion, and plantarflexion of the forefoot, respectively. The bifurcate ligament ruptures and the talocalcaneal ligament remains intact; therefore the talocalcaneal joint does not dislocate.

Diagnosis and Initial Management

History and Physical Examination

There is a history of either twisting or direct trauma to the midfoot and pain localized to the midfoot.

Radiographic Examination

The radiographic examination starts with anteroposterior, lateral, and oblique views of the foot. Stress views, obtained while inverting, everting, abducting, or adducting the forefoot, demonstrate instability of the Chopart joint. In cases of suspected stress fracture, bone scan is helpful for diagnosis and CT for preoperative planning.

Fracture of the navicular tuberosity can be confused with the os tibiale externum, an accessory ossicle. Distinguishing features are that the os tibiale externum is frequently bilateral and its edges are rounded.

Initial Management

Initial management consists of splinting, ice, and elevation. Dislocations of the Chopart joint are usually reduced by axial traction and manipulation of the forefoot under sedation. If closed reduction is not accomplished, immediate open reduction is indicated. Subluxations of the first cuneiform are usually not significantly displaced. In cases where the soft tissue is not at risk, these injuries are splinted in situ.

Associated Injuries

There are no specific injuries associated with injuries of the midfoot.

Definitive Management

Dorsal chip fractures of the **navicular** are managed symptomatically with a short leg cast and weight bearing as tolerated for approximately 4 weeks. Minimally displaced (2 mm or less) fractures of the tuberosity of the navicular are managed with a short leg cast with the forefoot inverted. At 4 weeks, the cast is changed and the foot is positioned in neutral; a short leg cast is applied and maintained for an additional 2 weeks. Displaced fractures of the navicular are managed with open reduction and internal fixation. The surgical exposure is through an incision centered over the navicular, parallel to the anterior tibial tendon. The talonavicular joint is exposed and the navicular is reduced under direct vision as the joint is distracted with longitudinal traction. Interfragmentary screws or pins are used for fixation.

Postoperatively, a short leg cast is applied. In unstable situations, temporary fixation with smooth Kirschner wires into the talus or primary arthrodesis with cuneiforms are options. Combined injuries and significant instability of the medial column are stabilized by temporary bridge plating (talus to medial cuneiform), which will preserve anatomy until healing occurs.

Incomplete stress fractures can be successfully treated with casting and avoidance of weight bearing for 6 weeks, but complete stress fractures require internal fixation and bone grafting.

Fractures of the cuneiforms are usually combined with other midfoot injuries. In case of a displaced or unstable isolated fracture of the **medial** cuneiform, the articulations between the first cuneiform and the navicular and intermediate cuneiform are involved. The **intermediate** cuneiform is the cornerstone of the transverse arch. It is necessary to restore its anatomy and stability by screw or Kirschner-wire temporary fixation or permanent fusion with spared cuneiforms or metatarsals. Splinting and non-weight-bearing period of 6 to 8 weeks is required for secure healing.

Cuboid injuries usually result from an indirect mechanism, compression between the calcaneus proximally and the fourth and fifth metatarsal base, distally resulting in a "nutcracker" fracture. Significant shortening will adversely affect the lateral foot column. Bone grafting and plating, including calcaneocuboid fusion, is indicated. It is important to preserve mobility at cuboidometatarsal joints.

Dislocations of the Chopart joint are managed operatively. Dislocations without associated fractures are stabilized with a minimum of two pins inserted under fluoroscopy. The first pin crosses the calcaneocuboid joint and the second pin crosses the talonavicular joint. A short leg cast is applied and weight bearing avoided for 6 weeks. At 6 weeks, the pins are removed and a stiff-soled shoe and arch support are worn.

Complications

The complication of midfoot injuries is arthritis. Management is anti-inflammatory drugs and alterations in footwear. If necessary, injections of local anesthetic agents and steroids can be done. Arthrodesis of an arthritic joint (e.g., talonavicular) is a last resort.

INJURIES OF THE FOREFOOT

Injuries of the forefoot are the Lisfranc dislocation, fractures of the metatarsals and phalanges, and dislocations of the metatarsophalangeal and interphalangeal joints. The forefoot is a platform during weight-bearing activities: it must have full contact, to be flat on the ground for even distribution of weight, and to propel the body forward with plantarflexion of the tibiotalar joint.

The **Lisfranc joint**, or tarsometatarsal joint, consists of a series of plane joints (Fig. 27-11). The greatest degree of motion occurs through the first metatarsal medial cuneiform articulation. Motion through the remainder of the joint is restricted by dorsal and volar ligaments and the bony architecture (i.e., the second metatarsal is inset between the first and third cuneiforms). The five metatarsal heads are connected by strong interosseous ligaments, but only the lateral four metatarsal bases have strong interosseous ligaments. In place of the interosseous ligament between the first and second metatarsal bases there is the Lisfranc ligament, connecting the medial cuneiform and the base of the second metatarsal. Because of this structural anatomy, dislocations of the Lisfranc joint are frequently limited to the lateral side (i.e., second through fifth metatarsals) or the medial side (i.e., first metatarsal).

The **metatarsophalangeal joints** function as hinge joints to tension the plantar aponeurosis.

The **interphalangeal joints** are hinge joints. They actively flex but extend actively only to neutral.

Classification

The mechanism of injury of the **Lisfranc dislocation** is hyperextension. Lisfranc dislocations are classified into one of three groups: total incongruity, partial incongruity, and divergent (Fig. 27-12). **Total incongruity (type I)** is characterized by involvement of the entire joint and displacement in one direction (usually laterally). **Partial incongruity (type II)** is characterized by involvement of only part of the joint, usually either the first metatarsal or the second through fifth metatarsals. This break between the first and second metatarsals occurs because there is no stabilizing ligament between their bases, as there is between the bases of the other metatarsals. **Divergent dislocations (type III)** are characterized by involvement of the entire joint. Displacement is in two directions (usually the first metatarsal is displaced medially and the second through fifth metatarsals laterally).

Metatarsal fractures are classified as traumatic or stress fractures. Two types of traumatic fractures bear special mention: the Jones's fracture and avulsion fractures of the base of the fifth metatarsal. The **Jones's fracture** is a transverse fracture of the fifth metatarsal at the junction of the proximal metaphysis and diaphysis and has characteristics of a stress fracture in that it may initially be incomplete, involving only the lateral cortex of the metatarsal. Jones's fractures frequently fail to heal when managed nonoperatively. **Avulsion fractures of the base (tuberosity) of the fifth metatarsal** are caused by the lateral cord of plantar aponeurosis rather than by the peroneus brevis.

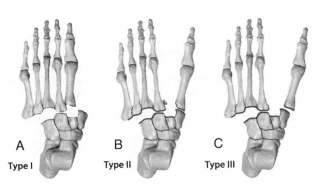

A   Type I   B   Type II   C   Type III

FIG. 27-12   Total (*A*), partial (*B*), and divergent (*C*) incongruities at a Lisfranc joint.

This fracture is distinguished from the Jones's fracture by its metaphyseal location and its tendency to heal when managed with immobilization.

Fractures of the **phalanges** are classified as intraarticular, extraarticular, or tuft fractures.

Dislocations of the metatarsal phalangeal and interphalangeal joints are classified, according to the direction of displacement, as dorsal or volar.

Diagnosis and Initial Management

History and Physical Examination

The patient complains of pain localized to the injured structure. The dorsum of the forefoot quickly becomes swollen and ecchymotic. Shortening of the forefoot indicates an unreduced Lisfranc dislocation or displaced fractures of all five metatarsals. Apparent hyperflexion or hyperextension of a metatarsophalangeal or interphalangeal joint indicates dislocation.

Radiographic Examination

Anteroposterior, oblique, and lateral radiographs are obtained.

The medial border of the second and fourth metatarsals should align with the medial border of the middle cuneiform and cuboid. A fracture of the base of the second metatarsal indicates that the Lisfranc joint is disrupted. Loss of congruity between articular surfaces and double densities (i.e., one articular surface superimposed on another) indicates subluxation. Dorsal subluxation of the second metatarsal base on the lateral view signifies Lisfranc ligament rupture (Fig. 27-13).

If there is no obvious displacement on non-weight-bearing x-rays, then weight bearing as tolerated is permitted after a week or two. Repeat radiographs should be obtained within 7 to 14 days if symptoms warrant. Any dorsal subluxation of the metatarsal bases, displacement of 2 mm between bones, or more than 15 degrees of angulation of any joint articulation should be corrected surgically. Forefoot abduction and adduction stress radiographs with anesthesia may help make the final determination about Lisfranc joint stability.

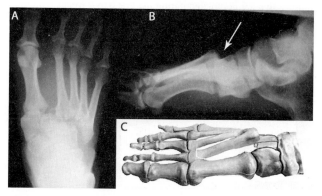

FIG. 27-13   Anteroposterior (*A*) and lateral (*B*) radiographs of partial Lisfranc injury with a drawing of easily recognizable dorsal subluxation of the second metatarsal base on the lateral view (*C*).

A CT scan will show occult fractures and a bone scan will help diagnose stress fractures of the metatarsals prior to their radiographic appearance.

Initial Management

Initial management consists of alignment of severely displaced fractures, reduction of dislocations, immobilization, elevation, and ice.

Dislocations of the Lisfranc joint with an absent dorsalis pedis or posterior tibial pulse or compromised overlying skin are reduced immediately as emergencies. General anesthesia is administered, and axial traction is applied to the involved rays by suspending the foot by the toes with finger traps. Inability to obtain a closed reduction is an indication for immediate open reduction.

Associated Injuries

Significant foot swelling, disproportionate pain, lost two-point discrimination, and pain made worse by passive toe motion are the cardinal signs of **compartment syndrome**. The diagnosis is confirmed by measuring the compartment pressures and finding an elevation greater than 30 mmHg or a difference of less than 30 mmHg between the diastolic pressure and the compartment pressure. Management is surgical release of the four dorsal osseofascial spaces and the five plantar and deep adductor compartments.

Involved compartments are released through incisions in the second and fourth webspaces dorsally and a separate medial incision. It is crucial to do this in a timely manner, as irreversible damage (after 12 h) will cause contractures, pain, scarring, and nerve dysfunction.

Definitive Management

The definitive management of a **Lisfranc dislocation** is reduction and stabilization with pins or screws (Fig. 27-14). We prefer open reduction because we have been impressed by the amount of displacement and comminution that is routinely present. Longitudinal incisions parallel to the second and fourth metatarsals will allow good access to the whole joint. Medial tarsometatarsal joints are cleaned and transfixed with screws and the cuboidometatarsal joints with Kirschner wires (removed after 6 to 10 weeks to preserve mobility). Lisfranc injuries that are not treated during the first 6 to 8 weeks require first-to-third tarsometatarsal joint arthrodesis and resection hemiarthroplasty of the fourth and fifth tarsometatarsal joints.

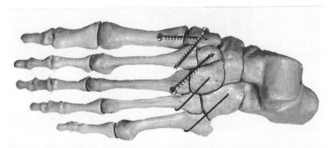

FIG. 27-14   Fixation of Lisfranc joint disruptions. Cuboidometatarsal joints are fixed with temporary K wires.

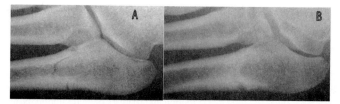

FIG. 27-15   Jones's fracture in a young person. *A*. Initial radiograph. *B*. Non-operatively treated healed fracture.

The **first metatarsal** bears the most weight and must be anatomically reduced and fixed, usually with plates. Isolated fractures of the lesser metatarsal with displacement of more than 3 mm and sagittal-plane angulation of more than 10 degrees require surgery. Multiple metatarsal fractures indicate instability and should be fixed with intramedullary Kirschner wires (antegrade through the distal fragment and the base of the proximal phalanx and then realigned with the proximal fragment and pinned retrograde).

Metaphyseal-diaphyseal junction fractures of the **fifth metatarsal base** have a tenuous blood supply and a poor tendency to heal (dancer's or Jones's fracture (Fig. 27-15). These fractures are treated with a non-weight-bearing cast for 6 weeks and with cast-protected weight bearing for an additional 6 weeks. If healing is delayed, an intramedullary screw with bone grafting is indicated.

Athletes can have primary screw fixation in order to return to their sport sooner. Minimally displaced avulsion fractures of the fifth metatarsal base are treated with protected (cam walker) weight bearing for 3 to 6 weeks. If displacement is more than 1 cm in a young person, reattachment with a lag screw or Kirschner wires and a tension band will improve healing.

Fractures of the **phalanges** are usually caused by direct trauma. Displaced shaft fractures of proximal and middle phalanges are aligned with the aid of a digital block, and the toe is buddy taped to the neighboring toe (with cotton roll between the toes). Protected weight bearing (supporting hard-soled shoes) for a few weeks will allow mobility and improve comfort. Subungual hematomas are decompressed with a battery-heated wire. Nail bed lacerations are repaired

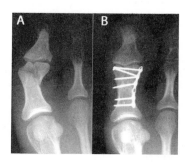

FIG. 27-16   Displaced intercondylar fracture of the proximal phalanx of the great toe in a 17-year-old girl. *A*. Initial radiograph. *B*. The fracture healed in anatomic position following fixation with a plate.

and the nail preserved as a splint. Displaced intraarticular or intercondylar fractures of the great toe's proximal phalanx need anatomic reduction and fixation (Fig. 27-16).

Dislocations of metatarsophalangeal and interphalangeal joints are managed with closed reduction under hematoma or regional blocks. Simple axial traction and gentle correction of the deformity will reduce the dislocation. Occasionally, an interphalangeal dislocation of the great toe is irreducible because of interposition of the long flexor tendon and requires open reduction through a dorsal incision.

Lawn-mower injuries are severe and dirty, often requiring multiple trips to the operating room or amputation. Primary wound closure should not be done. Gas gangrene can result from inadequate debridement.

Complications

Posttraumatic arthritis of the Lisfranc joint is managed with arch supports, anti-inflammatory medication, and local injections of steroids. If these measures fail, the joint is arthrodesed.

Malunion of a metatarsal fracture results in a localized area of increased pressure on the plantar aspect of the foot. A metatarsal bar or custom-molded shoe insert may compensate for the malunion and resolve the pain. If conservative measures are not effective, a corrective osteotomy is performed. Fixation is not required, and the patient is encouraged to bear weight postoperatively so that the involved metatarsal head will heal in the proper location.

SELECTED READINGS

Injuries of the Hindfoot

Buckley R, Tough S, McCormack R, et al. Operative compared with nonoperative treatment of displaced intra-articular calcaneal fractures: a prospective, randomized, controlled multicenter trial. *J Bone Joint Surg* 84A:1733–1744, 2002.

Canale ST, Kelly FB Jr. Fractures of the neck of the talus. Long-term evaluation of seventy-one cases. *J Bone Joint Surg* 60A:143–156, 1978.

Daniels TR, Smith JW. Varus talar neck malunion. Its influence on foot position and subtalar motion. *Foot Ankle* 14:302, 1993.

DeLee JC, Curtis R. Subtalar dislocation of the foot. *J Bone Joint Surg* 64A:433–437, 1982.

Hawkins LG. Fractures of the neck of the talus. *J Bone Joint Surg* 52A:991–1002, 1970.

Mann RA, Holmes GB Jr, Seale KS, Collins DN. Chronic rupture of Achilles tendon: a new technique of repair. *J Bone Joint Surg* 73A:214–219, 1991.

Nistor L. Surgical and non-surgical treatment of Achilles tendon rupture: a prospective randomized study. *J Bone Joint Surg* 63A:394–399, 1981.

Rammelt S, Gavlik JM, Barthel S, Zwipp H. The value of subtalar arthroscopy in the management of intraarticular calcaneus fractures. *Foot Ankle Int* 23:906–916, 2002.

Sanders R, Fortin P, DiPasquale T, Walling A. Operative treatment in 120 displaced intraarticular calcaneal fractures. Results using a prognostic computed tomography scan classification. *Clin Orthop* 290:87–95, 1993.

Szyskowitz R, Reschauer R, Seggl W. Eighty-five talus fractures treated by ORIF with five to eight years of follow-up study of 69 patients. *Clin Orthop* 199:97–107, 1985.

Injuries of the Midfoot

Komenda GA, Myerson MS, Biddinger KR. Results of arthrodesis of the tarsometatarsal joints after traumatic injury. *J Bone Joint Surg* 78A:1665–1676, 1996.

Mulier T, Reynders P, Dereymacker G, Broos P. Severe Lisfranc injuries: primary arthrodesis or ORIF? *Foot Ankle Int* 23:902–905, 2002.

Pinney SJ, Sangeorzan BJ. Fractures of the tarsal bones. In Sangeorzan BJ (ed). *The Traumatized Foot.* Rosemont, IL: American Academy of Orthopaedic Surgeons, 2001:41–53.

Richter M, Wippermann B, Krettek C, et al. Fractures and fracture dislocations of mid-foot. Occurrence, causes and long-term results. *Foot Ankle Int* 22:392–398, 2001.

Injuries of the Forefoot

Floyd DW, Heckman JD, Rockwood CA Jr. Tendon lacerations in the foot. *Foot Ankle Int* 4:8–14, 1983.

Kavanaugh JH, Brower TD, Mann RV. The Jones fracture revisited. *J Bone Joint Surg* 60A:776–782, 1978.

Richli WR, Rosenthal DI. Avulsion fracture of the fifth metatarsal: experimental study of pathomechanics. *Am J Roentgenol* 143:889–891, 1984.

Wiener BD, Linder JF, Giattini JF. Treatment of fractures of the fifth metatarsal: a prospective study. *Foot Ankle Int* 18:267–269, 1997.

General

DiGiovanni CW, Benirschke SK, Hansen ST Jr. Foot injuries. In Browner BD, Jupiter JB, Levin AM, Trafton PG (eds): *Skeletal Trauma*, 3d ed. Philadelphia: Saunders, 2003:2375–2492.

Sangeorzan BJ (ed). *The Traumatized Foot.* AAOS monograph series. Rosemont, IL: American Academy of Orthopaedic Surgeons, 2001.

28 | Fracture and Bone Injury Related to Athletic Participation

Mark R. Hutchinson   Raymond Klug

The term *sport-specific injury* is something of a misnomer. A fracture of any bone or dislocation of any joint can occur during athletic activity (Fig. 28-1). Indeed, it has been said that the playing fields of collision sports are perhaps the best-controlled incubators of human trauma. You could sit for years at a given intersection waiting for a vehicle accident to occur, but attendance at a high school football game guarantees the observation of multiple collisions every few minutes. Perhaps the primary advantage to the clinician in evaluating sports-related fractures and bone injuries is a well-defined mechanism of injury. For example, it is not difficult to understand the valgus angulation of a tibial fracture when a soccer player is kicked from the side by an opposing player, or how the ischium was avulsed in a gymnast who falls and hyperflexes the hip with the leg extended at the knee. An understanding of the mechanism can also alert the clinician to other associated injuries.

Working with athletes requires special attention to details. Certain fracture patterns occur more commonly during athletic activity. Care of athletes with bone injuries introduces the additional dilemma of return-to-play decisions. The goal of this chapter is to emphasize these variations and special challenges of caring for the athletic population; evaluate special populations and injury patterns in specific sports, such as avulsions and stress fractures; and clarify the unique aspects of athletic participation on bone injury.

PATTERNS OF SPORTS-SPECIFIC INJURY

Each sport is unique and offers distinctive physical challenges and musculoskeletal risks to participants; therefore each sport has a specific injury pattern. Evaluating injury risk and injury patterns is fundamentally a study of the mechanism of injury. Sports can be grouped into categories that help to subdivide the patterns. For example, collision sports of American football, ice hockey, and rugby pose a greater risk of acute fractures and dislocations. Throwing and overhead sports—such as baseball, javelin, swimming, tennis, and racquetball—pose an increased risk of overuse injuries of the upper extremity and stress fractures. Running, sprinting, and jumping sports—including soccer, track and field, and basketball—tend to risk overuse and failure in the lower extremity. Increased training intensity, poor nutritional habits, and repetitive submaximal load during practice of certain elements elevate the risk of stress fractures in athletes. The use of steroids in the athletic population increases the risk of tendon failure and avulsion injuries. Knowledge of common injuries or risks in a given sport can help the clinician to make an accurate diagnosis and choose the correct treatment (Table 28-1). Some sports-specific injury patterns are rare; others are so common that they have pseudonyms related to their specific sport (boxer's fracture, snowboarder's fracture, Little Leaguer's shoulder, etc.).

410

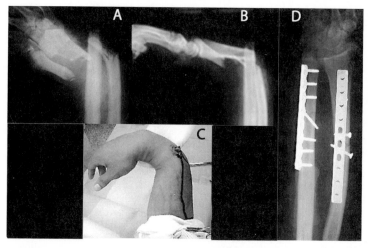

FIG. 28-1   Open both-bone forearm fracture in a gymnast whose grip locked on a high-bar routine. *A.* AP radiograph. *B.* Lateral radiograph. *C.* Clinical photograph. *D.* Postoperative AP radiograph.

SPECIAL POPULATIONS

Female Athletes

Beyond the specific sport, the participating population can affect bone injury patterns. Various studies have revealed that female athletes tend to be at greater risk for stress fractures and overuse injuries than their male counterparts. Prospective and retrospective studies of stress fractures among military recruits report a cumulative incidence of 0.99 to 2.0% for males. Female recruits generally sustain stress fractures at rates over three times that of their male counterparts. In running sports, women develop stress fractures at rates up to 10 times greater than men on the same training course. Other retrospective studies have documented stress fracture rates of 23 to 52% among female distance runners and 22 to 45% among ballet dancers. When women are followed prospectively, high recurrence rates are seen as well. When female recruits or athletes undergo a period of preconditioning or when "conditioned" male and female athletes are compared, the relative risk of stress fracture is more equal.

Additional factors affecting the risk of bone stress injury in female athletes include hormonal and nutritional issues. Competitive female athletes tend to have later menarche, menstrual irregularities, and diminished circulating estrogen levels. With relative estrogen deficiency comes reduced peak bone mass and a reduction in the ability to remodel bone in response to mechanical loading. This is thought to predispose women to stress fractures as well as osteoporosis later in life. Inadequate energy intake relative to calories burned also increases the risk of stress injuries to the bone. The "female athlete triad" describes the association between menstrual irregularities, disordered eating, and osteoporosis. It is relatively common among elite female athletes, with

TABLE 28-1   Fractures Commonly Associated with Specific Sports and Activities

Sport/Activity	Fracture
Arm wrestling	Humeral and forearm fracture
Ballet	Stress fracture (pelvis, femur, metatarsal), os trigonum
Baseball	Fingertip injuries, mallet finger, volar plate avulsion, spiral humerus fracture, medial epicondylar avulsion Stress fracture of the olecranon Hook of hamate fracture
Basketball	Base of fifth metacarpal, navicular stress fracture
Boxing	Boxer's fracture, facial fractures
Cheerleading	Spondylolysis, stress fractures
Cross-country running	Stress fracture (pelvis, femur, tibia, metatarsal)
Cycling	Spoke injuries in children, fractures from falls
Diving	Spondylolysis
Fencing	Pubic stress fracture
Football	Acute fracture, spondylolysis, navicular stress fracture
Gymnastics	Spondylolysis, distal radial physeal fractures, both-bone forearm grip injuries, forearm stress fracture
Handball	Metacarpal stress fracture
Ice hockey	Clavicular fracture
Martial arts	Clavicular fracture
Rollerblading	Distal radial fracture, scaphoid fracture
Rowing	Rib fractures
Shooting sports	Coracoid fracture, hamate fracture (hand guns)
Skateboarding	Distal radial fracture, scaphoid fracture
Snowboarding	Talus fractures
Snow skiing	Boot-top fractures, gamekeeper's thumb
Soccer	Tibial stress fracture, pubic stress fracture
Swimming	Stress fracture of the humerus
Tennis	Hook of hamate fracture Stress fracture (ulna, metacarpal, metatarsal)
Track (sprint)	Avulsion injuries
Volleyball	Distal fibular stress fracture
Water skiing	Spondylolysis
Weight lifting	Avulsions, tendon injuries, spondylolysis
Wrestling	Clavicular fracture

SOURCE: Modified from Bennett KL, Brukner PD. Epidemiology and site specificity of stress fractures. *Clin Sports Med* 16:179, 1997.

an incidence as high as 15 to 62%. While athletic trainers, coaches, or fellow players may be witness to abnormal eating behaviors, the stress fracture is commonly the athlete's initial contact with the physician.

There should be a high index of suspicion for this condition in female competitors of all sports but especially in sports with a significant advantage to low weight or where judging includes the athlete's esthetic presentation. The physician should automatically screen for the female athlete triad in any female athlete who presents with a stress fracture in crew, distance running, gymnastics, rhythmic gymnastics, cheerleading, figure skating, and ballet. The athlete may be in denial; therefore the physician must be on the alert and be willing to perform additional evaluation for confirmation of the diagnosis. Once the diagnosis is confirmed, a multidisciplinary approach should be undertaken to address gynecologic, psychological, and nutritional issues as well as the orthopedic care of the stress fracture. Anorexia or bulimia has high mortality rates. Occasionally in these cases the best treatment for the stress fracture may be to disqualify the athlete from sports until the eating disorder is under control.

Child Athletes

Child athletes introduce the risk of injury to the open physis and actively growing skeleton. In general, the weak link in the skeletally immature athlete is the physis. Ligamentous injuries are less common than growth plate injuries and avulsion injuries of an apophysis. A high degree of suspicion is encouraged in evaluating the child athlete. Inadequate treatment or an unrecognized physeal injury can lead to permanent deformity and disability. Physical examination should always include palpation of the physis. If instability is appreciated, stress radiographs should be obtained to clarify a ligamentous or physeal source. Imaging should often include comparison views of the contralateral side.

Chronic repetitive overuse can cause repetitive microtrauma at the level of the physis, which leads to adaptive changes in the bone. The microtrauma may be painful for the child but is frequently subclinical, with little pain. Children should not play through pain. Examples commonly associated with mild pain include repetitive loading of the tibial tubercle in jumpers, leading to Osgood-Schlatter disease; repetitive loading of the medial epicondyle in pitchers, leading to hypertrophy or avulsion; or repetitive loading of the anterosuperior iliac spine in hurdlers, leading to chronic apophysitis. Examples commonly associated with little or no pain include repetitive loading of the proximal humeral physis in child pitchers, leading to increased external rotation; repetitive loading of the proximal femoral physis in ballet dancers, leading to increased turn-out; and repetitive loading of the lateral compartment of the elbow in young throwers, leading to hypertrophy of the radial head or capitellum.

Master's Athletes

The athletically active older patient has only recently become the subject of research regarding injury patterns. Bone density is decreased in both male and female athletes, slightly increasing the risk of fracture. A majority of the fractures in older people are complete fractures, with fewer stress fractures as compared with a younger population. The reduced incidence of stress fractures may be secondary to less total repetition in training, a reduced likelihood of ramping up intensity too quickly, and some metabolic factors in bone healing. When fractures occur in the mature athlete, bone densitometry to look for possible osteoporosis may be indicated.

Perhaps the most interesting aspect of sport in the elderly is not the treatment or identification of specific patterns but rather prevention. A number of studies have instituted the use of Tai Chi to maximize proprioception and reduce the risk of falls in the elderly. Weight-lifting and weight-bearing activities increase load and allow the elderly to build new bone and offset the effect of osteoporosis.

Elite Athletes

When elite and competitive athletes sustain fractures, they introduce special challenges in decision making. As in all fractures, the clinician should look for associated injuries and treat the fracture appropriately and with indicated reha-bilitation. The bones do not heal any quicker in athletes than in an age-compara-ble group of nonathletes. Nonetheless athletes often demand an expedited reha-bilitation program and an early return to sport. The physician should never compromise fracture care for time of the season, the possibility of winning a scholarship, the financial impact on the athlete or the club, or the approach of "the big game." Medicolegal considerations may also come into play, as athletes have sued both for not being allowed to play and for being returned to play too quickly. Ultimately, the athlete is a patient first and must be treated as such; however, in treating competitive athletes, it behooves the treating physician to be aware that not all fracture patterns and bone stress injuries need to be treated with tentative conservatism. There is ample literature to support early return to play with vari-ous levels of immobilization in the case of certain fracture and bone stress pat-terns. For example, pneumatic braces can safely be used to treat tibial stress frac-tures of the mid- to lower thirds and allow athletes to return to sport. Some sports (football, soccer) will allow return to play with a soft or padded cast for hand in-juries as long as there is no risk of injury to others. Each athlete's treatment must be individualized, and each must be aware of the additional risk incurred in at-tempting to return to play prior to complete healing of the fracture.

STRESS FRACTURES

The evaluation and treatment of complete single trauma fractures related to athletics is not significantly different from the approach to those presented elsewhere in this text. In contrast, stress injury to bone and stress fractures are much more common in the athletic population than in the general popula-tion. Stress fractures (fatigue fractures) are caused by repetitive submaximal stresses that exceed a bone's adaptive capability. The stress injury to bone is actually a continuum of pathology ranging from mild bone edema or stress reaction to an incomplete fracture or stress fracture that in the worst-case sce-nario can catastrophically fail and become a complete fracture. Stress fractures were originally described in exercise-active military recruits (i.e., *march frac-ture, Deutschlander's fracture*), the common theme being repetitive activity in a relatively underconditioned individual. Patients commonly complain of lo-calized pain with activity, pain with impact, and pain that is relieved by rest and returns on resumption of the inciting activity. Associated factors can be an alteration in the intensity or frequency of training, new or different equip-ment (especially shoe wear), rigidity of the playing surface, inadequate energy intake, or menstrual irregularities.

Physical examination may be nonspecific, with local point tenderness being the most consistent physical finding in bones. Superficial locations may also ex-hibit localized swelling or palpable periosteal thickening. Pain with passive range of motion or stresses on extremes of motion may also exacerbate the pain. The involved bone tends to be hypersensitive to vibration, and the patient is unable to tolerate ultrasound treatment. A tuning fork is an inexpensive tool available in the clinic or training room. When the vibrating tuning fork is placed in contact with the bone, pain may also be exacerbated.

Plain radiographs obtained within the first 2 to 3 weeks after injury are usu-ally negative. Periosteal reactions, cortical lucency, fracture lines, or callus formation may take several months to appear if at all. In suspicious cases with negative plain films, radionuclide bone scanning or magnetic resonance imag-ing should be used.

Radionuclide bone scanning is the most sensitive and earliest indicator of stress fracture but lacks specificity. Bone scanning also has the advantage of being able to detect distant or multiple lesions and to distinguish bipartite bones from stress fractures.

Acute stress fractures are visualized as discrete areas of increased uptake on all three phases of the bone scan. Soft tissue injuries characteristically have increased uptake in only the first two phases. Bone scans are usually positive within the first 2 to 7 days after the patient becomes symptomatic. After symptoms have persisted for at least this amount of time, a negative bone scan virtually eliminates the diagnosis of stress fracture. Single-photon emission computed tomography (SPECT) scanning has the advantage of increased resolution by eliminating surrounding soft tissue structures. This may be particularly advantageous with subtle stress fractures and especially those of the spine and pelvis. While bone scans are helpful in confirming the diagnosis, they should not be used to dictate return to play for athletes, as the scan may continue to be positive for nearly 2 years.

Magnetic resonance imaging (MRI) has more recently emerged for early and specific identification of stress fractures in high-level athletes. The MRI is specific and can rule out other potential differential diagnoses, but perhaps its greatest value in the treatment of athletic bone stress injury is its ability to provide predictive value in estimating the duration of disability. Grade I injuries have negative radiographs but positive short tau inversion recovery (STIR) images but negative T2 images on MRI. Grade I injuries generally improve with 3 weeks of rest. Grade II injuries have negative radiographs but are positive on both STIR and T2 images. Grade II images require 3 to 6 weeks of rest. Grade III injuries may or may not have positive radiographs but MRI reveals no cortical break. MRI is positive on STIR, T2, and T1 images. Grade III injuries require 12 to 16 weeks of rest. Grade IV injuries have a radiolucent line and periosteal reaction on radiographs with a cortical crack on T2 and T1 MRI images. Grade IV stress injuries have a guarded prognosis and may require 16 weeks of rest. Grade III and IV stress fractures are considered high-risk fractures, and algorithms for their treatment have been proposed (Fig. 28-2).

The majority of stress fractures occur in weight-bearing bones such as the lower extremity in runners and jumpers or the upper extremity in gymnasts. Matheson reported on 320 bone scan–positive stress fractures in 145 males and 175 females and showed, in decreasing order of frequency, stress fractures of the tibia (49.1%), tarsal bones (25.3%), metatarsals (8.8%), femur (7.2%), fibula (6.6%), pelvis (1.6%), sesamoids (0.9%), and back (0.6%). Femoral and tarsal stress fractures were more common in older athletes and tibial and fibular stress fractures were more common in younger athletes. Bilateral stress fractures occurred in 16.6%. Other studies have shown variations in frequency if plain radiographs were used for diagnosis: metatarsal (35.2%), calcaneus (28.0%), tibia (24%), ribs (5.6%), femur (3.2%), fibula (3.2%), spine (0.4%), and pubic ramus (0.4%). Among runners, up to 76% of stress fractures occur in the tibia, fibula, and metatarsals.

SPECIFIC FRACTURES RELATED TO SPORTS

Athletic participation improves general fitness, muscular strength, heart health, and coordination as well as offering opportunities to experience leadership, team play, a sense of achievement, and social interaction with friends and teammates.

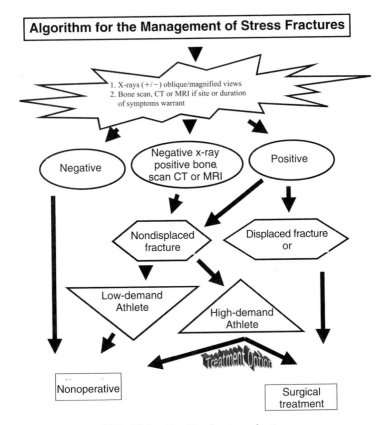

FIG. 28-2 Algorithm for stress fracture.

With all of the positives, the risk of injury, including fracture, is pervasive in sports, especially in contact and collision sports. The following section briefly discusses the unique aspects of specific injuries of bone and their relationship to sports participation. For the treatment of specific fractures, the reader is referred to the relevant chapter in this text.

Cervical Spine

Injuries to the cervical spine, including fractures and dislocations, are thankfully rare in sports. Nonetheless, sideline management requires a high level of suspicion. Any athlete with midline neck pain or a head injury with abnormal sensorium must be assumed to have a cervical spine injury. This requires immobilization and full radiographic evaluation. The most common cause of catastrophic cervical spine injury in the United States is football. Rule changes (1976) penalizing spear tackling have had a significant effect on reducing the number of cervical spine injuries. The next most common risky sport for male athletes is ice hockey. The most common mechanism is a check from behind, sending the athlete head-first into the boards. Rule changes with significant penalties for unsafe checking have helped to reduce the incidence of neck injuries in hockey. For female athletes, the most common cause of catastrophic cervical spine injury is cheerleading, followed by gymnastics. The mechanism in both instances is a fall from a height.

Thoracic Spine and Ribs

The thoracic spine is relatively protected by the rib cage and associated musculature, making sports-related fractures of the thoracic spine exceedingly rare. Rib fractures can occur with collision sports. Stress injuries to the second through tenth ribs are correlated with rowing, crew, and kayaking. Stress fractures of the first rib have been reported in pitchers and throwers.

Upper Extremity

Bone injury to the upper extremity can be correlated to sports involving contact/collision, throwing, or weight bearing/weight lifting. The recoil of the gun stock in shooting sports has been associated with stress injuries of the coracoid. The recoil of the bat or stick in stick sports has been associated with fractures of the hook of the hamate. Clavicular fractures occur more commonly in collision sports such as ice hockey, when a player is checked into the boards, or in martial arts/wrestling, when a participant is being driven into the mat. Clavicular fractures may also occur in stick sports such as ice hockey, field hockey, and lacrosse from being hit by the equipment. Scapular fractures have been reported secondary to direct trauma in football as well as secondary to chronic microtrauma from carrying hand weights while running. Falls onto the extended wrist should raise suspicion of a scaphoid fracture, the most common carpal fracture in sports. Ball-catching and tackling sports increase the incidence of fractures of the fingers and hands.

Weight-bearing and weight-lifting activities tend to lead to chronic overuse injuries of the upper extremities. Arm wrestlers place significant force across their humeri and forearms, thus increasing their risk of a fracture at either location. The epidemic use of steroids in competitive weight lifters or body builders increases the risk of avulsion injuries. Gymnastics is the classic upper extremity weight-bearing sport. Gymnasts are at risk for a variety of overuse stress injuries up and down the upper extremity, including forearm stress fractures, scaphoid stress fractures, dorsal wrist impingement, and physeal stress syndrome of the distal radius. This syndrome occurs in young, skeletally immature gymnasts and appears radiographically as widening and irregularity of the distal radial physis with marginal sclerosis. The athlete should be rested until pain-free. Dorsiflexion block braces ("tiger paws") can be used to prevent recurrence on return to sport. If left untreated, radial shortening can occur, with a positive ulnar variance and chronic wrist pain in adulthood.

Throwing and racquet sports provide the next common thread of bone-related injuries in athletes. Throwing and racquet sports both impose chronic repetitive loading on the shoulder and elbow. In the skeletally immature, this can lead to "Little Leaguer's shoulder," which is usually a minimally or nondisplaced injury to the proximal humeral physis. In general, it is treated with rest for 3 to 6 weeks, but the athlete is not allowed to return to throwing for 2 to 3 months for fear of recurrence. Chronic subclinical loading of the proximal humeral physis has been correlated with the increased external rotation, as seen in professional and collegiate pitchers. When a complete spiral fracture of the proximal humerus is seen in a young pitcher, an underlying pathology such as a bone cyst or tumor should be considered.

Throwing sports also place chronic repetitive loads about the elbow. Stress fractures of the olecranon have been reported in mature throwers secondary to triceps traction or valgus-extension overload. Most will respond to a period of rest; however, a single screw placed across the olecranon down the ulnar shaft can expedite an athlete's return to sport. In the skeletally immature thrower, too many pitches can lead to traction apophysitis or complete avulsion of the medial epicondyle. Virtually all avulsions of the medial epicondyle (which are not entrapped in the joint) will heal uneventfully with fibrous tissue and scarring. In elite athletes, open reduction and internal fixation (ORIF) of avulsions separated by more than 3 mm may be offered to reduce the fragment, with the expectation of better motor power. Valgus extension overload may also contribute to subchondral bone changes of the capitellum (osteochondritis dissecans), hypertrophy of the radial head, and/or stress fractures of the olecranon physis.

Lumbar Spine and Pelvis

Golf and baseball are sports that make significant rotational demands of the trunk. Ballet dancers, artistic gymnasts, rhythmic gymnasts, cheerleaders, and football linemen all have chronic repetitive demands of extension on the lumbar spine. These two mechanisms load the pars interarticularis of the lumbar spine and increase the risk of a spondylolysis (a stress fracture of the pars interarticularis). Chronic low back pain in young athletes deserves an appropriate workup and diagnosis. Radiographs including obliques are rarely diagnostic. SPECT bone scans can confirm the diagnosis. When a spondylolysis can be identified in the acute phase (first 3 months), the goal is cure, and the most common treatment is a thoracolumbosacral orthosis until the patient is pain-free. In chronic cases, pain is treated symptomatically. If the pain is intractable, local fusion can provide relief, with a guarded prognosis regarding return to sport.

Bone injuries about the pelvis related to sports can be due to direct trauma, avulsions, or overuse. Collision sports can lead to pelvic fractures and hip dislocations, with associated acetabular fractures. These are treated no differently than general orthopedic trauma. Avulsions of the anterosuperior iliac spine (sartorius), anteroinferior iliac spine (rectus), inferior pubis (gracilis), and ischium (hamstrings) occur more commonly in sprinters and speed sports but have been seen traumatically in football, soccer, and gymnastics. The accepted treatment for avulsions with less than 2 cm of separation is conservative. In athletes, consideration should be given to ORIF to place the muscle back at length and optimize the strength recovered. Chronic overuse at the level of the pelvis increases the risk of stress fractures, particularly of the symphysis pubis. This is more commonly seen in runners with a crossover gait and is treated nonoperatively.

Proximal Femur

Stress fractures of the femoral neck are uncommon but have a potential for serious morbidity. They are more common in runners and endurance athletes. Because of their rarity, diagnosis is commonly delayed. Patients often present with anterior groin pain, which is exacerbated with weight bearing. Tenderness is difficult to elicit, but pain with passive motion or at the extremes of motion (especially rotation) is common. An antalgic gait may also be present.

Compressive-side (inferior) stress fractures are more common and begin at the inferior cortex of the femoral neck. Complete displacement of compression-sided fractures is rare; therefore nonoperative treatment, including protected weight bearing with close radiographic follow-up, is appropriate. Of greater concern and less common are tension-sided (superior) or transverse femoral neck stress fractures. These fractures start at the superior cortex and travel across the femoral neck relatively perpendicular to its axis. Because of the mechanical moments imparted across the proximal femur, this fracture pattern has a greater propensity to displace and therefore requires operative fixation with three parallel screws.

Knee

Sports-related bone injuries about the knee may be traumatic, associated with other injuries, or secondary to overuse. The clinician caring for the skeletally immature athlete must always be alert for the potential of an injury of the distal femoral physis rather than a ligamentous injury. Indeed, another concern for the young athlete who presents with knee pain is the potential of referred pain from the hip (slipped capital femoral epiphysis). Appropriate radiographic workup including the joint above and below the area of interest, comparison views, and stress views when indicated will help to secure the diagnosis.

Twisting and cutting sports, including basketball, soccer, team handball, etc., have an increased risk of injury to the anterior cruciate ligament, especially in women. Care should be taken to identify associated injuries such as avulsions or bone bruises so as to best advise the athlete regarding prognosis. In most cases, avulsion injuries of the medial collateral ligament, lateral collateral ligament, or posterior cruciate ligament will be repaired primarily.

Chronic repetitive loading related to jumping and sprinting, as seen in track and field, volleyball, and basketball, increases the load along the extensor mechanism of the knee and in turn increases the risk of patellar stress fracture or avulsion of the patellar or quadriceps tendon. In the skeletally immature, chronic loading can lead to apophysitis of the distal pole of the patella (Sinding-Larson-Johanson) or of the tibial tubercle (Osgood-Schlatter's). If avulsion occurs, anatomic repair is necessary for optimal function of the extensor mechanism.

Leg and Ankle

In athletes, the tibial shaft is the most common location of stress fracture. Such fractures are usually transverse, at the posteromedial cortex (compression side). Posterior tibial stress fractures respond well to relative rest, with gradual return to activity. Since the injury usually involves the mid- to distal third, tibial stress fractures are highly amenable to long leg pneumatic braces. Indeed, the use of such braces can safely speed an athlete's return to play from 3 months to about 1 month. The athlete is rested for a short period and then allowed to return to play, wearing the brace for all impact activities. As long as there is no increase in pain, the athlete can continue to compete. To date, there have been no reported progressions of the stress injury to a complete fracture.

Less common but more worrisome are anterior cortex (tension-sided) stress fractures. Radiographic findings may be subtle, if present, which can lead to delay in diagnosis. Focused views or magnification may help. Relative hypovascularity and tension on the anterior cortex are thought to contribute to progression to complete fracture or nonunion. Initial treatment is rest for 4 to

6 months. Ultrasonic bone stimulation may be used as an adjunct to promote healing in stress fractures (magnetic and electrical devices have not been approved for this purpose by the U.S. Food and Drug Administration). If radiographs show signs of chronic changes (the "dreaded black line"), excision and bone grafting or intramedullary fixation may be necessary. Expeditious surgical treatment of anterior cortex stress fractures may allow an earlier return to sport. Tibial stress fractures are more common in distance runners and distal fibular stress fractures appear to be common in ballet, aerobics, race walking, and volleyball.

About the ankle, athletes can sustain avulsion injuries of the ligaments or osteochondral injuries of the talar dome secondary to severe ankle sprains. Stress fractures of the medial malleolus in adults and physeal injuries of the distal fibula and distal tibia in children can present as ankle sprains. Avulsion injuries and stress fractures are generally treated with immobilization and resolve in 6 to 8 weeks.

Foot

Navicular stress fractures are relatively uncommon, representing 0.7 to 2.4% of all stress fractures; however, the risk they pose of nonunion and ultimately career-ending disability is greater than with most other stress fractures (Fig. 28-3). Navicular stress fractures can occur in athletes in any sport with repetitive loading, including basketball, long jump, triple jump, football, and running. A high index of suspicion is required to make the diagnosis. Stress fractures of the tarsal navicular bone are difficult to detect on plain films due to the orientation of the bone. An anatomic anteroposterior view with the foot inverted may help. The diagnosis is commonly made with a bone scan, CT, or MRI. Navicular stress fractures occur at the relatively avascular central third in the sagittal plane. Due to the relatively increased risk of nonunion, these fractures are treated with cast immobilization and the avoidance of weight bearing for 6 to 8 weeks. When nonunion or displacement occurs, internal fixation with bone grafting may be necessary.

Stress fractures of the metatarsal shaft are found among runners and military recruits (*march fracture, Deutschlander's fracture*), typically occurring in the diaphysis of the second and third metatarsals. Treatment is symptomatic and immobilization is rarely necessary. The most important consideration in athletes is an assessment of why the fracture occurred in the first place, in order

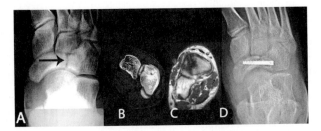

FIG. 28-3 Female basketball player with gradual onset of midfoot pain. *A.* AP radiograph. *B.* CT scan. *C.* MRI scan showing a nondisplaced stress fracture of the tarsal navicular with sclerosis. *D.* Postoperative fixation with headless compression screw after 4 months of conservative treatment had failed.

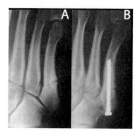

FIG. 28-4   Male basketball player with acute onset of lateral foot pain while rebounding. *A.* Oblique radiograph shows a nondisplaced fracture of the base of the fifth metatarsal (Jones's fracture). *B.* Surgical fixation with a cannulated

to reduce the risk of a recurrence. Review of the training history, assessment of shoe wear and lower extremity alignment, evaluation of nutritional history, and screening of women for risk of the "female athlete triad" may identify an underlying treatable cause.

The fifth metatarsal may introduce unique treatment considerations in the athletic population (Fig. 28-4). As in the case of metatarsals two through four, avulsion injuries of the tuberosity or diaphyseal fractures of the fifth metatarsal are treated symptomatically with a removable "cam-walker boot" or a stiff-soled shoe with crutches followed by progressive weight bearing. Fractures at the avascular junction of the proximal metaphysis and diaphysis (Jones's fractures) carry an elevated risk of delayed union, nonunion, or recurrent fracture. Symptomatic patients with positive bone scans but negative radiographs are treated nonoperatively with weight bearing avoided and a semirigid orthosis. With greater than 3 weeks of symptoms or radiographic confirmation, avoidance of weight bearing and cast immobilization for 6 to 8 weeks is recommended. In elite athletes who desire a quicker return to sport and reduced risk of recurrence, intramedullary screw fixation is performed. This may be the first line of treatment in elite basketball players.

SUMMARY

Virtually every bone in the body can be injured secondary to athletic participation. Fundamentally, treatment is not different than it is in other fractures, and the clinician must always treat the athlete as a patient first. Certain fracture patterns are more commonly seen in sports, especially overuse and stress injuries of the bone. Attention to these patterns will assist the clinician in making accurate diagnoses.

Most of these injuries will respond to a conservative course of treatment; however, associated factors including injury mechanism, alignment, nutritional issues, gender-related issues, and issues related to training intensity must be understood in order to optimize care. The athlete's desire to return to play must be balanced against the possibility of further injury and of permanent impairment as well as the athlete's (or parents') ability to live with the consequences. In situations where the athlete can offer an informed consent, more aggressive treatment options can be selected that will allow the athlete to return to play sooner. Ultimately, caring for sports-related fractures calls for a holistic approach in which the clinician understands and responds to the patient's needs and desires with enough information that the athlete can make an informed decision.

SELECTED READINGS

Bennell KL, Brukner PD. Epidemiology and site specificity of stress fractures. *Clin Sports Med* 16:179, 1997.

Caine D, Roy S, Singer KM, Broekhof J. Stress changes of the distal radial growth plate: a radiographic survey and review of the literature. *Am J Sports Med* 20:290, 1992.

Fredericson, Bergman AG, Hoffman KL, et al. Tibial stress reaction in runners: correlation of clinical symptoms and scintigraphy with a new magnetic resonance grading system. *Am J Sports Med* 3:472, 1995.

Knapp TP, Garrett WE Jr. Stress fractures: general concepts. *Clin Sports Med* 16:339, 1997.

McBryde AM. Stress fractures in athletes. *J Sport Med* 3:212–217, 1995.

Myburgh KH, Hutchins J, Fataar AB, et al. Low bone density is an etiologic factor for stress fractures in athletes. *Ann Intern Med* 113:754, 1990.

Pentacost RL, Murray R, Brindley H, et al. Fatigue, insufficiency and pathological fractures. *JAMA* 187:1001, 1964.

Protzman RR, Griffis CG. Stress fractures in men and women undergoing military training. *J Bone Joint Surg* 59A:825, 1977.

Teitz C. Stress fractures. In Teitz C (ed). *The Female Athlete*. AAOS Monograph Series. Rosemont, IL: American Association of Orthopaedic Surgeons, 1997:81.

Tuan K, Wu S, Sennett B. Stress fractures in athletes: risk factors, diagnosis, and management. *Orthopaedics* 27:583–591, 2004.

Index

NOTE: Page numbers followed by *f* indicate figures; those followed by *t* indicate tables.